HERE'S AMERICA'S MOST ACCURATE AND DEPENDABLE DIET GUIDE

CALORIES AND CARBOHYDRATES

THE BOOK THAT MAKES IT FUN TO TRIM DOWN— AND STAY THAT WAY

Whether you aim to lose five pounds or fifty, the only safe, healthy way is to eat an adequate, well-balanced diet, choosing your calories from many different kinds of foods in order to ensure that you're getting sufficient vitamins, minerals, and other nutrients. CALORIES AND CARBOHYDRATES contains the most accurate and dependable calorie and carbohydrate counts for practically everything you will eat and drink—thousands and thousands of brand names and basic foods, such as your favorites from TACO BELL and WENDY'S.

SO DIET WITH EASE— AND LOSE LIKE NEVER BEFORE!

BARBARA KRAUS

CALORIES AND CARBOHYDRATES

NINTH REVISED EDITION

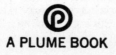

A PLUME BOOK

PLUME
Published by the Penguin Group
Penguin Books USA Inc., 375 Hudson Street,
New York, New York 10014, U.S.A.
Penguin Books Ltd, 27 Wrights Lane,
London W8 5TZ, England
Penguin Books Australia Ltd, Ringwood,
Victoria, Australia
Penguin Books Canada Ltd, 2801 John Street,
Markham, Ontario, Canada L3R 1B4
Penguin Books (N.Z.) Ltd, 182–190 Wairau Road,
Auckland 10, New Zealand

Penguin Books Ltd, Registered Offices:
Harmondsworth, Middlesex, England

First published by Plume, an imprint of New American Library, a
division of Penguin Books USA Inc.

Ninth Revised Edition [Sixteenth Plume Printing,] January, 1991
24 23 22 21 20 19 18 17 16

REGISTERED TRADEMARK—MARCA REGISTRADA

Printed in the United States of America

BOOKS ARE AVAILABLE AT QUANTITY DISCOUNTS WHEN USED TO PROMOTE
PRODUCTS OR SERVICES. FOR INFORMATION PLEASE WRITE TO PREMIUM
MARKETING DIVISION, PENGUIN BOOKS USA INC., 375 HUDSON STREET, NEW
YORK, NEW YORK 10014.

For Helen and Chet Osiecky

Contents

Introduction

This dictionary of foods lists several thousand brand-name products and basic foods with their caloric and carbohydrate content. The calorie yield of your diet versus the amount of energy you expend is the key to whether you maintain your ideal weight, gain too many pounds or lose weight.

Because of the relationship of weight to health, many individuals are "counting calories" at every meal. Interest has also been directed to the carbohydrate content of the diet in relation to weight control. Comprehensive information on these values in basic foods and brand-name products is not readily available in any one source. Nor is the information regularly supplied in single-serving portions. (For example, the United States Department of Agriculture supplies counts primarily in bulk-sized portions.) To compound the problem, hundreds of new food items appear in our stores every year.

Analyses of foods to provide information on nutritive values are extremely expensive to conduct. Many small companies have not been able to afford to have their products analyzed and thus were unable to provide data for this book or were able to provide only the calories or only the carbohydrates. Other companies have simply never gotten around to having the analysis done. Other companies simply refuse to supply nutritional information. New requirements for labeling nutritive values of products may provide information on additional items in the future. Therefore, wherever data for carbohydrates were unavailable, blank spaces were left which may be filled in by the reader at a later time.

Arrangement of This Book

Foods are listed alphabetically by brand name or by the name of the food. The singular form is used for most entries—that is, Blackberry instead of Blackberries. Most items are listed individually though a few are grouped under the general food category. For example, all candies are listed together so that if you are looking for *Mars* bar, you look first under Candy, then under *M* in alphabetical order; but, if you are looking for a breakfast food such as oatmeal, you will find it under *O* in the main alphabet. Other foods that are grouped include Baby Food, Gravy, Ice Cream, Marinade Mix, Pie, Sauce, Soft Drinks, Soup, and "Vegetarian Foods." Many cross references are included to assist in finding items called by different names.

Under the main headings, it was often not possible or even desirable to follow an alphabetical arrangement. For basic foods such as apricots, for example, the first entries are for the fresh product weighed with seeds as it is purchased in the store, then the fruit in small portions as they may be eaten or measured. These entries are followed by the processed products, canned (although it may actually be a bottle or jar), dehydrated, dried and frozen. This basic plan, with adaptations where necessary, was followed for fruits, vegetables and meats.

In almost all entries where data were available the U.S. Department of Agriculture figures are shown first. The Department values represent averages from several manufacturers and are shown for comparison with the values from individual companies or for use where particular brands are not available.

All brand-name products have been italicized and company names appear in parentheses.

Portions Used

The portion column is a most important one to read and note. Common household measures are used insofar as possible. For some items, the amounts given are those commonly purchased in the store, such as 1 pound of meat. These quantities can be divided into the number of servings used in the home and the nutritive values available to each person served can then be readily determined. Of course, any ingredients added when preparing such products must also be taken into account.

The smaller portions given are for foods as served or measured in moderate amounts, such as ½ cup of juice reconstituted, or 4 ounces of meat. Be sure to adjust the calories and carbohydrates to the actual portions you use. For example, if you serve 1 cup of juice instead of ½ cup, multiply the calories and carbohydrates shown for the smaller amount by 2.

Don't fool yourself about the size of portions you use. If you are serious about controlling the calories and carbohydrates in your diet, weigh your foods until you can accurately gauge the weight visually. Remember, the calories and carbohydrates go up with any increase in the weight of foods. Remember, too, that 4 ounces by weight may be very different from 4 fluid ounces or ½ cup. Ounces in the table are always ounces by weight unless specified as fluid ounces, or fractions of a cup or other volumetric measure. Foods that are fluffy in texture, such as flaked coconut and bean sprouts, vary greatly in weight per cup depending on how tightly they are packed into the cup. Such foods as canned green beans also vary when weighed with or without liquid; for example, canned green beans with liquid weigh 4.2 ounces for ½ cup, but drained beans weigh 2.5 ounces for the same ½ cup. Check the weights of your serving portions regularly. Bear in mind that you can cut calories and carbohydrates by cutting the serving size.

It was impossible to convert all the portions to a uniform basis. Some sources were only able to report data in terms of weights with no information on cup or other volumetric measures. I have shown small portions in quantities that might reasonably be expected to be served or measured in the home. Package sizes are useful to show the composition of products as they are purchased and may be divided into the number of serving portions prepared from the entire product, taking into account any added ingredients.

You will find in the portion column the phrases "weighed with bone," or "weighed with skin and seeds" or other inedible parts. These descriptions apply to the products as you purchase them in the markets, but the caloric values and the carbohydrate content as shown are for the amount of edible food after you discard the bone, skin, seed or other inedible part. The weight given in the "measure or quantity" column is to the nearest gram or fraction of an ounce.

Data on the composition of foods are constantly changing for many reasons. Better sampling and analytical methods, improvements in marketing procedures and changes in for-

mulas of mixed products, all may alter values for carbohydrates and other nutrients as well as caloric values. Weights
of packaged foods are frequently changed. It is essential to
read label information to be informed about these matters
and to make intelligent use of food tables.

This book, along with the individual calorie annual guide
(*The Barbara Kraus 1991 Calorie Guide to Brand Names
and Basic Foods*), is constantly revised and updated to help
keep you as up-to-date as possible.

Calories

What is a calorie? It is not a nutrient nor is it a good
guide to the nutritive value of food. It is more like a yard-
stick to measure the energy that a food will yield in the
body. You need energy for your body functions as well as
for exercise. If your diet contains more calories than your
body uses for these purposes, the extra "energy" will be
stored as fat.

If your plan is to cut down on calories, the easiest way to
do so is to consult the calorie column of this counter and
keep an accurate count of your total intake of food and
beverages for a period of seven days. If you have not gained
or lost weight during that week divide that number by
seven and you'll have your maintenance diet expressed in
calories. To lose weight, you must reduce your daily or
weekly intake of calories below this maintenance level. (To
gain, increase the intake.)

One pound of fat is equal to 3,500 calories. Add this
number of calories to those you need to balance your energy
requirements and you will gain one pound; subtract it, and
you will lose a pound.

Carbohydrates

The carbohydrate column shows the amount of this nutrient in grams for the quantities of foods indicated in the
portion column. Some dietitians are giving special attention
to this nutrient at present in connection with weight control.
Carbohydrates include sugars, starches, some acids and other
nutrients. The values in this book are total carbohydrates

by difference, the basis on which calories from carbohydrates are calculated in the U.S. diet.

Other Nutrients

Do not forget that other nutrients are extremely important in diet planning—protein, fat, minerals and vitamins. Calories yielded by alcohol must also be taken into consideration. From a nutrition viewpoint, perhaps the best advice that can be given to the dieter is to eat a varied diet with all classes of foods represented. Meat, fish, chicken, fats and oils, milk, vegetables, fruits and grain products are all important sources of essential nutrients and some foods from each of these classes of foods should be included in the diet every day. With the great abundance and variety of foods on the grocer's shelves, there is no reason why the dieter should not enjoy a tasty, nutritious and attractive diet. Just eat in moderation and there is no need to eliminate any one food altogether, except in special conditions under a doctor's directions. Choose wisely and eat well.

Sources of Data

Values in this dictionary are based on publications issued by the U.S. Department of Agriculture and on data submitted by manufacturers and processors. The U.S. Department of Agriculture issues basic tables on food composition for use in the United States. The commercial products from USDA publications represent average values obtained on products of more than one company. The figures designated "home recipe" are based on recipes on file with the Department of Agriculture. Data on commercial products listed by brand name in this publication are based on values supplied by manufacturers and processors for their own individual products. Very few supermarket brand names, such as Pathmark or private labels, were included in this book because they are not usually analyzed under these trade names. Every care has been taken to interpret the data and the descriptions supplied by the companies as fully and accurately as possible. Many values have been recalculated to different portions from those submitted in order to bring about greater uniformity among similar items.

Calories in these different sources are not always on a strictly uniform basis. In the Department of Agriculture, calories are calculated using specific factors, which make allowances for losses in digestion and metabolism. The technical explanation of these factors is given in Handbook 74 of the USDA. Most manufacturers use average factors of 4, 9 and 4 for calories yielded by each gram of protein, fat and carbohydrate respectively; a factor of 7 is used as an average value to calculate the calories from one gram of alcohol. These differences in procedure will give somewhat different results for products of similar composition. Some manufacturers have adopted the values from U.S. Department of Agriculture publications as representative of their own products. In these cases, it will be apparent in the table that the data from the companies match exactly those from USDA publications.

Bear in mind that small differences in calorie values on similar products of the same weight are not important in diet planning. They may be due to different methods of calculating the calories or to small differences in the nutritive values of the samples analyzed because no two foods ever have exactly the same composition. Some differences may also be due to the way the food was measured, as noted in the case of green beans earlier.

Carbohydrates in this book are usually total carbohydrates by difference. A few manufacturers reported only "available carbohydrates." These values were omitted.

Abbreviations and Symbols

(USDA) = United States Department of Agriculture
(HEW/FAO) = Health, Education and Welfare/Food and Agriculture Organization
* = prepared as package directs[1]
< = less than
& = and
" = inch
canned = bottles or jars as well as cans
dia. = diameter

fl. = fluid
liq. = liquid
lb. = pound
med. = medium
oz. = ounce
pkg. = package
pt. = pint
qt. = quart
sq. = square
T. = tablespoon
Tr. = trace
tsp. = teaspoon
wt. = weight

italics or name in parentheses = registered trademark, ®
the letters DNA indicate that data are not available.

Equivalents

By Weight
1 pound = 16 ounces
1 ounce = 28.35 grams
3.52 ounces = 100 grams

By Volume
1 quart = 4 cups
1 cup = 8 fluid ounces
1 cup = ½ pint
1 cup = 16 tablespoons
2 tablespoons = 1 fluid ounce
1 tablespoon = 3 teaspoons

[1]If the package directions call for whole or skim milk, the data given here are for whole milk, unless otherwise stated.

CALORIES
AND
CARBOHYDRATES

Food and Description	Measure or Quantity	Calories	Carbo-hydrates (grams)

A

ABALONE (USDA):
Raw, meat only	4 oz.	111	3.9
Canned	4 oz.	91	2.6

AC'CENT
	¼ tsp.	3	0.

ACEROLA, fresh fruit
	¼ lb. (weighed with seeds)	52	12.6

AGNOLETTI, frozen (Buitoni):
Cheese filled	2-oz. serving	196	33.4
Meat filled	2-oz. serving	206	31.7

ALBACORE, raw, meat only (USDA)
	4 oz.	201	0.

ALCOHOL (See **DISTILLED LIQUOR**)

ALE (See **BEER**)

ALFALFA SEEDS (USDA) sprouted
	1 cup	10	1.0

ALLSPICE (French's)
	1 tsp.	6	1.3

ALMOND:
Fresh (USDA):
In shell	10 nuts	60	2.0
Shelled, raw, natural, with skins	1 oz.	170	5.5

Roasted:
Dry (Planters)	1 oz.	170	6.0

(USDA): United States Department of Agriculture
(HEW/FAO):   Health, Education and Welfare/Food and Agriculture
                    Organization
* Prepared as Package Directs

Food and Description	Measure or Quantity	Calories	Carbo-hydrates (grams)
Honey roast (Eagle)	1 oz.	150	10.0
Oil:			
(Fisher)	1 oz.	178	5.5
(Tom's)	1 oz.	180	6.0
ALMOND EXTRACT (Virginia Dare) pure	1 tsp.	10	0.
ALPHA-BITS, cereal (Post)	1 cup (1 oz.)	113	24.6
AMARANTH, raw, trimmed (USDA)	4 oz.	41	7.4
AMARETTO DI SARONNO, 28% alcohol	1 fl. oz.	82	9.0
ANCHOVY, PICKLED, canned:			
(USDA) flat or rolled, not heavily salted, drained	2-oz. can	79	.1
(Granadaisor)	2-oz. can	80	Tr.
ANISE EXTRACT (Virginia Dare) 76% alcohol	1 tsp.	22	0.
ANISE SEEDS (USDA)	1 T.	21	3.0
ANISETTE:			
(DeKuyper)	1 fl. oz.	95	11.4
(Mr. Boston)	1 fl. oz.	87	10.8
APPLE:			
Fresh (USDA):			
Eaten with skin	2½" dia. (4.1 oz.)	61	15.3
Eaten without skin	2½" dia. (4.1 oz.)	53	13.9
Canned:			
(Comstock):			
Rings, drained	1 ring (1.1 oz.)	30	7.0
Sliced	⅙ of 21-oz. can	45	10.0
(White House):			
Rings, spiced	.7-oz. ring	11	8.0
Sliced	½ cup (4 oz.)	54	14.0
Dried:			
(Del Monte)	2-oz. serving	140	37.0
(Sun-Maid/Sunsweet) chunks	2-oz. serving	150	42.0
Frozen (USDA), sweetened, slices	10-oz. pkg.	264	68.9

Food and Description	Measure or Quantity	Calories	Carbo-hydrates (grams)
APPLE BROWN BETTY, home recipe (USDA)	1 cup	325	63.9
APPLE BUTTER:			
(Bama)	1 T.	36	9.0
(Home Brands)	1 T.	51	13.5
(White House)	1 T.	75	18.0
APPLE CHERRY BERRY DRINK, canned (Lincoln)	6 fl. oz.	90	23.0
APPLE-CHERRY JUICE COCKTAIL, canned, *Musselman's*	8 fl. oz.	110	28.0
APPLE CIDER:			
Canned:			
(Johanna Farms)	½ cup	56	14.5
(Mott's) sweet	½ cup	59	14.6
(Tree Top)	6 fl. oz.	90	22.0
*Mix:			
Country Time	8 fl. oz.	98	24.5
(Hi-C)	6 fl. oz.	72	18.0
APPLE CINNAMON SQUARES, cereal (Kellogg's)	½ cup (1 oz.)	90	23.0
APPLE-CRANBERRY JUICE, canned (Lincoln)	6 fl. oz.	100	25.0
APPLE DRINK:			
Canned:			
Capri Sun, natural	6¾ fl. oz.	90	22.7
(Hi-C)	6 fl. oz.	92	23.0
(Johanna Farms) *Ssips*	8.45-fl.-oz. container	130	32.0
*Mix (Hi-C)	6 fl. oz.	72	18.0
APPLE DUMPLINGS, frozen (Pepperidge Farm)	1 dumpling (3.1 oz.)	260	33.0

(USDA): United States Department of Agriculture
(HEW/FAO):   Health, Education and Welfare/Food and Agriculture
            Organization
* Prepared as Package Directs

Food and Description	Measure or Quantity	Calories	Carbohydrates (grams)
APPLE, ESCALLOPED:			
Canned (White House)	½ cup (4.5 oz.)	1.63	39.0
Frozen (Stouffer's)	4-oz. serving	130	27.0
APPLE-GRAPE JUICE, canned:			
Musselman's	6 fl. oz.	82	21.0
(Red Cheek)	6 fl. oz.	69	22.6
APPLE JACKS, cereal (Kellogg's)	1 cup (1 oz.)	110	26.0
APPLE JAM (Smucker's)	1 T.	53	13.5
APPLE JELLY:			
Sweetened (Smucker's)	1 T. (.7 oz.)	57	14.0
Dietetic:			
(Featherweight; Louis Sherry)	1 T. (.6 oz.)	6	0.
(Diet Delight)	1 T. (.6 oz.)	12	3.0
(Estee)	1 T. (.6 oz.)	6	0.
APPLE JUICE:			
Canned:			
(Ardmore Farms)	6 fl. oz.	90	22.2
(Borden) *Sippin' Pak*	8.45-fl.-oz. container	110	28.0
(Johanna Farms)	6 fl. oz.	85	21.0
(Johanna Farms) *Tree Ripe*	8.45-fl.-oz. container	121	29.7
(Lincoln) cocktail	6 fl. oz.	90	22.0
(Mott's)	6 fl. oz.	88	22.0
Musselman's	6 fl. oz.	80	21.0
(Ocean Spray)	6 fl. oz.	90	23.0
(Red Cheek)	6 fl. oz.	83	21.2
(Tree Top):			
Regular	6 fl. oz.	90	22.0
Sparkling	6 fl. oz.	80	21.0
(White House)	6 fl. oz.	87	22.0
Chilled (Minute Maid)	6 fl. oz.	91	22.7
*Frozen:			
(Minute Maid)	6 fl. oz.	91	22.7
(Sunkist)	6 fl. oz.	59	14.5
(Tree Top):			
Regular	6 fl. oz.	90	22.0
Unfiltered	6 fl. oz.	90	23.0

Food and Description	Measure or Quantity	Calories	Carbo-hydrates (grams)
APPLE JUICE DRINK, canned			
(Sunkist)	8.45 fl. oz.	140	34.0
APPLE RAISIN CRISP, cereal			
(Kellogg's)	⅔ cup (1 oz.)	130	32.0
APPLE PIE (See **PIE,** Apple)			
APPLE SAUCE, canned:			
Regular:			
(Comstock)	½ cup (4.4 oz.)	100	25.0
(Hunt's) *Snack Pack*:			
Regular	4¼ oz.	80	19.0
Natural	4¼ oz.	50	12.0
Raspberry	4¼ oz.	80	21.0
Strawberry	4¼ oz.	80	20.0
(Mott's):			
Regular, jarred:			
Plain	6 oz.	150	36.0
Chunky	6 oz.	86	21.0
Cinnamon	6 oz.	152	36.0
Single-serve cups:			
Regular	4 oz.	100	24.0
Cherry	3¾ oz.	72	17.0
Cinnamon	4 oz.	101	24.0
Peach	3¾ oz.	75	18.0
Pineapple	3¾ oz.	86	21.0
Strawberry	3¾ oz.	76	18.0
(Thank You Brand)	½ cup (4.5 oz.)	87	21.7
(Tree Top):			
Cinnamon or original	½ cup	80	20.0
Natural	½ cup	60	14.0
(White House)	½ cup (5 oz.)	80	22.0
Dietetic:			
(Del Monte, Lite; Diet Delight)	½ cup	50	13.0
(Mott's):			
Jarred	6 oz.	80	20.0
Single-serve cups	4 oz.	53	15.0
(S&W) *Nutradiet,* white or blue label	½ cup	55	14.0

(USDA): United States Department of Agriculture
(HEW/FAO): Health, Education and Welfare/Food and Agriculture
Organization
* Prepared as Package Directs

Food and Description	Measure or Quantity	Calories	Carbo-hydrates (grams)
(Thank You Brand)	½ cup (4.3 oz.)	54	13.4
(White House):			
Regular	½ cup (4.7 oz.)	50	12.0
Apple juice added	½ cup (4.7 oz.)	50	13.0
APPLE STRUDEL, frozen			
(Pepperidge Farm)	3-oz. serving	240	35.0
APRICOT:			
Fresh (USDA):			
Whole	1 lb. (weighed with pits)	217	54.6
Whole	3 apricots (about 12 per lb.)	55	13.7
Halves	1 cup (5½ oz.)	79	19.8
Canned, regular pack, solids & liq.:			
(USDA):			
Juice pack	4 oz.	61	15.4
Extra heavy syrup	4 oz.	115	29.5
(Del Monte):			
Whole	½ cup (4¼ oz.)	100	26.0
Halves, peeled	½ cup	200	27.0
(Stokely-Van Camp)	½ cup (4.6 oz.)	110	27.0
Canned, dietetic, solids & liq.:			
(Del Monte) Lite	½ cup (4¼ oz.)	60	16.0
(Diet Delight):			
Juice pack	½ cup (4.4 oz.)	60	15.0
Water pack	½ cup (4.3 oz.)	35	9.0
(Featherweight):			
Juice pack	½ cup	50	12.0
Water pack	½ cup	35	9.0
(Libby's) Lite	½ cup (4.4 oz.)	60	15.0
(S&W) *Nutradiet:*			
Halves, white or blue label	½ cup	35	9.0
Whole, juice pack	½ cup	28	7.0
Dried (Del Monte; Sun-Maid; Sunsweet) uncooked	2-oz. serving	140	35.0
APRICOT, CANDIED (USDA)	1 oz.	96	24.5
APRICOT LIQUEUR			
(DeKuyper) 60 proof	1 fl. oz.	82	8.3

Food and Description	Measure or Quantity	Calories	Carbo-hydrates (grams)
APRICOT NECTAR, canned:			
(Ardmore Farms)	6 fl. oz.	94	24.2
(Del Monte)	6 fl. oz.	100	26.0
APRICOT-PINEAPPLE NECTAR, canned, dietetic			
(S&W) *Nutradiet,* blue label	6 oz.	35	12.0
APRICOT & PINEAPPLE PRESERVE or JAM:			
Sweetened (Smucker's)	1 T. (.7 oz.)	53	13.5
Dietetic:			
(Diet Delight; Louis Sherry)	1 T. (.6 oz.)	6	3.0
(Featherweight)	1 T.	6	1.0
(S&W) *Nutradiet,* red label	1 T.	12	3.0
(Tillie Lewis) *Tasti Diet*	1 T.	12	3.0
APRICOT PRESERVE, dietetic			
(Estee)	1 T.	6	0.
APRICOT, STRAINED, canned			
(Larsen) no salt added	½ cup	55	14.5
ARBY'S:			
Bac'n Cheddar Deluxe	1 sandwich	561	36.0
Beef & Cheddar Sandwich	1 sandwich	490	51.0
Chicken breast sandwich	7¼-oz. sandwich	592	56.0
Croissant:			
Bacon & egg	1 order	420	32.0
Butter	1 piece	220	28.0
Chicken salad	1 order	460	16.0
Ham & swiss	1 order	330	33.0
Mushroom & swiss	1 order	340	34.0
Sausage & egg	1 order	530	31.0
French fries	1½-oz. serving	211	33.0
Ham 'N Cheese	1 sandwich	353	33.0
Potato cakes	2 pieces	201	22.0
Potato, stuffed:			
Broccoli & cheese	1 potato	541	72.0
Deluxe	1 potato	648	59.0

(USDA): United States Department of Agriculture
(HEW/FAO):   Health, Education and Welfare/Food and Agriculture
Organization
* Prepared as Package Directs

Food and Description	Measure or Quantity	Calories	Carbo- hydrates (grams)
Mushroom & cheese	1 potato	506	61.0
Taco	1 potato	619	73.0
Roast Beef:			
Regular	5-oz. sandwich	353	32.0
Junior	3-oz. sandwich	218	22.0
King	6.7-oz sandwich	467	44.0
Super	8.3-oz. sandwich	501	50.0
Turkey deluxe	7-oz. sandwich	375	32.0
Shake:			
Chocolate	10.6-oz. serving	314	62.0
Jamocha	10.8-oz. serving	424	76.0
Vanilla	8.8-oz. serving	295	44.0
ARTICHOKE:			
Fresh (USDA):			
Raw, whole	1 lb. (weighed untrimmed)	85	19.2
Boiled, without salt, drained	15-oz. artichoke	187	42.1
Canned (Cara Mia) marinated, drained	6-oz. jar	175	12.6
Frozen (Birds Eye) hearts, deluxe	⅓ pkg. (3 oz.)	33	6.6
ASPARAGUS:			
Fresh (USDA):			
Raw, spears	1 lb. (weighed untrimmed)	66	12.7
Boiled, without salt, drained	1 spear (½" dia. at base)	3	.5
Canned, regular pack, solids & liq.:			
(Del Monte) spears, green or white	½ cup (4 oz.)	20	3.0
(Green Giant) cuts or spears	½ cup (4 oz.)	20	3.0
(Le Sueur) green spears	½ of 8-oz. can	30	4.0
Mussleman's	½ cup (4.5 oz.)	20	3.0
Canned, dietetic pack (USDA) drained solids, cut	1 cup (8.3 oz.)	47	7.3
Canned, dietetic pack, solids & liq.:			
(Diet Delight)	½ cup	16	2.0
(S&W) *Nutradiet,* green label	½ cup	17	3.0
Frozen:			
(USDA) cuts & tips, boiled,			

Food and Description	Measure or Quantity	Calories	Carbo-hydrates (grams)
drained	1 cup (6.3 oz.)	40	6.3
(Birds Eye):			
Cuts	⅓ pkg. (3.3 oz.)	22	3.8
Spears	⅓ pkg. (3.3 oz.)	23	3.9
(Frosty Acres)	3.3-oz. serving	25	4.0
(McKenzie)	⅓ pkg. (3.3 oz.)	25	4.0
ASPARAGUS PUREE, canned			
(Larsen) no salt added	½ cup (4.4 oz.)	22	3.5
AUNT JEMIMA SYRUP (See **SYRUP**)			
AVOCADO, all varieties (USDA):			
Whole	1 fruit (10.7 oz.)	378	14.3
Cubed	1 cup (5.3 oz.)	251	9.5
AVOCADO PUREE			
(Calavo)	½ cup (8.1 oz.)	411	15.9
AWAKE (Birds Eye)	6 fl. oz. (6.5 oz.)	84	20.5

Food and Description	Measure or Quantity	Calories	Carbo- hydrates (grams)

B

BABY FOOD:

Advance (*Similac*)	1 fl. oz.	15	1.5
Apple & apricot (Beech-Nut):			
Junior	7¾-oz. jar	93	24.4
Strained	4¾-oz. jar	57	14.0
Apple-apricot juice (Gerber)			
strained	4.2 oz.	60	15.0
Apple-banana juice (Gerber)			
strained	4.2 fl. oz.	70	16.0
Apple-betty (Beech-Nut):			
Junior	7¾-oz. jar	173	41.4
Strained	4¾-oz. jar	106	25.4
Apple-blueberry (Gerber):			
Junior	7½-oz. jar	110	24.0
Strained	4½-oz. jar	60	14.0
Apple-cherry juice:			
Strained:			
(Beech-Nut)	4⅕ fl. oz.	50	14.0
(Gerber)	4.2 fl. oz.	60	15.0
Toddler (Gerber)	4 fl. oz.	52	12.7
Apple-cranberry juice (Beech-Nut) strained	4½ fl. oz.	55	13.6
Apple dessert, Dutch (Gerber):			
Junior	7½-oz. jar	160	36.0
Strained	4½-oz. jar	100	21.0
Apple-grape juice:			
Strained:			
(Beech-Nut)	4⅕ fl. oz.	56	13.9
(Gerber)	4.2 fl. oz.	60	15.0
Toddler (Gerber)	4 fl. oz.	60	15.0
Apple juice:			
Strained:			
(Beech-Nut)	4⅕ fl. oz.	54	13.6
(Gerber)	4.2 fl. oz.	60	15.0
Toddler (Gerber)	4 fl. oz.	60	15.0
Apple-peach juice, strained:			
(Beech-Nut)	4⅕ fl. oz.	59	14.6

Food and Description	Measure or Quantity	Calories	Carbo-hydrates (grams)
(Gerber)	4.2 fl. oz.	60	14.0
Apple-pineapple juice (Gerber) strained	4.2 fl. oz.	60	15.0
Apple-plum juice (Gerber) strained	4.2 fl. oz.	60	15.0
Apple-prune juice (Gerber) strained	4.2 fl. oz.	70	17.0
Applesauce:			
Junior:			
(Beech-Nut)	7¾-oz. jar	97	24.1
(Gerber)	7½-oz. jar	100	23.0
Strained:			
(Beech-Nut)	4¾-oz. jar	60	14.8
(Gerber):			
Regular	4½-oz. jar	60	14.0
First Foods	2½-oz. jar	30	7.0
Applesauce & apricots (Gerber):			
Junior	7½-oz. jar	110	24.0
Strained	4½-oz. jar	70	15.0
Applesauce & bananas (Beech-Nut) strained	4¾-oz. jar	63	15.4
Applesauce & cherries (Beech-Nut):			
Junior	7¾-oz. jar	115	28.4
Strained	4¾-oz. jar	61	15.1
Applesauce with pineapple (Gerber) strained	4½-oz. jar	60	14.0
Applesauce & raspberries (Beech-Nut):			
Junior	7¾-oz. jar	102	24.6
Strained	4¾-oz. jar	61	15.1
Apricot with tapioca:			
Junior:			
(Beech-Nut)	7½-oz. jar	113	27.9
(Gerber)	7¾-oz. jar	160	39.0
Strained (Gerber)	4½-oz. jar	90	20.0
Apricot with tapioca & apple juice (Beech-Nut) strained	4¾-oz. jar	72	17.6
Banana (Gerber) *First Foods*	2½-oz. jar	60	15.0

(USDA): United States Department of Agriculture
(HEW/FAO): Health, Education and Welfare/Food and Agriculture
Organization
* Prepared as Package Directs

Food and Description	Measure or Quantity	Calories	Carbo-hydrates (grams)
Banana-apple dessert (Gerber):			
Junior	7½-oz. jar	150	34.0
Strained	4½-oz. jar	90	21.0
Banana dessert (Beech-Nut)			
Junior	7½-oz. jar	165	40.1
Banana with pineapple & tapioca (Gerber):			
Junior	7½-oz. jar	110	25.0
Strained	4½-oz. jar	70	15.0
Banana & pineapple with tapioca & apple juice (Beech-Nut):			
Junior	7¾-oz. jar	109	26.6
Strained	4¾-oz. jar	67	16.3
Banana with tapioca:			
Junior:			
(Beech-Nut)	7½-oz. jar	72	27.5
(Gerber)	7½-oz. jar	160	39.0
Strained:			
(Beech-Nut)	4¾-oz. jar	72	16.9
(Gerber)	4½-oz. jar	100	24.0
Bean, green:			
Junior (Beech-Nut)	7¼-oz. jar	62	13.0
Strained:			
(Beech-Nut)	4½-oz. jar	38	8.1
(Gerber):			
Regular	4½-oz. jar	50	8.0
First Foods	2½-oz. jar	20	5.0
Bean, green, creamed (Gerber)			
Junior	7½-oz. jar	100	20.0
Beef (Gerber):			
Junior	3½-oz. jar	110	1.0
Strained	3½-oz. jar	100	0.
Beef & beef broth (Beech-Nut):			
Junior	7½-oz. jar	235	.4
Strained	4½-oz. jar	152	.3
Beef dinner, high meat, with vegetables (Gerber):			
Junior	4½-oz. jar	130	10.0
Strained	4½-oz. jar	120	8.0
Beef & egg noodle (Beech-Nut):			
Junior	7½-oz. jar	122	17.0
Strained	4½-oz. jar	72	9.9

Food and Description	Measure or Quantity	Calories	Carbo-hydrates (grams)
Beef & egg noodle with vegetables (Gerber) toddler, chunky	6-oz. jar	130	16.0
Beef with vegetables & cereal, high meat (Beech-Nut):			
Junior	4½-oz. jar	132	8.0
Strained	4½-oz. jar	132	8.1
Beef liver (Gerber) strained	3½-oz. jar	100	3.0
Beet (Gerber) strained	4½-oz. jar	50	11.0
Carrot:			
Junior:			
(Beech-Nut)	7½-oz. jar	67	13.8
(Gerber)	7½-oz. jar	60	12.0
Strained:			
(Beech-Nut)	4½-oz. jar	40	8.3
(Gerber):			
Regular	4½-oz. jar	40	7.0
First Foods	2½-oz. jar	30	5.0
Cereal, dry:			
Barley:			
(Beech-Nut)	½-oz. serving	54	9.9
(Gerber)	4 T. (½ oz.)	60	11.0
High protein:			
(Beech-Nut)	½-oz. serving	55	7.1
(Gerber)	4 T. (½ oz.)	50	5.0
High protein with apple & orange (Gerber)	4 T. (½ oz.)	60	4.0
Mixed:			
(Beech-Nut)	½-oz. serving	55	9.9
(Gerber)	4 T. (½ oz.)	50	10.0
Mixed with banana (Gerber)	4 T. (½ oz.)	60	11.0
Oatmeal:			
(Beech-Nut)	½-oz. serving	56	9.7
(Gerber)	4 T. (½ oz.)	50	9.0
Oatmeal & banana (Gerber)	4 T. (½ oz.)	60	10.0
Oat rings, toasted (Gerber) toddler	½ oz. serving	60	10.0
Rice:			
(Beech-Nut)	½-oz. serving	49	9.9
(Gerber)	4 T. (½ oz.)	60	11.0

(USDA): United States Department of Agriculture
(HEW/FAO):   Health, Education and Welfare/Food and Agriculture
                        Organization
* Prepared as Package Directs

Food and Description	Measure or Quantity	Calories	Carbo- hydrates (grams)
Rice with banana (Gerber)	4 T. (½ oz.)	56	10.7
Cereal or mixed cereal:			
With applesauce & banana:			
Junior (Gerber)	7½-oz. jar	131	26.4
Strained:			
(Beech-Nut)	4½-oz. jar	80	17.3
(Gerber)	4½-oz. jar	100	22.0
With egg yolks & bacon (Beech-Nut):			
Junior	7½-oz. jar	163	14.9
Strained	4½-oz. jar	113	8.9
Oatmeal with applesauce & banana (Gerber):			
Junior	7½-oz. jar	119	23.0
Strained	4½-oz. jar	100	21.0
Rice with applesauce & banana, strained:			
(Beech-Nut)	4¾-oz. jar	96	21.4
(Gerber)	4¾-oz. jar	100	23.0
Cherry vanilla pudding (Gerber):			
Junior	7½-oz. jar	150	35.0
Strained	4½-oz. jar	87	18.9
Chicken (Gerber):			
Junior	3½-oz. jar	140	0.
Strained	3½-oz. jar	140	1.0
Chicken & chicken broth (Beech-Nut):			
Junior	7½-oz. jar	228	.4
Strained	4½-oz. jar	128	.3
Chicken & noodle:			
Junior:			
(Beech-Nut)	7½-oz. jar	86	16.6
(Gerber)	7½-oz. jar	120	18.0
Strained:			
(Beech-Nut)	4½-oz. jar	59	10.5
(Gerber)	4½-oz. jar	80	12.0
Chicken & rice (Beech-Nut) strained	4½-oz. jar	72	12.0
Chicken soup, cream of (Gerber) strained	4½-oz. jar	70	11.0
Chicken stew (Gerber) toddler	6-oz. jar	145	12.3
Chicken sticks (Gerber) toddler	2½-oz. jar	120	1.0

Food and Description	Measure or Quantity	Calories	Carbo-hydrates (grams)
Chicken with vegetables, high meat (Gerber):			
Junior	4½-oz. jar	130	8.0
Strained	4½-oz. jar	140	8.0
Chicken with vegetables & cereal (Beech-Nut):			
Junior	7½-oz. jar	150	14.9
Strained	4½-oz. jar	90	8.9
Cookie (Gerber):			
Animal-shaped	6½-gram piece	25	4.0
Arrowroot	5½-gram piece	25	4.0
Corn, creamed:			
Junior:			
(Beech-Nut)	7½-oz. jar	142	30.9
(Gerber)	7½-oz. jar	130	27.0
Strained:			
(Beech-Nut)	4½-oz. jar	85	18.5
(Gerber)	4½-oz. jar	80	17.0
Cottage cheese with pineapple juice (Beech-Nut):			
Junior	7¾-oz. jar	178	32.1
Strained	4¾-oz. jar	111	22.3
Custard:			
Apple (Beech-Nut):			
Junior	7½-oz. jar	132	27.7
Strained	4½-oz. jar	79	16.6
Chocolate (Gerber) strained	4½-oz. jar	110	3.0
Vanilla:			
Junior:			
(Beech-Nut)	7½-oz. jar	166	29.0
(Gerber)	7½-oz. jar	190	38.0
Strained:			
(Beech-Nut)	4½-oz. jar	92	15.7
(Gerber)	4½-oz. jar	100	22.0
Egg yolk (Gerber):			
Junior	3⅓-oz. jar	184	.2
Strained	3⅓-oz. jar	190	1.0
Fruit dessert:			
Junior:			
(Beech-Nut):			

(USDA): United States Department of Agriculture
(HEW/FAO):   Health, Education and Welfare/Food and Agriculture
                    Organization
* Prepared as Package Directs

Food and Description	Measure or Quantity	Calories	Carbo-hydrates (grams)
Regular	7¾-oz. jar	162	40.3
Tropical	7¾-oz. jar	137	34.1
(Gerber)	7½-oz. jar	160	38.0
Strained:			
(Beech-Nut)	4½-oz. jar	97	24.0
(Gerber)	4½-oz. jar	100	22.0
Fruit juice, mixed:			
Strained:			
(Beech-Nut)	4⅕ fl. oz.	59	14.5
(Gerber)	4.2 fl. oz.	70	15.0
Toddler (Gerber)	4 fl. oz.	60	14.0
Fruit, mixed with yogurt:			
Junior (Beech-Nut)	7½-oz. jar	120	27.3
Strained:			
(Beech-Nut)	4¾-oz. jar	76	17.3
(Gerber)	4½-oz. jar	100	21.6
Guava (Gerber) strained	4½-oz. jar	84	19.9
Guava & tapioca (Gerber) strained	4½-oz. jar	90	20.0
Ham (Gerber):			
Junior	3½-oz. jar	120	0.
Strained	3½-oz. jar	110	1.0
Ham & ham broth (Beech-Nut) strained	4½-oz. jar	143	.3
Ham with vegetables, high meat (Gerber):			
Junior	4½-oz. jar	110	10.0
Strained	4½-oz. jar	100	9.0
Ham with vegetables & cereal (Beech-Nut):			
Junior	4½-oz. jar	126	7.9
Strained	4½-oz. jar	126	7.9
Hawaiian Delight (Gerber):			
Junior	7½-oz. jar	190	42.0
Strained	4½-oz. jar	120	25.0
Isomil (*Similac*) ready-to-feed	1 fl. oz.	20	1.9
Lamb (Gerber):			
Junior	3½-oz. jar	100	0.
Strained	3½-oz. jar	100	1.0
Lamb & lamb broth (Beech-Nut):			
Junior	7½-oz. jar	265	.4
Strained	4½-oz. jar	157	.2

Food and Description	Measure or Quantity	Calories	Carbo-hydrates (grams)
Macaroni alphabets with beef & tomato sauce (Gerber) toddler, chunky	6¼-oz. jar	130	20.0
Macaroni & cheese (Gerber):			
Junior	7½-oz. jar	135	18.8
Strained	4½-oz. jar	90	12.0
Macaroni & tomato with beef:			
Junior:			
(Beech-Nut)	7½-oz. jar	117	16.4
(Gerber)	7½-oz. jar	130	22.0
Strained:			
(Beech-Nut)	4½-oz. jar	81	10.7
(Gerber)	4½-oz. jar	80	12.0
Mango with tapioca (Gerber) strained	4¾-oz. jar	90	21.0
MBF (Gerber):			
Concentrate	1 fl. oz. (2 T.)	39	3.7
Concentrate	15 fl. oz. can	598	56.6
*Diluted, 1 to 1	1 fl. oz. (2 T.)	20	1.9
Meat sticks (Gerber) toddler	2½-oz. jar	110	1.0
Noodle & chicken with carrots & peas (Gerber) toddler, chunky	6-oz. jar	100	15.0
Orange-apple juice, strained:			
(Beech-Nut)	4½ fl. oz.	55	13.5
(Gerber)	4.2 fl. oz.	70	14.0
Orange-apricot juice (Beech-Nut) strained	4.2 fl. oz.	60	13.2
Orange-banana juice (Beech-Nut) strained	4⅕ fl. oz.	58	13.9
Orange juice, strained:			
(Beech-Nut)	4⅕ fl. oz.	56	13.2
(Gerber)	4.2 fl. oz.	70	14.0
Orange-pineapple dessert (Beech-Nut) strained	4¾-oz. jar	107	26.4
Orange-pineapple juice (Beech-Nut) strained	4⅕ fl. oz.	57	13.6
Orange pudding (Gerber) strained	4½-oz. jar	110	24.0

(USDA): United States Department of Agriculture
(HEW/FAO):   Health, Education and Welfare/Food and Agriculture
Organization
* Prepared as Package Directs

Food and Description	Measure or Quantity	Calories	Carbo-hydrates (grams)
Pea:			
Junior:			
(Beech-Nut)	7¼-oz. jar	114	19.1
(Gerber)	7½-oz. jar	110	20.0
Strained:			
(Beech-Nut)	4½-oz. jar	67	11.2
(Gerber)	4½-oz. jar	60	10.0
Pea & carrot (Beech-Nut) strained	4½-oz. jar	61	11.1
Peach:			
Junior:			
(Beech-Nut)	7¾-oz. jar	97	22.9
(Gerber)	7½-oz. jar	140	32.0
Strained:			
(Beech-Nut)	4¾-oz. jar	59	14.0
(Gerber):			
Regular	4½-oz. jar	90	19.0
First Foods	2½-oz. jar	30	7.0
Peach & apple with yogurt (Beech-Nut):			
Junior	7½-oz. jar	113	25.1
Strained	4½-oz. jar	68	15.1
Peach cobbler (Gerber):			
Junior	7½-oz. jar	160	38.0
Strained	4½-oz. jar	100	23.0
Peach melba (Beech-Nut):			
Junior	7¾-oz. jar	161	39.4
Strained	4¾-oz. jar	99	24.2
Pear:			
Junior:			
(Beech-Nut)	7½-oz. jar	106	26.2
(Gerber)	7½-oz. jar	120	27.0
Strained:			
(Beech-Nut)	4½-oz. jar	64	15.7
(Gerber):			
Regular	4½-oz. jar	80	16.0
First Foods	2½-oz. jar	40	11.0
Pear & pineapple:			
Junior:			
(Beech-Nut)	7½-oz. jar	121	29.6
(Gerber)	7½-oz. jar	109	25.4
Strained:			
(Beech-Nut)	4½-oz. serving	73	17.8
(Gerber)	4½-oz. jar	80	16.0
Pineapple dessert (Beech-Nut) strained	4¾-oz. jar	107	26.4

Food and Description	*Measure or Quantity*	*Calories*	*Carbo-hydrates (grams)*
Pineapple with yogurt (Beech-Nut):			
Junior	7½-oz. jar	133	30.0
Strained	4¾-oz. jar	84	19.0
Plum with tapioca (Gerber):			
Junior	7½-oz. jar	160	37.0
Strained	4¾-oz. jar	100	22.0
Plum with tapioca & apple juice (Beech-Nut):			
Junior	7¾-oz. jar	120	29.3
Strained	4¾-oz. jar	73	17.9
Pork (Gerber) strained	3½-oz. jar	110	0.
Potato & ham (Gerber) toddler, chunky	6-oz. jar	110	15.0
Pretzel (Gerber)	6-gram piece	25	5.0
Prune-orange juice (Beech-Nut) strained	4⅕ fl. oz.	66	15.7
Prune with tapioca:			
Junior (Beech-Nut)	7¾-oz. jar	174	40.5
Strained:			
(Beech-Nut)	4¾-oz. jar	107	24.8
(Gerber)	4¾-oz. jar	100	21.0
Rice & beef & tomato sauce (Gerber) toddler, chunky	6-oz. jar	150	20.0
Rice, saucy, & chicken (Gerber) toddler, chunky	6-oz. jar	110	17.0
Similac:			
Ready-to-feed or concentrated liquid, with or without added iron	1 fl. oz.	20	2.0
*Powder, regular or with iron	1 fl. oz.	20	2.0
Spaghetti, tomato & beef (Beech-Nut) junior	7½-oz. jar	131	19.4
Spaghetti with tomato sauce & beef (Gerber) junior	7½-oz. jar	140	25.0
Spinach, creamed (Gerber) strained	4½-oz. jar	60	9.0
Split pea & ham, junior:			
(Beech-Nut)	7½-oz. jar	149	23.4
(Gerber)	7½-oz. jar	150	24.0

(USDA): United States Department of Agriculture
(HEW/FAO): Health, Education and Welfare/Food and Agriculture Organization
* Prepared as Package Directs

Food and Description	Measure or Quantity	Calories	Carbo-hydrates (grams)
Squash:			
Junior:			
(Beech-Nut)	7½-oz. jar	57	11.7
(Gerber)	7½-oz. jar	70	13.0
Strained:			
(Beech-Nut)	4½-oz. jar	34	7.0
(Gerber):			
Regular	4½-oz. jar	40	8.0
First Foods	2½-oz. jar	20	4.0
Sweet potato:			
Junior:			
(Beech-Nut)	7¾-oz. jar	118	27.5
(Gerber)	7½-oz. jar	140	30.0
Strained:			
(Beech-Nut)	4½-oz. jar	68	15.9
(Gerber)	4½-oz. jar	80	18.0
Turkey (Gerber):			
Junior	3½-oz. jar	130	0.
Strained	3½-oz. jar	130	0.
Turkey & rice (Beech-Nut):			
Junior	7½-oz. jar	83	16.6
Strained	4½-oz. jar	59	12.0
Turkey with vegetables & cereal (Beech-Nut) high meat:			
Junior	4½-oz. jar	112	8.9
Strained	4½-oz. jar	112	8.9
Turkey sticks (Gerber) toddler	2½-oz. jar	120	1.0
Turkey & turkey broth (Beech-Nut) strained	4½-oz. jar	140	.2
Veal (Gerber):			
Junior	3½-oz. jar	100	0.
Strained	3½-oz. jar	100	0.
Veal & vegetables (Gerber):			
Junior	4½-oz. jar	110	10.0
Strained	4½-oz. jar	100	9.0
Veal & veal broth (Beech-Nut) strained	4½-oz. jar	143	.2
Vegetable & bacon:			
Junior:			
(Beech-Nut)	7½-oz. jar	141	18.9
(Gerber)	7½-oz. jar	180	21.0
Strained:			
(Beech-Nut)	4½-oz. jar	83	9.9
(Gerber)	4½-oz. jar	100	11.0

Food and Description	Measure or Quantity	Calories	Carbo-hydrates (grams)
Vegetable & beef:			
Junior:			
(Beech-Nut)	7½-oz. jar	123	18.1
(Gerber)	7½-oz. jar	140	20.0
Strained:			
(Beech-Nut)	4½-oz. jar	79	10.9
(Gerber)	4½-oz. jar	80	11.0
Vegetable & chicken:			
Junior:			
(Beech-Nut)	7½-oz. jar	89	15.9
(Gerber)	7½-oz. jar	120	18.0
Strained:			
(Beech-Nut)	4½-oz. jar	58	9.9
(Gerber)	4½-oz. jar	80	12.0
Vegetable & ham:			
Junior (Gerber)	4½-oz. jar	110	10.0
Strained:			
(Beech-Nut)	4½-oz. jar	75	10.9
(Gerber)	4½-oz. jar	80	11.0
Vegetable & lamb with rice & barley (Beech-Nut):			
Junior	7½-oz. jar	120	17.0
Strained	4½-oz. jar	74	10.0
Vegetable & liver (Gerber):			
Junior	7½-oz. jar	90	16.4
Strained	4½-oz. jar	60	11.0
Vegetable & liver with rice & barley (Beech-Nut):			
Junior	7½-oz. jar	91	16.8
Strained	4½-oz. jar	58	9.8
Vegetable, mixed:			
Junior:			
(Beech-Nut)	7½-oz. jar	79	17.0
(Gerber)	7½-oz. jar	90	17.0
Strained:			
(Beech-Nut):			
Regular	4½-oz. jar	55	12.0
Garden	4½-oz. jar	66	12.5
(Gerber):			
Regular	4½-oz. jar	50	10.0

(USDA): United States Department of Agriculture
(HEW/FAO):   Health, Education and Welfare/Food and Agriculture
                        Organization
* Prepared as Package Directs

Food and Description	Measure or Quantity	Calories	Carbo-hydrates (grams)
Garden	4½-oz. jar	50	8.0
Vegetable & turkey:			
Junior (Gerber)	7½-oz. jar	120	19.0
Strained:			
(Beech-Nut)	4½-oz. jar	77	12.1
(Gerber)	4½-oz. jar	70	10.0
Vegetable & turkey casserole			
(Gerber) toddler	6¼-oz. jar	147	14.2
BACON, broiled:			
(USDA):			
Medium slice	1 slice (7½ grams)	43	.1
Thick slice	1 slice (12 grams)	64	.2
Thin slice	1 slice (5 grams)	30	.2
(Hormel):			
Black Label	1 slice	30	0.
Range Brand	1 slice	55	0.
(Oscar Mayer):			
Center cut	1 slice (4 grams)	25	.1
Lower salt	1 slice	32	.1
Regular slice	6-gram slice	35	.1
Thick slice	1 slice (11 grams)	64	.2
BACON BITS:			
*Bac*Os* (Betty Crocker)	1 tsp.	13	.6
(French's) imitation	1 tsp.	6	Tr.
(Hormel)	1 tsp.	10	0.
(Libby's) crumbles	1 tsp.	8	.7
(McCormick) imitation	1 tsp.	9	.7
(Oscar Mayer) real	1 tsp.	6	.1
BACON, CANADIAN,			
unheated:			
(USDA)	1 oz.	61	Tr.
(Eckrich)	1-oz. slice	35	1.0
(Hormel):			
Regular	1 oz	45	0.
Light & Lean	1 slice	17	0.
(Oscar Mayer):			
Thin	.7-oz. slice	30	0.
Thick	1-oz. slice	35	.1

Food and Description	Measure or Quantity	Calories	Carbo-hydrates (grams)
BACON, SIMULATED,			
cooked:			
(Oscar Mayer) *Lean 'N Tasty:*			
Beef	1 slice (.4 oz.)	48	.2
Pork	1 slice (.4 oz.)	54	.1
(Swift's) *Sizzlean:*			
Beef	1 strip (4 oz.)	25	Tr.
Pork	1 strip	35	0.
BAGEL:			
(USDA):			
Egg	3″-dia. bagel, 1.9 oz.	162	28.3
Water	3″-dia. bagel, (1.9 oz.)	163	30.5
(Lender's):			
Plain	2-oz. bagel	150	30.0
Bagelettes	.9-oz. bagel	70	13.0
Egg	2-oz. bagel	150	29.0
Onion	1 bagel	160	31.0
Raisin & honey	2½-oz. bagel	200	40.0
Wheat & raisin with honey	2½-oz. bagel	190	39.0
BAKING POWDER:			
(USDA):			
Phosphate	1 tsp. (3.8 grams)	5	1.1
SAS	1 tsp. (3 grams)	4	.9
Tartrate	1 tsp. (2.8 grams)	2	.5
(Calumet)	1 tsp. (3.6 grams)	2	1.0
(Davis)	1 tsp. (3 grams)	7	1.7
(Featherweight) low sodium, cereal free	1 tsp.	8	2.0
BALSAMPEAR, fresh			
(Hew/FAO):			
Whole	1 lb. (weighed with cavity contents)	69	16.3
Flesh only	4 oz.	22	5.1

(USDA): United States Department of Agriculture
(HEW/FAO): Health, Education and Welfare/Food and Agriculture Organization
* Prepared as Package Directs

Food and Description	Measure or Quantity	Calories	Carbo-hydrates (grams)
BAMBOO SHOOTS:			
Raw, trimmed (USDA)	4 oz.	31	5.9
Canned, drained			
(Chun King)	8½-oz. can	65	12.5
(La Choy)	¼ cup	6	1.0
BANANA (USDA):			
Common yellow:			
Fresh:			
Whole	1 lb. (weighed with skin)	262	68.5
Small size	5.9-oz. banana (7¾" × 1¹¹⁄₃₂")	81	21.1
Medium size	6.3-oz. banana (8¾" × 1¹³⁄₃₂")	101	26.4
Large size	7-oz. banana (9¾" × 1⁷⁄₁₆")	116	30.2
Mashed	1 cup (about 2 med.)	191	50.0
Sliced	1 cup (about 1¼ med.)	128	33.3
Dehydrated flakes	½ cup (1.8 oz.)	170	44.3
Red, fresh, whole	1 lb. (weighed with skin)	278	72.2
BANANA EXTRACT (Durkee) imitation	1 tsp.	15	DNA
BANANA NECTAR, canned (Libby's)	6 fl. oz.	60	14.0
BANANA PIE (See **PIE,** Banana)			
BARBECUE SAUCE (See **SAUCE,** Barbecue)			
BARBECUE SEASONING (French's)	1 tsp. (.1 oz.)	6	1.0
BARBERA WINE (Louis M. Martini) 12½% alcohol	3 fl. oz.	65	.2

Food and Description	Measure or Quantity	Calories	Carbo- hydrates (grams)
BARDOLINO WINE (Antinori)			
12% alcohol	3 fl. oz.	84	6.3
BARLEY, pearl, dry:			
Light (USDA)	¼ cup (1.8 oz.)	174	39.4
Pot or Scotch:			
(USDA)	2 oz.	197	43.8
(Quaker) Scotch	¼ cup (1.7 oz.)	172	36.3
BASIL:			
Fresh (HEW/FAO) sweet, leaves	½ oz.	6	1.0
Dried (French's)	1 tsp.	3	.7
BASS (USDA):			
Black Sea:			
Raw, whole	1 lb. (weighed whole)	165	0.
Baked, stuffed, home recipe	4 oz.	294	12.9
Smallmouth & largemouth, raw:			
Whole	1 lb. (weighed whole)	146	0.
Meat only	4 oz.	118	0.
Striped:			
Raw, whole	1 lb. (weighed whole)	205	0.
Raw, meat only	4 oz.	119	0.
Oven-fried	4 oz.	222	7.6
White, raw, meat only	4 oz.	111	0.
BAY LEAF (French's)	1 tsp.	5	1.0
B & B LIQUEUR, 86 proof	1 fl. oz.	94	5.7
B.B.Q. SAUCE & BEEF, frozen (Banquet) *Cookin' Bag,* sliced	4-oz. pkg.	133	13.0
BEAN, BAKED:			
(USDA):			
With pork & molasses sauce	1 cup (9 oz.)	382	53.8

(USDA): United States Department of Agriculture
(HEW/FAO):   Health, Education and Welfare/Food and Agriculture
Organization
* Prepared as Package Directs

Food and Description	Measure or Quantity	Calories	Carbo-hydrates (grams)
With pork & tomato sauce	1 cup (9 oz.)	311	48.5
With tomato sauce	1 cup (9 oz.)	306	58.7
Canned:			
(Allen's) *Wagon Master*	1 cup	260	48.0
(B&M) *Brick Oven:*			
Barbecue style	8 oz.	310	48.0
Pea bean with pork in brown sugar sauce	8 oz.	300	42.0
Red kidney or yellow eye bean in brown sugar sauce	8 oz.	290	42.0
Vegetarian	8 oz.	250	42.0
(Campbell):			
Home style	8-oz. can	270	48.0
With pork & tomato sauce	8-oz. can	270	49.0
Old fashioned, in molasses & brown sugar sauce	8-oz. can	240	42.0
(Friend's):			
Pea	9-oz. serving	360	62.0
Red kidney	9-oz. serving	340	57.0
Yellow eye	9-oz. serving	360	60.0
(Furman's) & pork, in tomato sauce	8-oz. serving	245	46.4
(Grandma Brown's) home baked	8-oz. serving	289	54.1
(Hormel) *Short Orders:*			
With bacon	7½-oz. serving	330	40.0
With ham	7½-oz. serving	360	32.0
(Hunt's) & pork	8-oz. serving	280	52.0
(Van Camp):			
& pork	8-oz. serving	226	41.3
Vegetarian	8-oz. serving	216	41.9
BEAN, BARBECUE (Campbell)	7⅞-oz. can	250	43.0
BEAN & BEEF BURRITO DINNER, frozen (Swanson) 4-compartment	15¼-oz. dinner	720	88.0
BEAN, BLACK OR BROWN:			
Dry (USDA)	1 cup	678	122.4
canned (Goya)	1 cup	250	42.0
BEAN, FAVA, canned (Progresso)	4 oz. serving	90	15.5

Food and Description	Measure or Quantity	Calories	Carbo- hydrates (grams)
BEANS 'N FIXIN'S, canned (Hunt's) *Big John's:*			
Beans	3 oz.	100	21.0
Fixin's	1 oz.	50	7.0
BEAN & FRANKFURTER, canned:			
(USDA)	1 cup (9 oz.)	367	32.1
(Campbell) in tomato and molasses sauce	7⅞-oz. can	360	43.0
(Hormel) *Short Orders,* 'n wieners	7½-oz. can	280	39.0
BEAN & FRANKFURTER DINNER, frozen:			
(Banquet)	10-oz. dinner	510	57.0
(Morton)	10-oz. dinner	343	46.0
(Swanson) 3-compartment	12½-oz. dinner	550	75.0
BEAN, GARBANZO (See **CHICK-PEAS**)			
BEAN, GREEN: Fresh (USDA):			
Whole	1 lb. (weighed untrimmed)	128	28.3
French style	½ cup (1.4 oz.)	13	2.8
Boiled (USDA):			
Whole, drained	½ cup (2.2 oz.)	16	3.3
Boiled, 1½" to 2" pieces, drained	½ cup (2.4 oz.)	17	3.7
Canned, regular pack: (USDA):			
Whole, solids & liq.	½ cup (4.2 oz.)	22	5.0
Whole, drained solids	4 oz.	27	5.9
Cut, drained solids	½ cup (2.5 oz.)	17	3.6
Drained liquid only	4 oz.	11	2.7
(Allen's) solids & liq:			
Whole	½ cup (4.2 oz.)	21	4.0

(USDA): United States Department of Agriculture
(HEW/FAO):   Health, Education and Welfare/Food and Agriculture
Organization
* Prepared as Package Directs

Food and Description	Measure or Quantity	Calories	Carbo-hydrates (grams)
Cut	½ cup (4 oz.)	25	4.0
French	½ cup (4.1 oz.)	25	4.0
(Comstock) solids & liq.	½ cup (4 oz.)	25	5.0
(Del Monte) solids & liq.	4 oz.	20	4.0
(Green Giant) french or whole, solids & liq.	½ cup	20	4.0
(Larsen) *Freshlike*, solids & liq.	½ cup	20	4.0
(Sunshine) solids & liq.	½ cup (4.2 oz.)	20	3.8
Canned, dietetic or low calorie: (USDA):			
Solids & liq.	4 oz.	18	4.1
Drained solids	4 oz.	25	5.4
(Del Monte) No Salt Added, solids & liq.	½ cup (4 oz.)	19	4.0
(Diet Delight) solids & liq.	½ cup (4.2 oz.)	20	3.0
(Featherweight) solids & liq.	½ cup (4 oz.)	25	5.0
(Larsen) *Fresh-Lite*, water pack	½ cup (4.2 oz.)	20	4.0
(S&W) *Nutradiet* green label, solids & liq.	½ cup	20	4.0
Frozen:			
(Birds Eye):			
Cut:			
Plain	¼ of 12-oz. pkg.	25	5.8
With mushrooms	5-oz. serving	70	9.4
French:			
Plain	⅓ of 9-oz. pkg.	26	6.0
With toasted almonds	⅓ of 9-oz. pkg.	52	8.4
Petite, deluxe	⅓ of 8-oz. pkg.	20	4.6
Whole	⅓ of 9-oz. pkg.	23	5.1
(Frosty Acres)	3-oz. serving	25	6.0
(Green Giant):			
Cut or french, with butter sauce	½ cup	30	4.0
Cut, *Harvest Fresh*	½ cup	16	4.0
With mushroom in cream sauce	½ cup	80	10.0
Polybag	½ cup	14	4.0
(Larsen)	3 oz.	25	6.0
(McKenzie)	3 oz.	30	6.0
(Southland) cut or French	⅓ of 16-oz. pkg.	25	6.0
BEAN, GREEN, & MUSHROOM CASSEROLE, frozen (Stouffer's)	½ of 9½-oz. pkg.	160	13.0

Food and Description	Measure or Quantity	Calories	Carbo-hydrates (grams)
BEAN, GREEN, WITH POTATO, canned			
(Sunshine) solids & liq.	½ cup (4.3 oz.)	34	7.0
BEAN, GREEN, PUREE,			
canned (Larsen) no salt added	½ cup (4.4 oz.)	35	7.5
BEAN, ITALIAN:			
Canned (Del Monte) cut,			
solids & liq.	4 oz.	25	6.0
Frozen:			
(Birds Eye)	⅓ of pkg. (3 oz.)	31	7.2
(Frosty Acres)	3-oz. serving	30	7.0
(Larsen)	3 oz.	30	7.0
BEAN, KIDNEY OR RED:			
(USDA):			
Dry	½ cup (3.3 oz.)	319	57.6
Cooked	½ cup (3.3 oz.)	109	19.8
Canned, regular pack,			
solids & liq.:			
(Allen's)	½ cup (4.1 oz.)	110	20.0
(Comstock)	½ cup (4.4 oz.)	120	20.0
(Furman) red, fancy, light	½ cup (4½ oz.)	121	21.2
(Goya):			
Red	½ cup	115	20.0
White	½ cup	100	18.5
(Hunt's):			
Regular	½ cup (3.5 oz.)	80	16.0
Small red	4 oz.	120	21.0
Canned, dietetic (S&W)			
Nutradiet, low sodium,			
green label	½ cup	90	16.0
BEAN, LIMA:			
Raw (USDA):			
Young, whole	1 lb.		
	(weighed in pod)	223	40.1
Mature, dry	½ cup (3.4 oz.)	331	61.4
Young, without shell	1 lb.		
	(weighed shelled)	558	100.2

(USDA): United States Department of Agriculture
(HEW/FAO):   Health, Education and Welfare/Food and Agriculture
                        Organization
* Prepared as Package Directs

Food and Description	Measure or Quantity	Calories	Carbo-hydrates (grams)
Boiled (USDA) drained	½ cup	94	16.8
Canned, regular pack:			
(USDA):			
Solids & liq.	4 oz.	81	15.2
Drained solids	4 oz.	109	20.8
(Allen's):			
Regular	½ cup	60	9.0
Butter	½ cup	105	19.0
(Comstock) solids & liq.:			
Regular	½ cup (4.4 oz.)	110	20.0
Butter	½ cup (4.2 oz.)	100	16.0
(Del Monte) solids & liq.	4 oz.	70	14.0
(Furman's)	½ cup	92	16.7
(Larsen) *Freshlike*, solids & liq.	½ cup (4 oz.)	80	16.0
Canned, dietetic, solids & liq.:			
(Featherweight)	½ cup	80	16.0
(Larsen) *Fresh-Lite*, water pack, no salt added	½ cup (4.4 oz.)	80	16.0
Frozen:			
(Birds Eye):			
Baby	⅓ of 10-oz. pkg.	126	24.1
Fordhook	⅓ of 10-oz. pkg.	99	18.5
(Frosty Acres):			
Baby	3.3 oz.	130	24.0
Butter	3.3 oz.	140	26.0
Fordhook	3.3 oz.	100	19.0
(Green Giant):			
In butter sauce	½ cup	83	20.4
Harvest Fresh, or polybag	½ cup	60	15.0
(Larsen) baby	3.3 oz.	130	24.0
(McKenzie):			
Baby	3.3 oz.	130	24.0
Fordhook	3.3 oz.	100	19.0
Speckled butter	3.3 oz.	130	24.0
(Southland) speckled butter	⅕ of 16-oz. pkg.	120	22.0
BEAN, MUNG (USDA) dry	½ cup (3.7 oz.)	357	63.3
BEAN, PINK, canned (Goya) solids & liq.	½ cup	115	20.5
BEAN, PINTO:			
Dry (USDA)	4 oz.	396	72.2

Food and Description	Measure or Quantity	Calories	Carbo-hydrates (grams)
Canned:			
(Gebhardt)	½ of 15-oz. can	370	67.0
(Goya)	½ cup (4 oz.)	100	13.0
(Progresso)	½ cup (4 oz.)	82	16.5
Frozen (McKenzie)	3.2-oz. serving	160	29.0
BEAN, REFRIED, canned:			
(Del Monte) regular or spicy	½ cup (4.3 oz.)	130	20.0
(Gebhardt):			
Regular	4 oz.	130	20.0
Jalapeño	4 oz.	110	18.0
Little Pancho (Borden) & green chili	½ cup	80	15.0
Old El Paso:			
Plain	4 oz.	106	17.0
With green chili peppers	4 oz.	100	18.2
With sausage	4 oz.	224	14.8
(Rosarita):			
Regular	4 oz.	130	20.0
Bacon	4 oz.	132	19.6
With beans & onion	4 oz.	125	20.0
With green chilis	4 oz.	116	18.5
With nacho cheese & onion	4 oz.	135	21.1
Spicy	4 oz.	120	18.7
Vegetarian	4 oz.	120	18.7
BEAN SALAD, canned (Green Giant) three bean, solids & liq.	¼ of 17-oz. can	70	15.0
BEAN SOUP (See **SOUP,** Bean)			
BEAN SPROUT:			
Fresh (USDA):			
Mung, raw	½ lb.	80	15.0
Mung, boiled, drained	¼ lb.	32	5.9
Soy, raw	½ lb.	104	12.0
Soy, boiled, drained	¼ lb.	43	4.2
Canned, drained:			
(Chun King)	4 oz.	40	5.9
(La Choy)	⅔ cup (2 oz.)	6	1.4

(USDA): United States Department of Agriculture
(HEW/FAO): Health, Education and Welfare/Food and Agriculture
Organization
* Prepared as Package Directs

Food and Description	Measure or Quantity	Calories	Carbo-hydrates (grams)
BEAN, WHITE, canned (Goya) solids & liq.	½ cup	105	19.0
BEAN, YELLOW OR WAX:			
Raw, whole (USDA)	1 lb. (weighed untrimmed)	108	24.0
Boiled (USDA) 1″ pieces, drained	½ cup (2.9 oz.)	18	3.7
Canned, regular pack, solids & liq.:			
(Comstock)	½ cup (4.2 oz.)	20	4.0
(Del Monte) cut or french	½ cup (4 oz.)	20	4.0
(Larsen) *Freshlike,* cut, solids & liq.	½ cup (4.2 oz.)	25	5.0
Canned, dietetic, (Featherweight) cut stringless, solids & liq.	½ cup (4 oz.)	25	5.0
(Larsen) *Fresh-Lite,* cut, water pack, no salt added	½ cup (4.2 oz.)	18	4.0
Frozen:			
(Frosty Acres)	3 oz.	25	5.0
(Larsen) cut	3 oz.	25	5.0
BEAR CLAWS (Dolly Madison):			
Cherry	2¾-oz. piece	270	36.0
Cinnamon	2¾-oz. piece	290	39.0
BEEF. Values for beef cuts are given below for "leans and fat" and for "lean only." Beef purchased by the consumer at the retail store usually is trimmed to about one-half inch layer of fat. This is the meat described as "lean and fat." If all the fat that can be cut off with a knife is removed, the remainder is the "lean only." These cuts still contain flecks of fat known as "marbling" distributed through the meat. Cooked meats are medium done. Choice grade cuts (USDA):			
Brisket:			
Raw	1 lb. (weighed with bone)	1284	0.

Food and Description	Measure or Quantity	Calories	Carbo-hydrates (grams)
Braised:			
Lean & fat	4 oz.	467	0.
Lean only	4 oz.	252	0.
Chuck:			
Raw	1 lb. (weighed with bone)	984	0.
Braised or pot-roasted:			
Lean & fat	4 oz.	371	0.
Lean only	4 oz.	243	0.
Dried (see **BEEF, CHIPPED**)			
Fat, separable, cooked	1 oz.	207	0.
Filet mignon. There is no data available on its composition. For dietary estimates, the data for sirloin steak, lean only, afford the closest approximation.			
Flank:			
Raw	1 lb.	653	0.
Braised	4 oz.	222	0.
Foreshank:			
Raw	1 lb. (weighed with bone)	531	0.
Simmered:			
Lean & fat	4 oz.	310	0.
Lean only	4 oz.	209	0.
Ground:			
Lean:			
Raw	1 lb.	812	0.
Raw	1 cup (8 oz.)	405	0.
Broiled	4 oz.	248	0.
Regular:			
Raw	1 lb.	1216	0.
Raw	1 cup (8 oz.)	606	0.
Broiled	4 oz.	324	0.
Heal of round:			
Raw	1 lb.	966	0.
Roasted:			
Lean & fat	4 oz.	296	0.
Lean only	4 oz.	204	0.

(USDA): United States Department of Agriculture
(HEW/FAO):   Health, Education and Welfare/Food and Agriculture
                        Organization
* Prepared as Package Directs

Food and Description	Measure or Quantity	Calories	Carbo-hydrates (grams)
Hindshank:			
Raw	1 lb. (weighed with bone)	604	0.
Simmered:			
Lean & fat	4 oz.	409	0.
Lean only	4 oz.	209	0.
Neck:			
Raw	1 lb. (weighed with bone)	820	0.
Pot-roasted:			
Lean & fat	4 oz.	332	0.
Lean only	4 oz.	222	0.
Plate:			
Raw	1 lb. (weighed with bone)	1615	0.
Simmered:			
Lean & fat	4 oz.	538	0.
Lean only	4 oz.	252	0.
Rib roast:			
Raw	1 lb. (weighed with bone)	1673	0.
Roasted:			
Lean & fat	4 oz.	499	0.
Lean only	4 oz.	273	0.
Round:			
Raw	1 lb. (weighed with bone)	863	0.
Broiled:			
Lean & fat	4 oz.	296	0.
Lean only	4 oz.	214	0.
Rump:			
Raw	1 lb. (weighed with bone)	1167	0.
Roasted:			
Lean & fat	4 oz.	393	0.
Lean only	4 oz.	236	0.
Steak, club:			
Raw	1 lb. (weighed without bone)	1724	0.
Broiled:			
Lean & fat	4 oz.	515	0.
Lean only	4 oz.	277	0.
One 8-oz. steak (weighed without bone before cooking) will give you:			

Food and Description	Measure or Quantity	Calories	Carbo-hydrates (grams)
Lean & fat	5.9 oz.	754	0.
Lean only	3.4 oz.	234	0.
Steak, porterhouse:			
Raw	1 lb. (weighed with bone)	1603	0.
Broiled:			
Lean & fat	4 oz.	527	0.
Lean only	4 oz.	254	0.
One 16-oz. steak (weighed with bone before cooking) will give you:			
Lean & fat	10.2 oz.	1339	0.
Lean only	5.9 oz.	372	0.
Steak, ribeye, broiled:			
One 10-oz. steak (weighed before cooking without bone) will give you:			
Lean & fat	7.3 oz.	911	0.
Lean only	3.8 oz.	258	0.
Steak, sirloin, double-bone:			
Raw	1 lb. (weighed with bone)	1240	0.
Broiled:			
Lean & fat	4 oz.	463	0.
Lean only	4 oz.	245	0.
One 16-oz. steak (weighed before cooking with bone) will give you:			
Lean & fat	8.9 oz.	1028	0.
Lean only	5.9 oz.	359	0.
One 12-oz. steak (weighed before cooking with bone) will give you:			
Lean & fat	6.6 oz.	767	0.
Lean only	4.4 oz.	268	0.
Steak, sirloin, hipbone:			
Raw	1 lb. (weighed with bone)	1585	0.
Broiled:			
Lean & fat	4 oz.	552	0.

(USDA): United States Department of Agriculture
(HEW/FAO): Health, Education and Welfare/Food and Agriculture Organization
* Prepared as Package Directs

Food and Description	Measure or Quantity	Calories	Carbo-hydrates (grams)
Lean only	4 oz.	272	0.
Steak, sirloin, wedge & round-bone:			
Raw	1 lb. (weighed with bone)	1316	0.
Broiled:			
Lean & fat	4 oz.	439	0.
Lean only	4 oz.	235	0.
Steak, T-bone:			
Raw	1 lb. (weighed with bone)	1596	0.
Broiled:			
Lean & fat	4 oz.	536	0.
Lean only	4 oz.	253	0.
One 16-oz. steak (weighed before cooking with bone) will give you:			
Broiled:			
Lean & fat	4 oz.	463	0.
Lean only	4 oz.	245	0.
BEEF BOUILLON:			
(Borden) *Lite-Line*	1 tsp.	12	2.0
(Herb-Ox):			
Cube	1 cube	6	.7
Packet	1 packet	8	.9
(Wyler's)	1 cube	6	1.0
Low sodium (Featherweight)	1 tsp.	18	2.0
BEEF, CHIPPED:			
Cooked, creamed, home recipe (USDA)	½ cup (4.3 oz.)	188	8.7
Frozen, creamed:			
(Banquet)	4-oz. pkg.	100	9.0
(Stouffer's)	5½-oz. serving	230	9.0
BEEF DINNER or ENTREE:			
*Canned (Hunt's) *Entree Maker*, oriental	7.6-oz. serving	271	14.0
Frozen:			
(Armour):			
Classic Lite, Steak Diane	10-oz. meal	270	23.0
Dinner Classics:			
Sirloin roast	11-oz. meal	250	19.0
Sirloin tips	11-oz. meal	290	27.0

Food and Description	Measure or Quantity	Calories	Carbo-hydrates (grams)
(Banquet):			
American Favorites:			
Chopped	11-oz. dinner	434	23.0
With gravy	10-oz. dinner	345	19.0
Extra Helping:			
Regular	16-oz. dinner	864	72.0
Chopped	18-oz. dinner	1028	70.0
(Blue Star) *Dining Lite*, teriyaki with vegetables & rice	8⅝-oz. meal	230	33.0
(Chun King) Szechuan	13-oz. entree	331	57.0
(Conagra) *Light & Elegant*:			
Burgundy	9½-oz. entree	230	85.0
Julienne	8½-oz. entree	260	27.0
(La Choy) *Fresh & Light*, & broccoli, with rice	11-oz. meal	260	42.0
(Le Menu):			
Chopped sirloin	12¼-oz. dinner	440	28.0
Sirloin tips	11½-oz. dinner	390	26.0
Yankee pot roast	11-oz. dinner	360	28.0
(Morton) sliced	10-oz. dinner	215	19.0
(Stouffer's):			
Lean Cuisine:			
Oriental, with vegetable & rice	8⅝-oz. meal	250	28.0
Szechuan, with noodles & vegetables	9¼-oz. meal	260	22.0
Right Course:			
Dijon, with pasta & vegetables	9½-oz. meal	290	31.0
Fiesta, with corn & pasta	8⅞-oz. meal	270	23.0
Ragout, with rice pilaf	10-oz. meal	300	38.0
(Swanson):			
4-compartment dinner:			
Regular	11½-oz. dinner	320	35.0
Chopped sirloin	11½-oz. dinner	350	29.0
Hungry Man:			
Chopped	17¼-oz. dinner	600	48.0
Sliced	16-oz. dinner	470	49.0
Sliced	12¼-oz. entree	330	24.0

(USDA): United States Department of Agriculture
(HEW/FAO):   Health, Education and Welfare/Food and Agriculture
               Organization
* Prepared as Package Directs

Food and Description	Measure or Quantity	Calories	Carbo-hydrates (grams)
(Weight Watchers):			
Beefsteak, chopped	8¹⁵⁄₁₆-oz. pkg.	320	12.0
Oriental	10-oz. meal	260	32.1
BEEF, DRIED, packaged:			
(Carl Buddig) smoked	1 oz.	38	Tr.
(Hormel) sliced	1 oz.	45	0.
BEEF GOULASH (Hormel)			
Short Orders	7½-oz. can	230	17.0
BEEF, GROUND, SEASONING MIX:			
*(Durkee):			
Regular	1 cup	653	9.0
With onion	1 cup	659	6.5
(French's) with onion	1⅛-oz. pkg.	100	24.0
BEEF HASH, ROAST:			
Canned, *Mary Kitchen* (Hormel):			
Regular	7½-oz. serving	350	18.0
Short Orders	7½-oz. can	360	18.0
Frozen (Stouffer's)	10-oz. meal	380	16.0
BEEF, PACKAGED:			
(Carl Buddig) smoked	1 oz.	38	Tr.
(Hormel)	1 oz.	50	0.
BEEF, PEPPER, ORIENTAL:			
Canned (La Choy)	¾ cup	90	10.0
Frozen:			
(Chun King)	13-oz. entree	309	53.0
(La Choy)	12-oz. dinner	250	45.0
BEEF PIE, frozen:			
(Banquet)	8-oz. pie	449	44.0
(Empire Kosher)	8-oz. pie	540	51.0
(Morton)	7-oz. pie	430	27.0
(Stouffer's)	10-oz. pie	500	33.0
(Swanson):			
Regular	8-oz. pie	400	42.0
Chunky	10-oz. pie	530	53.0
Hungry Man:			
Regular	16-oz. pie	670	68.0

Food and Description	Measure or Quantity	Calories	Carbo-hydrates (grams)
Steak burger	16-oz. pie	750	61.0
BEEF, POTTED (USDA)	1 oz.	70	0.
BEEF ROLL (Hormel) Lumberjack	1 oz.	101	0.
BEEF, SHORT RIBS, frozen: (Armour) *Dinner Classics*, boneless	10½-oz. meal	390	35.0
(Stouffer's) boneless, with gravy	9-oz. entree	350	12.0
BEEF SOUP (See **SOUP**, Beef)			
BEEF SPREAD, ROAST, canned: (Hormel)	1 oz.	62	0.
(Underwood)	½ of 4¾-oz. can	140	Tr.
BEEF STEAK, BREADED (Hormel) frozen	4-oz. serving	370	13.0
BEEF STEW: Home recipe, made with lean beef chuck	1 cup (8.6 oz.)	218	15.2
Canned, regular pack: *Dinty Moore* (Hormel): Regular	⅓ of 24-oz. can	220	15.0
Short Orders	7½-oz. can	180	14.0
(Libby's)	7½-oz. serving	160	18.0
Canned, dietetic: (Estee)	7½-oz. serving	210	15.0
(Featherweight)	7½-oz. serving	220	24.0
Frozen, (Banquet) *Family Entrees*	2-lb. pkg.	1016	84.0
BEEF STEW SEASONING MIX: *(Durkee)	1 cup	379	16.7
(French's)	1⅛-oz. pkg.	150	30.0

(USDA): United States Department of Agriculture
(HEW/FAO): Health, Education and Welfare/Food and Agriculture Organization
* Prepared as Package Directs

Food and Description	Measure or Quantity	Calories	Carbo-hydrates (grams)
BEEF STOCK BASE (French's)	1 tsp (.13 oz.)	8	2.0
BEEF STROGANOFF, frozen:			
(Armour) *Dinner Classics*	10-oz. meal	320	22.0
(Conagra) *Light & Elegant*	9-oz. entree	260	27.0
(Green Giant) with noodles	9-oz. entree	380	35.0
(Le Menu)	9¼-oz. dinner	430	24.0
(Stouffer's) with parsley noodles	9¾-oz. pkg.	390	28.0
***BEEF STROGANOFF SEASONING MIX** (Durkee)	1 cup	820	71.2
BEER & ALE:			
Regular:			
Black Label	12 fl. oz.	136	11.2
Blatz	12 fl. oz.	142	11.8
Budweiser: Busch Bavarian	12 fl. oz.	148	12.4
Michelob	12 fl. oz.	162	14.3
Old Milwaukee	12 fl. oz.	142	13.4
Old Style	12 fl. oz.	146	11.5
Pearl Premium	12 fl. oz.	148	12.3
(Schlitz)	12 fl. oz.	150	13.2
(Schmidt)	12 fl. oz.	136	11.2
Stroh Bohemian	12 fl. oz.	148	13.6
Light or low carbohydrate:			
Budweiser Light	12 fl. oz.	108	6.7
Natural Light	12 fl. oz.	110	6.0
Michelob Light	12 fl. oz.	134	11.5
Old Milwaukee	12 fl. oz.	120	9.2
Pearl Light	12 fl. oz.	68	2.3
Schmidt Light	12 fl. oz.	96	3.2
Stroh Light	12 fl. oz.	115	7.1
BEER, NEAR:			
Goetz Pale	12 fl. oz.	78	3.9
(Metbrew)	12 fl. oz.	73	13.7
BEET:			
Raw (USDA):			
Whole	1 lb. (weighed with skins, without tops)	137	31.4
Diced	½ cup (2.4 oz.)	29	6.6
Boiled (USDA) drained:			

Food and Description	Measure or Quantity	Calories	Carbo-hydrates (grams)
Whole	2 beets (2″ dia., 3.5 oz.)	32	7.2
Diced	½ cup (3 oz.)	27	6.1
Sliced	½ cup (3.6 oz.)	33	7.3
Canned, regular pack, solids & liq.:			
(Blue Boy) Harvard	½ cup	100	23.0
(Comstock):			
Regular	½ cup	40	10.0
Pickled	½ cup	90	20.0
(Del Monte):			
Pickled	4 oz.	80	19.0
Sliced, tiny or whole	4 oz.	35	8.0
(Larsen) *Freshlike:*			
Pickled	½ cup (4.3 oz.)	100	25.0
Sliced or whole	½ cup (4.7 oz.)	40	9.0
Canned, dietetic, solids & liq.:			
(Del Monte) No Salt Added	½ cup (4 oz.)	35	8.0
(Featherweight) sliced	½ cup	45	10.0
(Larsen) *Fresh-Lite*, sliced, water pack, no salt added	½ cup (4.3 oz.)	40	9.0
(S&W) *Nutradiet*, sliced, green label	½ cup	35	9.0
BEET GREENS (USDA):			
Raw, whole	1 lb. (weighed untrimmed)	61	11.7
Boiled, halves & stems, drained	½ cup (2.6 oz.)	13	2.4
BEET PUREE, canned (Larsen) no salt added	½ cup (4.7 oz.)	45	10.0
BÉNÉDICTINE **LIQUEUR** (Julius Wile) 86 proof	1 fl. oz.	112	10.3
BERRY DRINK, MIXED, canned (Johanna Farms) *Ssips*	8.45-fl.-oz. container	130	32.0

(USDA): United States Department of Agriculture
(HEW/FAO):   Health, Education and Welfare/Food and Agriculture
            Organization
* Prepared as Package Directs

Food and Description	Measure or Quantity	Calories	Carbo-hydrates (grams)
BIG H, burger sauce			
(Hellmann's)	1 T. (.5 oz.)	71	1.6
BIG MAC (See **McDONALD'S**)			
BISCUIT DOUGH (Pillsbury):			
Baking Powder, *1869 Brand*	1 biscuit	100	12.0
Big Country	1 biscuit	95	15.5
Big Country, Good 'N Buttery	1 biscuit	100	14.0
Buttermilk:			
Regular	1 biscuit	50	10.0
Ballard, Oven Ready	1 biscuit	50	10.0
Butter Tastin', 1869 Brand	1 biscuit	100	12.0
Flaky, *Hungry Jack*, regular	1 biscuit	80	12.0
Oven Ready, Ballard	1 biscuit	50	10.0
BITTERS (Angostura)	1 tsp.	14	2.1
BLACKBERRY:			
Fresh (USDA) includes			
boysenberry, dewberry,			
youngsberry:			
With hulls	1 lb. (weighed		
	untrimmed)	250	55.6
Hulled	½ cup (2.6 oz.)	41	9.4
Canned, regular pack (USDA)			
solids & liq.:			
Juice pack	4-oz. serving	61	13.7
Light syrup	4-oz. serving	82	19.6
Heavy syrup	½ cup (4.6 oz.)	118	28.9
Extra heavy syrup	4-oz. serving	125	30.7
Frozen (USDA):			
Sweetened, unthawed	4-oz. serving	109	27.7
Unsweetened, unthawed	4-oz. serving	55	12.9
BLACKBERRY JELLY:			
Sweetened (Smucker's)	1 T. (.7 oz.)	53	13.5
Dietetic:			
(Diet Delight)	1 T. (.6 oz.)	12	3.0
(Featherweight) imitation	1 T.	16	4.0
BLACKBERRY LIQUEUR			
(Bols)	1 fl. oz.	95	8.9

Food and Description	Measure or Quantity	Calories	Carbo-hydrates (grams)
BLACKBERRY PRESERVE OR JAM:			
Sweetened (Smucker's)	1 T. (.7 oz.)	53	13.5
Dietetic:			
(Estee; Louis Sherry)	1 T. (.6 oz.)	6	0.
(Featherweight)	1 T.	16	4.0
(S&W) *Nutradiet*, red label	1 T.	12	3.0
BLACKBERRY WINE (Mogen David)	3 fl. oz.	135	18.7
BLACK-EYED PEAS:			
Canned, with pork, solids & liq:			
(Allen's) regular	½ cup	100	16.0
(Goya)	½ cup	105	19.5
Frozen:			
(Frosty Acres; McKenzie; Seabrook Farms)	⅓ of pkg. (3.3 oz.)	130	23.0
(Southland)	⅕ of 16-oz. pkg.	120	21.0
BLINTZE, frozen:			
(Empire Kosher):			
Apple	2½ oz.	100	24.0
Blueberry or cherry	2½ oz.	110	25.0
Cheese	2½ oz.	110	20.0
Potato	2½ oz.	130	21.0
(King Kold) cheese	2½ oz.	132	21.4
BLOODY MARY MIX:			
Dry (Bar-Tender's)	1 serving	26	5.7
Liquid (Sacramento)	5½-fl.-oz. can	39	9.1
BLUEBERRY:			
Fresh (USDA):			
Whole	1 lb. (weighed untrimmed)	259	63.8

(USDA): United States Department of Agriculture
(HEW/FAO):   Health, Education and Welfare/Food and Agriculture
                          Organization
* Prepared as Package Directs

Food and Description	Measure or Quantity	Calories	Carbo-hydrates (grams)
Trimmed	½ cup (2.6 oz.)	45	11.2
Canned, solids & liq.:			
(USDA):			
Syrup pack, extra heavy	½ cup (4.4 oz.)	126	32.5
Water pack	½ cup (4.3 oz.)	47	11.9
(Thank You Brand):			
Heavy syrup	½ cup (4.3 oz.)	102	25.4
Water pack	½ cup (4.2 oz.)	48	12.0
Frozen (USDA):			
Sweetened, solids & liq.	½ cup (4 oz.)	120	30.2
Unsweetened, solids & liq.	½ cup (2.9 oz.)	45	11.2
BLUEBERRY PIE (See PIE, Blueberry)			
BLUEBERRY PRESERVE OR JAM:			
Sweetened (Smucker's)	1 T.	53	13.5
Dietetic (Estee; Louis Sherry)	1 T.	6	0.
BLUEBERRY SQUARES, cereal (Kellogg's)	½ cup (1 oz.)	90	23.0
BLUEFISH (USDA):			
Raw:			
Whole	1 lb. (weighed whole)	271	0.
Meat only	4 oz.	133	0.
Baked or broiled	4.4-oz. piece (3½" × 3" × ½")	199	0.
Fried	5.3-oz. piece (3½" × 3" × ½")	308	7.0
BODY BUDDIES, cereal (General Mills):			
Brown sugar & honey	1 cup (1 oz.)	110	24.0
Natural fruit flavor	¾ cup (1 oz.)	110	24.0
BOLOGNA:			
(Eckrich):			
Beef:			
Regular	1 oz.	90	2.0
Smorgas Pak	¾-oz. slice	70	1.0

Food and Description	Measure or Quantity	Calories	Carbo-hydrates (grams)
Thick slice	1½-oz. slice	140	2.0
Thin slice	1 slice	55	1.0
Garlic	1-oz. slice	90	2.0
German brand, sliced or chub	1-oz. slice	80	1.0
Lunch chub	1-oz. serving	100	2.0
Meat:			
Regular	1-oz. slice	90	2.0
Thick slice	1.7-oz. slice	160	3.0
Thin slice	1 slice	55	1.0
Ring or sandwich	1-oz. slice	90	2.0
Hebrew National, beef	1 oz.	90	<1.0
(Hormel):			
Beef:			
Regular	1 slice	85	.5
Coarse grind	1 oz.	80	.5
Meat:			
Regular	1 slice	90	0.
Light & Lean:			
Regular	1 slice	70	1.0
Thin slice	1 slice	35	.5
(Ohse):			
Beef	1 oz.	85	1.0
Chicken, 15%	1 oz.	90	1.0
Chicken, beef & pork	1 oz.	75	3.0
(Oscar Mayer):			
Beef	.5-oz. slice	48	.5
Beef	1-oz. slice	90	.6
Beef Lebanon	.8-oz. slice	47	.3
Meat	1-oz. slice	90	.7
(Swift)	1-oz. slice	95	1.5
BOLOGNA & CHEESE:			
(Eckrich)	.7-oz. slice	90	2.0
(Oscar Mayer)	.8-oz. slice	74	.6
BONITO:			
Raw (USDA) meat only	4 oz.	191	0.
Canned (Star-Kist):			

(USDA): United States Department of Agriculture
(HEW/FAO): Health, Education and Welfare/Food and Agriculture
Organization
* Prepared as Package Directs

Food and Description	Measure or Quantity	Calories	Carbo-hydrates (grams)
Chunk	6½-oz. can	605	0.
Solid	7-oz. can	650	0.
BOO*BERRY, cereal			
(General Mills)	1 cup (1 oz.)	110	24.0
BORSCHT:			
Regular:			
(Gold's)	8-oz. serving	100	21.0
(Manischewitz)	8-oz. serving	80	20.0
(Rokeach)	1 cup (8 oz.)	96	21.5
Dietetic or low calorie:			
(Gold's)	8-oz. serving	24	17.5
(Manischewitz)	8-oz. serving	20	4.0
(Rokeach):	8-oz. serving	27	6.7
Diet	1 cup (8 oz.)	15	4.0
Unsalted	1 cup (8 oz.)	103	23.0
BOURBON (See **DISTILLED LIQUOR**)			
BOSCO (See **SYRUP**)			
BOYSENBERRY:			
Fresh (See **BLACKBERRY**)			
Frozen (USDA) sweetened	10-oz. pkg.	273	69.3
BOYSENBERRY JELLY:			
Sweetened (Smucker's)	1 T. (.7 oz.)	53	13.5
Dietetic (S&W) *Nutradiet,* red label	1 T.	12	3.0
BRAINS, all animals			
(USDA) raw	4 oz.	142	.9
BRAN:			
Crude (USDA)	1 oz.	60	17.5
Miller's (Elam's)	1 T. (.2 oz.)	17	2.8
BRAN BREAKFAST CEREAL:			
(General Mills) *Raisin Nut Bran*	½ cup (1 oz.)	110	20.0
(Kellogg's):			
All Bran or *Bran Buds*	⅓ cup (1 oz.)	70	22.0
Cracklin' Oat Bran	½ cup (1 oz.)	120	20.0
40% bran flakes	¾ cup (1 oz.)	90	23.0

Food and Description	Measure or Quantity	Calories	Carbohydrates (grams)
Fruitful Bran	¾ cup (1 oz.)	110	27.0
Raisin Bran	¾ cup	110	30.0
(Loma Linda)	1 oz.	90	19.0
(Nabisco)	½ cup (1 oz.)	70	21.0
(Post):			
40% bran flakes	⅔ cup (1 oz.)	107	22.5
With raisins	½ cup (1 oz.)	101	21.5
With raisins, *Honey Nut*			
Crunch	½ cup (1 oz.)	102	22.7
(Quaker) *Corn Bran*	⅔ cup (1 oz.)	109	23.3
(Ralston-Purina):			
Bran Chex	⅔ cup (1 oz.)	90	24.0
Bran News	¾ cup (1 oz.)	100	23.0
Oat	1 cup	130	32.0

BRANDY (See DISTILLED LIQUOR)

BRANDY, FLAVORED (Mr. Boston) 35% alcohol:

Apricot	1 fl. oz.	94	8.9
Blackberry	1 fl. oz.	92	8.6
Cherry	1 fl. oz.	87	8.4
Coffee	1 fl. oz.	72	10.6
Ginger	1 fl. oz.	72	3.5
Peach	1 fl. oz.	94	8.9

BRAUNSCHWEIGER:

(Eckrich) chub	1 oz.	70	1.0
(Hormel)	1 oz.	80	0.
(Oscar Mayer) tube	1 oz.	96	.9
(Swift) 8-oz. chub	1 oz.	109	1.4

BRAZIL NUT:
Raw (USDA):

Whole, in shell	1 cup (4.3 oz.)	383	6.4
Shelled	½ cup (2.5 oz.)	458	7.6
Shelled	4 nuts (.6 oz.)	114	1.9
Roasted (Fisher) salted	1 oz. (¼ cup)	193	3.1

(USDA): United States Department of Agriculture
(HEW/FAO): Health, Education and Welfare/Food and Agriculture Organization
* Prepared as Package Directs

Food and Description	Measure or Quantity	Calories	Carbo-hydrates (grams)
BREAD:			
Apple cinnamon (Pritikin)	1-oz. slice	80	14.0
Autumn grain (Interstate Brands) *Merita*	1-oz. slice	75	14.0
Barbecue, *Millbrook*	1.23-oz. slice	100	17.0
Boston Brown (USDA)	3″ × ¾″ slice (1.7 oz.)	101	21.9
Bran (Arnold) *Brannola*	1.2-oz. slice	90	16.0
Buttermilk, *Butternut*	1-oz. slice	80	13.0
Cinnamon (Pepperidge Farm)	.9-oz. slice	85	13.5
Cracked wheat:			
(Pepperidge Farm) thin sliced	.9-oz. slice	70	13.0
(Wonder)	1-oz. slice	75	13.6
Crispbread, *Wasa:*			
Mora	3.2-oz. slice	333	70.5
Rye:			
Golden	.3-oz. slice	37	7.8
Lite	.3-oz. slice	30	6.2
Sesame	.5-oz. slice	50	10.6
Sport	.4-oz. slice	42	9.1
Date nut roll (Dromedary)	1-oz. slice	80	13.0
Egg, *Millbrook*	1-oz. slice	70	14.0
Flatbread, *Ideal:*			
Bran	.2-oz. slice	19	4.1
Extra thin	.1-oz. slice	12	2.5
Whole grain	.2-oz. slice	19	4.0
French:			
(Arnold) *Francisco*	1/16 of loaf (1 oz.)	70	12.0
(Interstate Brands):			
Eddy's, sour	1.5-oz. slice	110	19.0
Sweetheart, regular	1-oz. slice	70	14.0
(Wonder)	1-oz. slice	71	13.6
Garlic (Arnold)	1-oz. slice	80	10.0
Hi-fibre (Monk's)	1-oz. slice	50	13.0
Hillbilly, Holsum	1-oz. slice	70	13.0
Hollywood:			
Dark	1-oz. slice	72	12.5
Light	1-oz. slice	71	13.1
Honey bran (Pepperidge Farm)	1 slice (1.2 oz.)	95	13.0
Honey wheat berry:			
(Arnold)	1.1-oz. slice	80	13.0
(Pepperidge Farm)	.9-oz. slice	70	13.5
Hunter's grain (Interstate Brands) *Country Farms*	1.5-oz. slice	120	22.0
Italian (Arnold) *Francisco*	1 slice	70	12.0

Food and Description	Measure or Quantity	Calories	Carbo-hydrates (grams)
Low sodium (Wonder)	1-oz. slice	71	13.6
Mountain oat (Interstate Brands) *Country Farms*	1.5-oz. slice	130	23.0
Multi-grain:			
(Arnold) *Milk & Honey*	1-oz. slice	70	14.0
(Pepperidge Farm) thin sliced	.5-oz. slice	40	7.0
(Pritikin)	1-oz. slice	70	12.0
Natural grains (Arnold)	.8-oz. slice	60	11.0
Oat (Arnold):			
Brannola	1.3-oz. slice	90	14.0
Milk & Honey	1-oz. slice	80	15.0
Oatmeal (Pepperidge Farm)	.9-oz. slice	70	12.5
Olympian meal (Interstate Brands) *Holsum*	1-oz. slice	70	13.0
Onion dill (Pritikin)	1-oz. slice	70	12.0
Potato (Interstate Brands) *Sweetheart*	1-oz. slice	70	14.0
Pita:			
Sahara (Thomas'):			
White:			
Regular	2-oz. piece	160	31.0
Mini	1-oz. piece	80	16.0
Large	3-oz. piece	240	48.0
Whole wheat:			
Regular	2-oz. piece	150	28.0
Mini	1-oz. piece	80	14.0
Poulsbo (Interstate Brands) *Eddy's*	1-oz. slice		
Protein (Thomas')	.7-oz. slice	46	7.4
Pumpernickel:			
(Arnold)	1.1-oz. slice	80	14.0
(Levy's)	1.1-oz. slice	80	14.0
(Pepperidge Farm):			
Regular	1.1-oz. slice	80	15.0
Party	.2-oz. slice	17	3.0
Raisin:			
(Arnold) tea	.9-oz. slice	70	13.0
(Interstate Brands) *Butternut*	1-oz. slice	80	15.0
(Monk's) & cinnamon	1-oz. slice	70	10.0
(Pepperidge Farm)	1 slice	75	14.0

(USDA): United States Department of Agriculture
(HEW/FAO):   Health, Education and Welfare/Food and Agriculture
                     Organization
* Prepared as Package Directs

Food and Description	Measure or Quantity	Calories	Carbo-hydrates (grams)
(Pritikin)	1-oz. slice	70	13.0
Sun-Maid (Interstate Brands)	1-oz. slice	80	15.0
Roman Meal	1-oz. slice	77	13.6
Rye:			
(Arnold):			
Jewish	1.1-oz. slice	80	14.0
Melba Thin	.7-oz. slice	40	8.0
(Levy's) real	1.1-oz. slice	80	14.5
(Pepperidge Farm):			
Family	1.1-oz. slice	85	15.5
Party	.2-oz. slice	17	3.2
(Pritikin)	1-oz. slice	70	12.0
(Wonder)	1-oz. slice	69	12.8
Salt Rising (USDA)	.9-oz. slice	67	13.0
7-Grain, Home Pride	1-oz. slice	72	12.8
Sourdough, *Di Carlo*	1-oz. slice	70	13.6
Split top (Interstate Brands)			
Merita	1-oz. slice	70	12.0
Sunflower & bran (Monk's)	1-oz. slice	70	12.0
Texas toast (Interstate Brands)			
Holsum	1.4-oz. slice	90	17.0
Wheat (see also Cracked Wheat or Whole Wheat):			
America's Own, cottage	1-oz. slice	70	13.0
(Arnold):			
Brannola:			
Dark	1.3-oz. slice	80	13.0
Hearty	1.3-oz. slice	90	13.0
Brick Oven	.8-oz. slice	60	9.0
Brick Oven	1.1-oz. slice	90	14.0
Country	1.3-oz. slice	80	13.0
Less or *Liteway*	.8-oz. slice	40	7.0
Milk & Honey	1-oz. slice	80	15.0
Very thin	.5-oz. slice	40	6.0
Fresh Horizons	1-oz. slice	54	9.6
Fresh & Natural	1-oz. slice	77	13.6
Home Pride	1-oz. slice	73	13.1
(Pepperidge Farm):			
Family	.9-oz. slice	85	17.5
Sandwich	.8-oz. slice	55	10.0
(Wonder) family	1-oz. slice	75	13.6
Wheatberry, *Home Pride:*			
Honey	1-oz. slice	74	13.3
Regular	1-oz. slice	70	12.5

Food and Description	Measure or Quantity	Calories	Carbo-hydrates (grams)
White:			
America's Own, cottage	1-oz. slice	70	15.0
(Arnold):			
Brick Oven	.8-oz. slice	60	11.0
Brick Oven	1.1-oz. slice	90	14.0
Country	1.3-oz. slice	100	18.0
Less or *Liteway*	.8-oz. slice	40	7.0
Milk & Honey	1-oz. slice	80	15.0
Very thin	.5-oz. slice	40	7.0
Fresh Horizons	1-oz. slice	54	10.0
Home Pride	1-oz. slice	72	13.1
(Interstate Brands):			
Butternut	1-oz. slice	70	14.0
Cookbook	1-oz. slice	75	14.0
Holsum	1-oz. slice	70	14.0
(Monk's)	1-oz. slice	60	10.0
(Pepperidge Farm):			
Regular	1.2-oz. slice	75	12.5
Toasting	1.2-oz. slice	85	16.0
Very thin slice	.6-oz. slice	40	8.0
(Wonder):			
Regular	1-oz. slice	70	13.4
Buttermilk	1-oz. slice	73	13.4
Whole wheat:			
(Arnold):			
Brick Oven	.8-oz. slice	60	9.5
Stone ground	.8-oz. slice	50	8.0
Home Pride	1-oz. slice	70	12.2
(Monk's) 100% stone ground	1-oz. slice	70	13.0
(Pepperidge Farm):			
Thin slice	.9-oz. slice	65	12.0
Very thin slice	.6-oz. slice	40	7.5
(Wonder) 100%	1-oz. slice	69	11.9
BREAD, CANNED, brown, plain or raisin:			
(B&M)	½" slice (1.6 oz.)	80	18.0
(Friend's)	½" slice	80	18.0
BREAD CRUMBS:			
(Contadina) seasoned	½ cup (2.1 oz.)	211	40.6

(USDA): United States Department of Agriculture
(HEW/FAO):   Health, Education and Welfare/Food and Agriculture
                        Organization
* Prepared as Package Directs

Food and Description	Measure or Quantity	Calories	Carbo-hydrates (grams)
(4C):			
Plain	4 oz.	405	85.2
Seasoned	4 oz.	384	77.3
(Pepperidge Farm) regular or seasoned	1 oz.	110	22.0
*BREAD DOUGH:			
Frozen:			
(Pepperidge Farm):			
Country rye or white	⅒ of loaf (1 oz.)	80	13.5
Stone ground wheat	⅒ of loaf (1 oz.)	75	13.0
(Rich's):			
French	½₀ of loaf	59	11.0
Italian	½₀ of loaf	60	11.0
Raisin	½₀ of loaf	66	12.3
Wheat	.5-oz. slice	60	10.5
White	.8-oz. slice	56	9.4
Refrigerated (Pillsbury) *Poppin' Fresh*:			
French	1″ slice	60	11.0
Wheat	1″ slice	80	12.0
White	1″ slice	80	13.0
*BREAD MIX:			
Home Hearth:			
French	⅜″ slice	85	14.5
Rye	⅜″ slice	75	14.0
White	⅜″ slice	75	14.5
(Pillsbury):			
Banana	½₁₂ of loaf	170	27.0
Blueberry nut	½₁₂ of loaf	150	26.0
Cherry nut	½₁₂ of loaf	180	29.0
Cranberry	½₁₂ of loaf	160	30.0
Date	½₁₂ of loaf	160	32.0
Nut	½₁₂ of loaf	170	28.0
BREAD PUDDING, with raisins, home recipe (USDA)	1 cup (9.3 oz.)	496	75.3
BREAD STICK (Stella D'Oro):			
Plain	1 piece	41	6.0
Sesame	1 piece	50	6.1
Wheat	1 piece	40	6.0
*BREAD STICK DOUGH (Pillsbury) *Pipin' Hot,* soft	1 piece	100	17.0

Food and Description	Measure or Quantity	Calories	Carbo-hydrates (grams)
*BREAKFAST DRINK (Pillsbury)	1 pouch	290	38.0
BREAKFAST SQUARES (General Mills) all flavors	1 bar (1.5 oz.)	190	22.5
BROCCOLI: Raw (USDA):			
Whole	1 lb. (weighed untrimmed)	69	16.3
Large leaves removed	1 lb.	113	20.9
Boiled (USDA):			
½" pieces, drained	½ cup (2.8 oz.)	20	3.5
Whole, drained	1 med. stalk (6.3 oz.)	47	8.1
Frozen: (Birds Eye):			
With almonds & selected seasonings	⅓ of pkg. (3.3 oz.)	62	5.7
In cheese sauce	⅓ of pkg. (3.3 oz.)	87	8.4
Chopped, cuts or florets	⅓ of pkg. (3.3 oz.)	26	4.9
Spears:			
Regular	⅓ of pkg. (3.3 oz.)	26	5.0
In butter sauce	⅓ of pkg. (3.3 oz.)	58	5.3
Deluxe	⅓ of pkg. (3.3 oz.)	29	5.0
& water chestnuts with selected seasonings	⅓ of pkg. (3.3 oz.)	35	5.8
(Frosty Acres)	3.3-oz. serving	25	5.0
(Green Giant):			
In cream sauce	3.3 oz.	0	7.4
Cuts, *Harvest Fresh*	3 oz.	16	3.0
Cuts, polybag	½ cup	12	3.0

(USDA): United States Department of Agriculture
(HEW/FAO): Health, Education and Welfare/Food and Agriculture Organization
* Prepared as Package Directs

Food and Description	Measure or Quantity	Calories	Carbo-hydrates (grams)
Spears:			
In butter sauce, regular	3⅓ oz.	40	6.0
Harvest Fresh	3 oz.	19	4.0
(McKenzie) chopped, cuts or spears	3.3 oz.	30	4.0
BROWNIE (See **COOKIE, Regular**)			
BROWNIE MIX (See **COOKIE MIX**)			
BRUNSWICK STEW, canned (Hormel) *Short Orders*	7½-oz. can	220	15.0
BRUSSELS SPROUT:			
Raw (USDA) trimmed	1 lb.	204	37.6
Boiled (USDA) drained	3-4 sprouts	28	4.9
Frozen:			
(USDA) boiled, drained	4 oz.	37	7.4
(Birds Eye):			
Regular	⅓ of 10-oz. pkg.	37	7.3
In butter sauce	⅓ of 10-oz. pkg.	59	7.2
Baby, with cheese sauce	⅓ of 10-oz. pkg.	84	8.7
Baby, deluxe	⅓ of 10-oz. pkg.	49	7.3
(Frosty Acres)	3-oz. serving	30	7.0
(Green Giant):			
In butter sauce	3.3 oz.	40	8.0
Polybag	½ cup	25	6.0
(Larsen)	3.3-oz. serving	35	7.0
(McKenzie)	3.3-oz. serving	35	7.0
BUCKWHEAT:			
Flour (See **FLOUR**)			
Groats (Pocono):			
Brown, whole	1 oz.	104	19.4
White, whole	1 oz.	102	20.1
BUC*WHEATS, cereal (General Mills)	1 oz. (¾ cup)	110	24.0

Food and Description	Measure or Quantity	Calories	Carbo-hydrates (grams)
BULGUR (form of hard red winter wheat) (USDA):			
Dry	1 lb.	1605	343.4
Canned:			
Unseasoned	4-oz. serving	191	39.7
Seasoned	4-oz. serving	206	37.2
BURGER KING:			
Apple pie	1 serving	305	44.0
Breakfast bagel sandwich:			
Plain	1 serving	387	46.0
Bacon	1 serving	438	46.0
Ham	1 serving	418	46.0
Sausage	1 serving	621	46.0
Breakfast Croissan'wich:			
Bacon	1 serving	355	20.0
Ham	1 serving	335	20.0
Sausage	1 serving	538	20.0
Cheeseburger:			
Regular	1 serving	304	27.0
Double:			
Plain	1 serving	464	27.0
Bacon	1 serving	510	27.0
Condiments:			
Ketchup	1 serving on sandwich	11	3.0
Mustard	1 serving on sandwich	2	0.
Pickles	1 serving on sandwich	0	0.
Chicken specialty sandwich:			
Plain	1 serving	492	54.0
Condiments:			
Lettuce	1 serving on sandwich	2	0.
Mayonnaise	1 serving on sandwich	194	2.0
Chicken Tenders	1 piece	34	1.7

(USDA): United States Department of Agriculture
(HEW/FAO):   Health, Education and Welfare/Food and Agriculture
          Organization
* Prepared as Package Directs

Food and Description	Measure or Quantity	Calories	Carbohydrates (grams)
Coffee, regular	1 serving	2	0.
Danish, great	1 piece	500	40.0
Egg platter, scrambled:			
Bacon	1 serving	68	0.
Croissant	1 serving	187	18.0
Eggs	1 serving	119	2.0
Hash browns	1 serving	162	13.0
Sausage	1 serving	234	0.
French fries	1 regular order	227	24.0
French toast sticks	1 serving	499	49.0
Hamburger:			
Plain	1 burger	262	26.0
Condiments:			
Ketchup	1 serving on burger	11	3.0
Mustard	1 serving on burger	2	0.
Pickles	1 serving on burger	0	0.
Ham & cheese specialty sandwich:			
Plain	1 sandwich	365	41.0
Condiments:			
Lettuce	1 serving on sandwich	3	1.0
Mayonnaise	1 serving on sandwich	97	1.0
Tomato	1 serving on sandwich	6	1.0
Milk:			
2% low fat	1 serving	121	12.0
Whole	1 serving	157	11.0
Onion rings	1 serving	274	28.0
Orange juice	1 serving	82	20.0
Salad:			
Chef	1 serving	180	7.0
Chicken	1 serving	140	8.0
Garden	1 serving	90	7.0
Side	1 serving	20	4.0
Salad dressing:			
Regular:			
Bleu cheese	1 serving	156	2.0
House	1 serving	130	3.0
1000 Island	1 serving	117	4.0
Dietetic, Italian	1 serving	14	2.0

Food and Description	Measure or Quantity	Calories	Carbo-hydrates (grams)
Shakes:			
Chocolate	1 shake	374	60.0
Vanilla	1 shake	334	51.0
Soft drink:			
Sweetened:			
Pepsi-Cola	1 regular size	159	40.0
7UP	1 regular size	144	38.0
Dietetic, *Pepsi*	1 regular size	1	0.
Whaler:			
Plain sandwich	1 sandwich	353	43.0
Condiments:			
Lettuce	1 serving on sandwich	1	0.
Tartar sauce	1 serving on sandwich	134	2.0
Whopper:			
Regular:			
Plain	1 burger	452	38.0
With cheese	1 burger	535	39.0
Condiments:			
Ketchup	1 serving on burger	17	4.0
Lettuce	1 serving on burger	1	0.
Mayonnaise	1 serving on burger	146	2.0
Onion	1 serving on burger	5	1.0
Pickle	1 serving on burger	1	0.
Tomato	1 serving on burger	6	1.0
Junior:			
Plain	1 burger	262	26.0
With cheese	1 burger	305	27.0
Condiments:			
Ketchup	1 serving on burger	8	2.0

(USDA): United States Department of Agriculture
(HEW/FAO): Health, Education and Welfare/Food and Agriculture
            Organization
* Prepared as Package Directs

Food and Description	Measure or Quantity	Calories	Carbo- hydrates (grams)
Lettuce	1 serving on burger	1	0.
Mayonnaise	1 serving on burger	48	1.0
Pickle	1 serving on burger	0	0.
Tomato	1 serving on burger	3	1.0
BURGUNDY WINE:			
(Carlo Rossi)	3 fl. oz.	69	1.2
(Louis M. Martini) 12½% alcohol	3 fl. oz.	60	.2
(Paul Masson) 12% alcohol	3 fl. oz.	70	2.2
(Taylor) 12½% alcohol	3 fl. oz.	75	3.3
BURGUNDY WINE, SPARKLING:			
(B&G) 12% alcohol	3 fl. oz.	69	2.2
(Great Western) 12% alcohol	3 fl. oz.	82	5.1
(Taylor) 12% of alcohol	3 fl. oz.	78	4.2
BURRITO:			
*Canned (Del Monte)	1 burrito	310	39.0
Frozen:			
(Fred's Frozen Foods) *Little Juan:*			
Bean & cheese	5-oz. serving	331	46.9
Beef & bean, spicy	10-oz. serving	814	92.2
Beef & potato	5-oz. serving	389	48.9
Chili:			
Green	10-oz. serving	741	87.6
Red	10-oz. serving	799	96.4
Chili dog	5-oz. serving	313	31.4
Red hot	5-oz. serving	433	47.7
(Hormel):			
Beef	1 burrito	205	31.0
Cheese	1 buritto	210	32.0
Chicken & rice	1 burrito	200	32.0
Grande	5½-oz. serving	380	45.0
Hot chili	1 burrito	240	33.0
(Patio):			
Dinner	12-oz. dinner	517	74.0

Food and Description	Measure or Quantity	Calories	Carbo-hydrates (grams)
Entree:			
Beef & bean:			
Regular	5-oz. serving	361	42.0
Green chili	5-oz. serving	330	42.0
Red chili	5-oz. serving	333	43.0
Red hot	5-oz. serving	352	43.0
(Swanson) with bean & beef	15¼-oz. dinner	720	88.0
(Van de Kamp's):			
Regular, crispy fried &			
guacamole sauce	6-oz. serving	365	40.0
Grande, with rice & corn	14¾-oz. pkg.	530	70.0
Sirloin	11-oz. pkg.	440	45.0
BURRITO FILLING MIX,			
canned (Del Monte)	½ cup (4.3 oz.)	110	20.0
BURRITO SEASONING MIX			
(Lawry's)	1½-oz. pkg.	132	23.3
BUTTER, salted or unsalted:			
Regular:			
(USDA)	¼ lb.	812	.5
(USDA)	1 T. (.5 oz.)	102	.1
(USDA)	1 pat (5 grams)	36	Tr.
(Breakstone)	1 T.	100	Tr.
(Meadow Gold)	1 tsp.	35	0.
Whipped (Breakstone)	1 T.	67	Tr.
BUTTERFISH, raw (USDA):			
Gulf:			
Whole	1 lb. (weighed whole)	220	0.
Meat only	4 oz.	108	0.
Northern:			
Whole	1 lb. (weighed whole)	391	0.
Meat only	4 oz.	192	0.
BUTTERSCOTCH MORSELS			
(Nestlé)	1 oz.	150	

(USDA): United States Department of Agriculture
(HEW/FAO):   Health, Education and Welfare/Food and Agriculture
                        Organization
* Prepared as Package Directs

Food and Description	Measure or Quantity	Calories	Carbohydrates (grams)
BUTTER SUBSTITUTE,			
Butter Buds:			
Dry	⅛ oz.	12	3.0
Liquid	1 fl. oz.	12	3.0
Sprinkles	1 tsp.	140	2.0

Food and Description	Measure or Quantity	Calories	Carbo- hydrates (grams)

C

CABBAGE:
White (USDA):
Raw:

Food and Description	Measure or Quantity	Calories	Carbo- hydrates (grams)
Whole	1 lb. (weighed untrimmed)	86	19.3
Finely shredded or chopped	1 cup (3.2 oz.)	22	4.9
Coarsely shredded or sliced	1 cup (2.5 oz.)	17	3.8
Wedge	3½" × 4½"	24	5.4
Boiled:			
Shredded, in small amount of water, short time drained	½ cup (2.6 oz.)	15	3.1
Wedges, in large amount of water, long time, drained	½ cup (3.2 oz.)	17	3.7
Dehydrated	1 oz.	87	20.9
Red:			
Raw (USDA) whole	1 lb. (weighed untrimmed)	111	24.7
Canned, solids & liq:			
(Comstock)	½ cup	60	13.0
(Greenwood)	½ cup	60	13.0
Savory (USDA) raw, whole	1 lb. (weighed untrimmed)	86	16.5
CABBAGE, STUFFED, frozen:			
(Green Giant)	½ of pkg.	220	19.0
(Stouffer's) *Lean Cuisine,* with meat, in tomato sauce	10¾-oz. pkg.	220	19.0

(USDA): United States Department of Agriculture
(HEW/FAO): Health, Education and Welfare/Food and Agriculture
                        Organization
* Prepared as Package Directs

Food and Description	Measure or Quantity	Calories	Carbo-hydrates (grams)
CABERNET SAUVIGNON:			
(Louis M. Martini) 12½% alcohol	3 fl. oz.	62	.2
(Paul Masson) 11.9% alcohol	3 fl. oz.	70	.2
***CAFE COMFORT,* 55 proof**	1 fl. oz.	79	8.8
CAKE:			
Non-Frozen:			
Plain:			
Home recipe, with butter & boiled white icing	⅑ of 9" square	401	70.5
Home recipe, with butter & chocolate icing	⅑ of 9" square	453	73.1
Angel food:			
Home recipe	1/12 of 8" cake	108	24.1
(Dolly Madison)	⅙ of 10½-oz. cake	120	17.0
Apple (Dolly Madison) Dutch, *Buttercrumb*	1½-oz. piece	170	28.0
Butter streusel (Dolly Madison) *Buttercrumb*	1½-oz. piece	150	23.0
Caramel, home recipe:			
Without icing	⅑ of 9" square	322	46.2
With caramel icing	⅑ of 9" square	331	50.2
Carrot (Dolly Madison) *Lunch Cake*	3¼-oz. serving	350	64.0
Chocolate, home recipe, with chocolate icing, 2-layer	1/12 of 9" cake	365	55.2
Chocolate (Dolly Madison) German, *Lunch Cake*	3¼-oz. serving	440	54.0
Cinnamon (Dolly Madison) *Buttercrumb*	1½-oz. piece	170	27.0
Creme (Dolly Madison) *Lunch Cake*	⅞-oz. piece	90	17.0
Crumb (see also **ROLL or BUN**) (Hostess)	1¼-oz. piece	131	21.7
Devil's food, home recipe:			
Without icing	3" × 2" × 1½" piece	201	28.6
With chocolate icing, 2-layer	1/16 of 9" cake	277	41.8
Fruit, home recipe:			
Dark	1/30 of 8" loaf	57	9.0
Light, made with butter	1/30 of 8" loaf	58	8.6
Hawaiian spice (Dolly Madison) *Lunch Cake*	3¼-oz. piece	350	58.0

Food and Description	Measure or Quantity	Calories	Carbo- hydrates (grams)
Honey (Holland Honey Cake)			
Low sodium:			
Fruit and raisin	½" slice (.9 oz.)	80	19.0
Orange and premium			
unsalted	½" slice (.9 oz.)	70	17.0
Honey 'n spice (Dolly			
Madison) *Lunch Cake*	3¼-oz. piece	330	57.0
Pound, home recipe:			
Equal weights flour, sugar			
butter and eggs	3½" × 3½" slice (1.1 oz.)	142	14.1
Pound (Dolly Madison)	⅙ of 14-oz. cake	220	33.0
Traditional, made with			
butter	3½" × 3½" slice (1.1 oz.)	123	16.4
Sponge, home recipe	1/12 of 10" cake	196	35.7
White, home recipe:			
Made with butter, without			
icing, 2-layer	⅑ of 9" wide, 3" high cake	353	50.8
Made with butter, with			
coconut icing, 2-layer	1/12 of 9" wide, 3" high cake	386	63.1
White & coconut (Dolly			
Madison), layer	1/12 of 30-oz. cake	220	37.0
Yellow, home recipe, made			
with butter, without icing,			
2-layer	⅑ of cake	351	56.3
Frozen:			
Apple walnut:			
(Pepperidge Farm) with			
cream cheese icing	⅛ of 11¾-oz. cake	150	18.0
(Sara Lee)	⅛ of 12½-oz. cake	165	21.6
Banana (Sara Lee)	⅛ of 13¾-oz. cake	175	26.9
Banana nut (Sara Lee)	⅛ of 20-oz. cake	232	26.5
Black Forest (Sara Lee)	⅛ of 21-oz. cake	203	27.9

(USDA): United States Department of Agriculture
(HEW/FAO): Health, Education and Welfare/Food and Agriculture Organization
* Prepared as Package Directs

Food and Description	Measure or Quantity	Calories	Carbo-hydrates (grams)
Boston Cream			
(Pepperidge Farm)	¼ of 11¾-oz. cake	290	39.0
Butterscotch pecan	⅒ of 17-oz. cake	160	23.0
Carrot:			
(Pepperidge Farm) with cream cheese icing	⅛ of 11¾-oz. cake	140	17.0
(Sara Lee)	⅛ of 12¼-oz. cake	152	18.9
(Weight Watchers)	3-oz. serving	180	27.0
Cheesecake:			
(Morton) *Great Little Desserts:*			
Cherry	6-oz. cake	460	47.0
Cream cheese	6-oz. cake	480	42.0
Pineapple	6-oz. cake	460	48.0
Strawberry	6-oz. cake	460	50.0
(Rich's) Viennese	⅟₁₄ of 42-oz. cake	230	24.1
(Sara Lee):			
Blueberry, *For 2*	½ of 11.3-oz. cake	425	66.6
Cream cheese:			
Regular	⅓ of 10-oz. cake	281	29.9
Large	⅙ of 17-oz. cake	231	25.9
Cherry	⅙ of 19-oz. cake	225	35.2
Cherry, *For 2*	½ of 11.3-oz. cake	423	69.3
French	⅛ of 23.5-oz. cake	274	24.9
Strawberry	⅙ of 19-oz. cake	223	33.6
Strawberry, *For 2*	½ of 11.3-oz. cake	420	67.9
(Weight Watchers):			
Regular	4-oz. serving	200	24.0
Black cherry	4-oz. serving	190	26.0
Strawberry	4-oz. serving	180	25.0
Chocolate:			
(Pepperidge Farm):			
Layer:			
Fudge	⅒ of 17-oz. cake	180	23.0
German	⅒ of 17-oz. cake	180	23.0
Mint	⅒ of 17-oz. cake	170	22.0
Supreme:			
Regular	¼ of 11½-oz. cake	310	37.0
Dutch	1¾-oz. serving	190	25.0

Food and Description	Measure or Quantity	Calories	Carbo- hydrates (grams)
(Sara Lee):			
Regular	⅛ of 13¼-oz. cake	199	28.1
Bavarian	⅛ of 22½-oz. cake	285	22.6
German	⅛ of 12¼-oz. cake	173	19.3
Layer:			
N'cream	⅛ of 18-oz. cake	215	23.8
Double	⅛ of 18-oz. cake	217	24.1
(Weight Watchers):			
Regular	2½-oz. serving	190	30.0
German	2½-oz. serving	200	31.0
Coconut (Pepperidge Farm) layer	¹⁄₁₀ of 17-oz. cake	180	25.0
Coffee (Sara Lee):			
Almond	⅛ of 11¾-oz. cake	165	20.2
Almond ring	⅛ of 9½-oz. cake	135	16.8
Apple	⅛ of 15-oz. cake	175	24.1
Apple, *For 2*	½ of 9-oz. cake	419	58.1
Blueberry ring	⅛ of 9¾-oz. cake	134	17.6
Butter, *For 2*	½ of 6½-oz. cake	356	41.9
Maple crunch ring	⅛ of 9¾-oz. cake	138	17.3
Pecan	⅛ of 11¼-oz. cake	163	19.1
Raspberry ring	⅛ of 9¾-oz. cake	133	18.5
Streusel, butter	⅛ of 11½-oz. cake	164	20.3
Streusel, cinnamon	⅛ of 10.9-oz. cake	154	19.0
Crumb (See **ROLL or BUN,** Crumb)			
Devil's food (Pepperidge Farm) layer	¹⁄₁₀ of 17-oz. cake	180	24.0

(USDA): United States Department of Agriculture
(HEW/FAO):   Health, Education and Welfare/Food and Agriculture
            Organization
* Prepared as Package Directs

Food and Description	Measure or Quantity	Calories	Carbo-hydrates (grams)
Golden (Pepperidge Farm) layer	1/10 of 17-oz. cake	180	24.0
Grand Marnier (Pepperidge Farm)	1½-oz. serving	160	22.0
Lemon coconut (Pepperidge Farm)	¼ of 12¼-oz. cake	280	38.0
Orange (Sara Lee)	⅛ of 13¾-oz. cake	179	25.3
Pineapple cream (Pepperidge Farm)	1/12 of 24-oz. cake	190	28.0
Pound:			
(Pepperidge Farm) butter	1/10 of 10¾-oz. cake	130	16.0
(Sara Lee):			
Regular	1/10 of 10¾-oz. cake	125	14.2
Banana nut	1/10 of 11-oz. cake	117	15.1
Chocolate	1/10 of 10¾-oz. cake	122	14.4
Chocolate swirl	1/10 of 11.8-oz. cake	116	16.0
Family size	1/15 of 16½-oz. cake	127	14.8
Homestyle	1/10 of 9½-oz. cake	114	13.1
Raisin	1/10 of 12.9-oz. cake	126	19.6
Spice (Weight Watchers)	3-oz. serving	170	24.0
Strawberry cream (Pepperidge Farm) Supreme	1/12 of 12-oz. cake	190	30.0
Strawberries'n cream, layer (Sara Lee)	⅛ of 20½-oz. cake	218	29.4
Strawberry shortcake (Sara Lee)	⅛ of 21-oz. cake	193	25.9
Torte (Sara Lee):			
Apples'n cream	⅛ of 21-oz. cake	203	26.2
Fudge & nut	⅛ of 15¾-oz. cake	200	21.0
Vanilla (Pepperidge Farm) layer	1/10 of 17-oz. cake	180	25.0
Walnut (Sara Lee) layer	⅛ of 18-oz. cake	210	22.8

Food and Description	Measure or Quantity	Calories	Carbo-hydrates (grams)
CAKE OR COOKIE ICING (Pillsbury):			
All flavors except chocolate	1 T.	70	12.0
Chocolate	1 T.	60	11.0
CAKE ICING:			
Amaretto almond (Betty Crocker) *Creamy Deluxe*	1/12 of can	170	26.0
Butter pecan (Betty Crocker) *Creamy Deluxe*	1/12 of can	160	25.0
Caramel, home recipe (USDA)	4 oz.	408	86.8
Caramel pecan (Pillsbury) *Frosting Supreme*	1/12 of can	160	21.0
Cherry (Betty Crocker) *Creamy Deluxe*	1/12 of can	160	26.0
Chocolate:			
(USDA) home recipe	1/2 cup (4.9 oz.)	519	93.0
(Betty Crocker) *Creamy Deluxe:*			
Regular	1/12 of can	170	23.0
Chip	1/12 of can	170	25.0
Fudge, dark dutch	1/12 of can	160	23.0
Nut	1/12 of can	160	22.0
Sour cream	1/12 of can	160	22.0
(Duncan Hines):			
Regular	1/12 of can	163	25.0
Fudge, dark dutch	1/12 of can	160	24.3
Milk	1/12 of can	162	24.7
(Pillsbury) *Frosting Supreme,* fudge, milk or mint	1/12 of can	150	24.0
Coconut almond (Pillsbury) *Frosting Supreme*	1/12 of can	150	17.0
Coconut pecan (Pillsbury) *Frosting Supreme*	1/12 of can	160	17.0
Cream cheese:			
(Betty Crocker) *Creamy Deluxe*	1/12 of can	170	26.0
(Pillsbury) *Frosting Supreme*	1/12 of can	160	26.0
Double dutch (Pillsbury) *Frosting Supreme*	1/12 of can	140	22.0

(USDA): United States Department of Agriculture
(HEW/FAO): Health, Education and Welfare/Food and Agriculture
            Organization
* Prepared as Package Directs

Food and Description	Measure or Quantity	Calories	Carbo-hydrates (grams)
Lemon:			
(Betty Crocker) *Creamy Deluxe*	1/12 of can	160	26.0
(Pillsbury) *Frosting Supreme*	1/12 of can	160	26.0
Orange (Betty Crocker)			
Creamy Deluxe	1/12 of can	160	26.0
Rocky road minimorsels (Betty			
Crocker) *Creamy Deluxe*	1/12 of can	160	20.0
Strawberry (Pillsbury) *Frosting*			
Supreme	1/12 of can	160	26.0
Vanilla:			
(Betty Crocker) *Creamy Deluxe*	1/12 of can	160	27.0
(Duncan Hines)	1/12 of can	163	25.5
(Pillsbury) *Frosting Supreme,*			
regular or sour cream	1/12 of can	160	27.0
White:			
Home recipe, boiled (USDA)	4 oz.	358	91.1
Home recipe, uncooked (USDA)	4 oz.	426	92.5
(Betty Crocker) *Creamy Deluxe,* sour cream	1/12 of can	160	26.0
*CAKE ICING MIX:			
Regular:			
Cherry (Betty Crocker) creamy	1/12 of pkg.	180	31.0
Chocolate:			
(Betty Crocker) creamy: Milk or sour cream	1/12 of pkg.	170	30.0
(Pillsbury) *Rich'n Easy* fudge or milk	1/12 of pkg.	150	26.0
Coconut almond:			
(Betty Crocker) creamy	1/12 of pkg.	140	18.0
(Pillsbury)	1/12 of pkg.	160	16.0
Coconut pecan:			
(Betty Crocker) creamy	1/12 of pkg.	160	19.0
(Pillsbury)	1/12 of pkg.	150	20.0
Cream cheese & nut (Betty			
Crocker) creamy	1/12 of pkg.	160	26.0
Double dutch (Pillsbury)			
Rich 'n Easy	1/12 of pkg.	150	26.0
Lemon:			
(Betty Crocker) creamy	1/12 of pkg.	180	31.0

Food and Description	Measure or Quantity	Calories	Carbo-hydrates (grams)
(Pillsbury) *Rich 'n Easy*	¹⁄₁₂ of pkg.	140	25.0
Strawberry (Pillsbury) *Rich 'n Easy*	¹⁄₁₂ of pkg.	140	25.0
Vanilla (Pillsbury) *Rich 'n Easy*	¹⁄₁₂ of pkg.	150	25.0
White:			
(Betty Crocker):			
Creamy	¹⁄₁₂ of pkg.	180	31.0
Fluffy	¹⁄₁₂ of pkg.	60	16.0
Sour cream, creamy	¹⁄₁₂ of pkg.	170	31.0
(Pillsbury) fluffy	¹⁄₁₂ of pkg.	60	15.0
CAKE MEAL (Manischewitz)	½ cup (2.6 oz.)	286	NA
CAKE MIX:			
Regular:			
Angel Food:			
(Betty Crocker):			
Chocolate or lemon custard	¹⁄₁₂ of pkg.	150	34.0
Confetti or strawberry	¹⁄₁₂ of pkg.	160	36.0
Traditional	¹⁄₁₂ of pkg.	130	30.0
(Duncan Hines)	¹⁄₁₂ of pkg.	124	28.9
*Apple (Betty Crocker) *Cake Lover's Collection,* Dutch	¹⁄₁₂ of cake	290	38.0
*Apple cinnamon (Betty Crocker) *Supermoist*	¹⁄₁₂ of cake	250	36.0
Applesauce raisin (Betty Crocker) *Snackin' Cake*	⅑ of pkg.	190	33.0
*Banana (Pillsbury):			
Pillsbury Plus	¹⁄₁₂ of cake	250	36.0
Streusel Swirl	¹⁄₁₂ of cake	260	38.0
*Banana walnut (Betty Crocker) *Snackin' Cake*	⅑ of cake	200	31.0
*Blackforest cherry (Pillsbury) *Bundt*	¹⁄₁₆ of cake	240	38.0
*Boston cream (Pillsbury) *Bundt*	¹⁄₁₆ of cake	270	43.0

(USDA): United States Department of Agriculture
(HEW/FAO):   Health, Education and Welfare/Food and Agriculture
Organization
* Prepared as Package Directs

Food and Description	Measure or Quantity	Calories	Carbohydrates (grams)
*Butter (Pillsbury)			
Pillsbury Plus	1/12 of cake	260	34.0
*Butter Brickle (Betty			
Crocker) Supermoist	1/12 of cake	260	38.0
Butter pecan (Betty Crocker)			
Supermoist	1/12 of cake	250	35.0
*Carrot (Betty Crocker):			
Cake Lover's Collection	1/12 of cake	320	40.0
Supermoist	1/12 of cake	260	34.0
*Carrot'n spice (Pillsbury)			
Pillsbury Plus	1/12 of cake	260	35.0
*Cheesecake:			
(Jello-O)	1/8 of cake	283	36.5
(Royal) No Bake:			
Lite	1/8 of cake	210	23.0
Real	1/8 of cake	280	31.0
*Cherry chip (Betty Crocker)			
Supermoist	1/12 of cake	190	37.0
Chocolate:			
(Betty Crocker):			
Cake Lover's Collection:			
Almond	1/12 of cake	360	41.0
Double	1/12 of cake	350	40.0
*Pudding	1/6 of cake	230	44.0
Snackin' Cake			
German coconut pecan	1/9 of pkg.	190	33.0
Stir 'N Frost:			
Chocolate chip, with			
chocolate frosting	1/6 of pkg.	230	41.0
Fudge, with vanilla			
frosting	1/6 of pkg.	230	43.0
*Supermoist:			
Butter recipe	1/12 of cake	270	35.0
Chip	1/12 of cake	280	36.0
Chocolate chip	1/12 of cake	250	34.0
Fudge	1/12 of cake	260	33.0
German	1/12 of cake	260	33.0
Milk	1/12 of cake	260	33.0
Sour cream	1/12 of cake	260	33.0
*(Duncan Hines):			
Deluxe	1/12 of cake	260	34.0
Devil's food	1/12 of cake	280	33.0
*(Pillsbury):			
Bundt:			
Tunnel of Fudge	1/16 of cake	260	37.0

Food and Description	Measure or Quantity	Calories	Carbo- hydrates (grams)
Macaroon	1/16 of cake	240	36.0
Microwave:			
Plain	1/8 of cake	210	23.0
Frosted:			
With chocolate frosting	1/8 of cake	300	35.0
With vanilla frosting	1/8 of cake	300	36.0
Supreme, double	1/8 of cake	330	39.0
Tunnel of Fudge	1/8 of cake	290	36.0
Pillsbury Plus:			
Chocolate chip	1/12 of cake	270	33.0
Fudge, dark	1/12 of cake	250	32.0
Fudge, marble	1/12 of cake	270	36.0
German	1/12 of cake	250	36.0
*Cinnamon (Pillsbury)			
Streusel Swirl	1/16 of cake	260	38.0
Coffee cake:			
*(Aunt Jemima)	1/8 of cake	170	29.0
*(Pillsbury) apple cinnamon	1/8 of cake	240	40.0
Devil's food:			
*(Betty Crocker)			
Supermoist	1/12 of cake	270	35.0
(Duncan Hines) deluxe	1/12 of pkg.	190	35.6
*(Pillsbury) *Pillsbury Plus*	1/12 of cake	270	32.0
Fudge (see Chocolate)			
Gingerbread (See **GINGERBREAD**)			
Golden chocolate chip (Betty Crocker) *Snackin' Cake*	1/9 of pkg.	190	34.0
Lemon:			
(Betty Crocker):			
*Chiffon	1/12 of cake	190	35.0
*Pudding	1/6 of cake	230	45.0
Supermoist	1/12 of cake	260	36.0
*(Pillsbury):			
Bundt, Tunnel of Lemon	1/16 of cake	270	45.0
Microwave:			
Plain	1/8 of cake	220	23.0
With lemon frosting	1/8 of cake	300	37.0
Supreme, double	1/8 of cake	300	40.0

(USDA): United States Department of Agriculture
(HEW/FAO): Health, Education and Welfare/Food and Agriculture Organization
* Prepared as Package Directs

Food and Description	Measure or Quantity	Calories	Carbo-hydrates (grams)
Pillsbury Plus	1/12 of cake	250	34.0
Streusel Swirl	1/16 of cake	270	39.0
*Lemon blueberry (Pillsbury) Bundt	1/16 of cake	200	28.0
*Marble (Betty Crocker) Supermoist	1/12 of cake	260	36.0
*Pineapple creme (Pillsbury) Bundt	1/16 of cake	260	41.0
Pound:			
*(Betty Crocker) golden	1/12 of cake	200	28.0
*(Dromedary)	1/2" slice (1/12 of pkg.)	150	21.0
Spice (Betty Crocker):			
Stir 'N Frost, with vanilla frosting	1/6 of pkg.	280	48.0
Supermoist	1/12 of cake	250	36.0
Strawberry:			
*(Betty Crocker) Supermoist	1/12 of cake	260	36.0
*(Pillsbury) Pillsbury Plus	1/12 of cake	260	37.0
*Upside down (Betty Crocker) pineapple	1/9 of cake	250	39.0
*Vanilla (Betty Crocker) golden, Supermoist	1/12 of cake	280	34.0
White:			
*(Betty Crocker) Supermoist	1/12 of cake	250	37.0
(Duncan Hines) deluxe	1/12 of pkg.	188	36.1
*(Pillsbury) Pillsbury Plus	1/12 of cake	240	35.0
Yellow:			
(Betty Crocker):			
Stir 'N Frost	1/6 of pkg.	230	37.0
*Supermoist	1/12 of cake	250	36.0
Supermoist, butter recipe	1/12 of cake	260	37.0
(Duncan Hines) deluxe	1/12 of pkg.	188	37.0
*(Pillsbury):			
Microwave:			
Plain	1/8 of cake	220	23.0
With chocolate frosting	1/8 of cake	300	36.0
Pillsbury Plus	1/12 of cake	260	36.0
*Dietetic (Estee)	1/10 of cake	100	18.0
CAMPARI, 45 proof	1 fl. oz.	66	7.1

Food and Description	Measure or Quantity	Calories	Carbo-hydrates (grams)
CANDY, GENERIC. The following values of candies from the U.S. Department of Agriculture are representative of the types sold commercially. These values may be useful when individual brands or sizes are not known:			
Almond:			
Chocolate-coated	1 cup (6.3 oz.)	1024	71.3
Chocolate-coated	1 oz.	161	11.2
Sugar-coated or Jordan	1 oz.	129	19.9
Butterscotch	1 oz.	113	26.9
Candy corn	1 oz.	103	25.4
Caramel:			
Plain	1 oz.	113	21.7
Plain with nuts	1 oz.	121	20.0
Chocolate	1 oz.	113	21.7
Chocolate with nuts	1 oz.	121	20.0
Chocolate-flavored roll	1 oz.	112	23.4
Chocolate:			
Bittersweet	1 oz.	135	13.3
Milk:			
Plain	1 oz.	147	16.1
With almonds	1 oz.	151	14.5
With peanuts	1 oz.	154	12.6
Semisweet	1 oz.	144	16.2
Sweet	1 oz.	150	16.4
Chocolate discs, sugar coated	1 oz.	132	20.6
Coconut center, chocolate-coated	1 oz.	124	20.4
Fondant, plain	1 oz.	103	25.4
Fondant, chocolate-covered	1 oz.	116	23.0
Fudge:			
Chocolate fudge	1 oz.	113	21.3
Chocolate fudge, chocolate-coated	1 oz.	122	20.7
Chocolate fudge with nuts	1 oz.	121	19.6
Chocolate fudge with nuts, chocolate-coated	1 oz.	128	19.1
Vanilla fudge	1 oz.	113	21.2

(USDA): United States Department of Agriculture
(HEW/FAO):   Health, Education and Welfare/Food and Agriculture
                        Organization
* Prepared as Package Directs

Food and Description	Measure or Quantity	Calories	Carbo-hydrates (grams)
Vanilla fudge with nuts	1 oz.	120	19.5
With peanuts & caramel, chocolate-coated	1 oz.	130	16.6
Gum drops	1 oz.	98	24.8
Hard	1 oz.	109	27.6
Honeycombed hard candy, with peanut butter, chocolate-covered	1 oz.	131	20.0
Jelly beans	1 oz.	104	26.4
Marshmallows	1 oz.	90	22.8
Mints, uncoated	1 oz.	103	25.4
Nougat & caramel, chocolate-covered,	1 oz.	118	20.6
Peanut bar	1 oz.	146	13.4
Peanut brittle	1 oz.	119	23.0
Peanuts, chocolate-covered	1 oz.	159	11.1
Raisins, chocolate-covered	1 oz.	120	20.0
Vanilla creams, chocolate-covered	1 oz.	123	19.9

CANDY, REGULAR:

Food and Description	Measure or Quantity	Calories	Carbo-hydrates (grams)
Almond, Jordan (Banner)	1¼-oz. box	154	27.9
Almond Joy (Peter Paul Cadbury)	1.5-oz. bar	220	26.0
Apricot Delight (Sahadi)	1 oz.	100	25.0
Baby Ruth	2-oz. piece	260	36.0
Bar None (Hershey's)	1½-oz. serving	240	23.0
Bonkers! (Nabisco)	1 piece	20	5.0
Breath Saver, any flavor	1 piece	8	2.0
Bridge Mix (Nabisco)	1 piece	10	2.0
Butterfinger	2-oz. bar	260	38.0
Butternut (Hollywood Brands)	2¼-oz. bar	310	36.0
Caramel Nip (Pearson)	1 piece	30	5.7
Charleston Chew	2-oz. bar	240	44.0
Cherry, chocolate-covered (Welchs):			
Dark	1 piece	90	16.0
Milk	1 piece	85	16.0
Chocolate bar:			
Brazil Nut (Cadbury's)	2-oz. serving	310	32.0
Caramello (Cadbury's)	2-oz. serving	280	37.0
Crunch (Nestlé)	1⅙-oz. bar	160	19.0
Fruit & nut (Cadbury's)	2-oz. serving	300	33.0
Hazelnut (Cadbury's)	2-oz. serving	310	32.0

Food and Description	Measure or Quantity	Calories	Carbo- hydrates (grams)
Milk:			
(Cadbury's)	2-oz. serving	300	34.0
(Hershey's)	1.65-oz. bar	250	27.0
(Nestlé)	.35-oz. bar	53	6.0
(Nestlé)	1¹⁄₁₆-oz. bar	159	18.1
Special Dark (Hershey's)	1.45-oz. bar	220	25.0
Chocolate bar with almonds:			
(Cadbury's)	2-oz. serving	310	31.0
(Hershey's) milk	1.55-oz. bar	250	22.0
(Nestlé)	1-oz.	160	15.0
Chocolate Parfait (Pearson)	1 piece		
	(6.5 grams)	30	5.7
Chocolate, Petite (Andes)	1 piece	26	2.6
Chuckles	1 oz.	100	23.0
Clark Bar	1.5-oz. bar	201	30.4
Coffee Nip (Pearson)	1 piece		
	(6.5 grams)	30	5.7
Coffioca (Pearson)	1 piece		
	(6.5 grams)	30	5.7
Creme De Menthe (Andes)	1 piece	25	2.6
Dutch Treat Bar (Clark)	1¹⁄₁₆-oz. bar	160	20.3
Eggs:			
(Nabisco) *Chuckles*	½ oz.	55	13.5
(Peter Paul Cadbury):			
Creme	1 oz.	136	19.2
Mini	1 oz.	140	20.0
5th Avenue (Hershey's)	1.93-oz. serving	270	41.0
Fruit bears (Flavor Tree) assorted	½ of 2.1-oz. pkg.	117	25.4
Fruit circus (Flavor Tree) assorted	½ of 2.1-oz. pkg.	117	25.4
Fruit roll (Flavor Tree):			
Apple, cherry, grape or raspberry	¾-oz. piece	75	18.5
Apricot	¾-oz. piece	76	17.7
Fruit punch or strawberry	¾-oz. piece	74	18.0
Fudge bar (Nabisco)	1 piece (.7 oz.)	85	14.5
Fun Fruit (Sunkist) any type	.9-oz. piece	100	21.8
Good & Plenty	1 oz.	100	24.8
Good Stuff (Nabisco)	1.8-oz. piece	250	29.0

(USDA): United States Department of Agriculture
(HEW/FAO): Health, Education and Welfare/Food and Agriculture
              Organization
* Prepared as Package Directs

Food and Description	Measure or Quantity	Calories	Carbo-hydrates (grams)
Halvah (Sahadi) original and marble	1 oz.	150	13.0
Hard (Jolly Rancher):			
All flavors except butterscotch	1 piece	23	5.7
Butterscotch	1 piece	25	5.6
Holidays (M&M/Mars):			
Plain	1 oz.	140	19.0
Peanut	1 oz.	140	16.0
Jelly bar, *Chuckles*	1 oz.	100	25.0
Jelly bean, *Chuckles*	½ oz.	55	13.0
Jelly rings, *Chuckles*	½ oz.	50	11.0
JuJubes, *Chuckles*	½ oz.	55	12.5
Kisses (Hershey's)	1 piece (.2 oz.)	24	2.5
Kit Kat	1.65-oz. bar	250	28.0
Krackle Bar	1.65-oz. bar	250	28.0
Licorice:			
Licorice Nips (Pearson)	1 piece (6.5 grams)	30	5.7
(Switzer) bars, bites or stix:			
Black	1 oz.	94	22.1
Cherry or strawberry	1 oz.	98	23.2
Chocolate	1 oz.	97	22.7
Life Savers	1 piece	7	3.0
Lollipops (Life Savers)	.1-oz. pop	45	11.0
Mallo Cup (Boyer)	.6-oz. piece	54	11.2
Mars Bar (M&M/Mars)	1.7-oz. bar	240	30.0
Marshmallow (Campfire)	1 oz.	111	24.9
Marshmallow Eggs, *Chuckles*	1 oz.	110	27.0
Mary Jane (Miller):			
Small size	¼-oz. piece	19	3.5
Large size	1½-oz. bar	110	20.3
Milk Duds (Clark)	¾-oz. bar	89	17.8
Milk Shake (Hollywood Brands)	2.4-oz. bar	300	51.0
Milky Way (M&M/Mars)	2.24-oz. bar	290	44.0
Mint Parfait:			
(Andes)	.2-oz. piece	27	2.7
(Pearson)	.2-oz. piece	30	5.7
Mint or peppermint:			
Junior mint pattie (Nabisco)	1 piece (.1 oz.)	10	2.0
Peppermint pattie:			
(Nabisco)	1 piece (.5 oz.)	55	12.5
York (Peter Paul Cadbury)	1¼-oz. serving	160	28.0
M & M's:			
Peanut	1.83-oz. pkg.	270	30.0
Plain	1.69-oz. pkg.	240	33.0

Food and Description	Measure or Quantity	Calories	Carbo-hydrates (grams)
Mounds (Peter Paul Cadbury)	1.65-oz. bar	230	28.0
Mr. Goodbar (Hershey's)	1.85-oz. bar	300	24.0
Munch bar (M&M/Mars)	1.42-oz. bar	220	19.0
My Buddy (Tom's)	1.8-oz. piece	250	30.0
Naturally Nut & Fruit Bar (Planters):			
Almond/apricot; almond/ pineapple; peanut/raisin	1 oz.	140	17.0
Walnut/apple	1 oz.	150	16.0
Nougat centers, *Chuckles*	1 oz.	110	26.0
$100,000 Bar (Nestlé)	1¼-oz. bar	175	23.8
Orange slices, *Chuckles*	1 oz.	110	24.0
Park Avenue (Tom's)	1.8-oz. piece	230	34.0
Payday (Hollywood Brands):			
Regular	1.9-oz. piece	250	28.0
Chocolate coated	2-oz. piece	290	30.0
Peanut bar (Planters)	1.6-oz. piece	240	21.0
Peanut, chocolate-covered:			
(Curtiss)	1 piece	5	1.0
(Nabisco)	1 piece (4.1 grams)	11	1.0
Peanut butter cup:			
(Boyer)	1.5-oz. pkg.	148	17.4
(Reese's)	.9-oz. cup	140	13.0
Peanut Butter Pals (Tom's)	1.3-oz. serving	200	19.0
Peanut crunch (Sahadi)	¾-oz. bar	110	9.0
Peanut Parfait:			
(Andes)	1 piece	28	2.5
(Pearson)	1 piece	30	5.7
Peanut Plank (Tom's)	1.7-oz. piece	230	28.0
Peanut Roll (Tom's)	1.7-oz. piece	230	29.0
Pom Poms (Nabisco)	1 oz.	100	15.0
Powerhouse (Peter Paul Cadbury)	2-oz. serving	260	38.0
Raisin, chocolate-covered (Nabisco)	1 piece	5	.7
Reese's Pieces (Hershey's)	1.95-oz. pkg.	270	31.0
Reggie Bar	2-oz. bar	290	29.0
Rolo (Hershey's)	1 piece (6 grams)	30	4.1

(USDA): United States Department of Agriculture
(HEW/FAO): Health, Education and Welfare/Food and Agriculture Organization
* Prepared as Package Directs

Food and Description	Measure or Quantity	Calories	Carbo-hydrates (grams)
Royals, mint chocolate (M&M/Mars)	1.52-oz. pkg.	212	29.5
Sesame Crunch (Sahadi)	¾-oz. bar	110	7.0
Sesame Tahini (Sahadi)	1 oz.	190	4.0
Skittles (M&M/Mars)	1 oz.	113	26.3
Skor (Hershey's)	1.4-oz. bar	220	22.0
Snickers (M&M/Mars)	2.16-oz. bar	290	36.0
Spearmint leaves (*Chuckles*)	1 oz.	110	15.0
Starburst (M&M/Mars)	1-oz. serving	120	24.0
Sugar Babies (Nabisco)	1⅝-oz. pkg.	180	40.0
Sugar Daddy (Nabisco) caramel sucker	1⅜-oz.	150	33.0
Sugar Mama (Nabisco)	1 piece (.8 oz.)	90	17.0
Taffy, Turkish (Bonomo)	1 oz.	108	24.4
3 Musketeers	2.13-oz. bar	260	46.0
Ting-A-Ling (Andes)	1 piece	24	2.8
Tootsie Roll:			
Chocolate	.23-oz. midgee	26	5.3
Chocolate	1/16-oz. bar	72	14.3
Chocolate	1-oz. bar	115	22.9
Flavored	.6-oz. square	19	3.8
Pop, all flavors	.49-oz. pop	55	12.5
Pop drop, all flavors	4.7-gram piece	19	4.2
Twizzler (Y & S) strawberry	1-oz. serving	100	23.0
Whatchamacallit (Hershey's)	1.8-oz. bar	260	30.0
Wispa (Peter Paul Cadbury)	1 oz.	150	17.0
Y & S Bites	1 oz.	100	23.0
Zagnut Bar (Clark)	.7-oz. bar	85	12.5
Zero (Hollywood Brands)	2-oz. bar	210	34.0
CANDY, DIETETIC:			
Carob bar, *Joan's Natural:*			
Coconut	3-oz. bar	516	28.4
Fruit & nut	3-oz. bar	559	31.2
Honey bran	3-oz. bar	487	34.0
Peanut	3-oz. bar	521	27.4
Chocolate or chocolate-flavored:			
(Estee) crunch or milk	.2-oz. square	30	2.5
(Louis Sherry):			
Coffee or orange flavored	.2-oz. square	22	2.0
Bittersweet or milk	.2-oz. square	30	2.5
Estee-ets, with peanuts (Estee)	1 piece (1.4 grams)	7	.8
Gum drops (Estee) any flavor	1 piece (1.8 grams)	3	.7

Food and Description	Measure or Quantity	Calories	Carbo-hydrates (grams)
Gummy Bears (Estee)	1 piece	5	1.0
Hard candy:			
(Estee) assorted fruit	1 piece (.1 oz.)	12	3.0
(Featherweight) assorted	1 piece	12	3.0
(Louis Sherry)	1 piece (.1 oz.)	12	3.0
Lollipop (Estee)	1 piece (.2 oz.)	25	3.0
Mint:			
(Estee)	1 piece (1.1 grams)	4	1.0
(Sunkist):			
Mini mint	1 piece (.2 grams)	<1	.2
Roll Mint	1 piece (.9 grams)	4	.9
Peanut brittle (Estee)	¼ oz.	35	5.0
Peanut butter cup (Estee)	1 cup (.3 oz.)	40	3.0
Raisins, chocolate-covered			
(Estee)	1 piece (1.2 grams)	5	.7
Rice crisp bar (Featherweight)	1 piece	50	4.5
CANNELONI, frozen:			
(Blue Star) *Dining Lite:*			
Cheese	9-oz. meal	261	35.5
Veal & vegetable	9-oz. meal	255	30.5
(Calentano) florentine	12-oz. pkg.	380	36.0
(Stouffer's) *Lean Cuisine:*			
Beef & pork with mornay sauce	9⅝-oz. pkg.	260	25.0
Cheese with tomato sauce	9⅛-oz. pkg.	260	22.0
(Weight Watchers) florentine, one-compartment meal	13-oz. meal	450	52.0
CANTALOUPE, fresh (USDA):			
Whole, medium	1 lb. (weighed with skin & cavity contents)	68	17.0
Cubed or diced	½ cup (2.9 oz.)	24	6.1

(USDA): United States Department of Agriculture
(HEW/FAO): Health, Education and Welfare/Food and Agriculture
            Organization
* Prepared as Package Directs

Food and Description	Measure or Quantity	Calories	Carbo-hydrates (grams)
CAP'N CRUNCH, cereal (Quaker):			
Regular	¾ cup (1 oz.)	121	22.9
Crunchberry	¾ cup (1 oz.)	120	22.9
Peanut butter	¾ cup (1 oz.)	127	20.9
CAPOCOLLO (Hormel)	1 oz.	80	0.
CARAWAY SEED (French's)	1 tsp (1.8 grams)	8	.8
CARL'S JR. RESTAURANT:			
Bacon	2 strips (10 grams)	50	0.
Cake, chocolate	3.2-oz. serving	380	43.0
California Roast Beef'n Swiss Sandwich	7.3-oz. serving	360	43.0
Cheese:			
American	.6-oz. serving	63	1.0
Swiss	.6-oz. serving	57	1.0
Chicken sandwich:			
Charbroiler BBQ	6.3-oz. serving	320	40.0
Charbroiler Club	8.2-oz. serving	510	53.0
Cookie, chocolate chip	2¼-oz. serving	330	44.0
Danish	3½-oz. piece	300	49.0
Eggs, scrambled	2.4-oz. serving	120	2.0
Fish sandwich, filet	7.9-oz. serving	550	58.0
French toast dips, excluding syrup	4.7-oz. serving	480	54.0
Hamburger:			
Plain:			
Famous Star	8.1-oz. serving	590	42.0
Happy Star	3.0-oz. serving	220	26.0
Old Time Star	6.9-oz. serving	400	38.0
Super Star	10.6-oz. serving	770	44.0
Cheeseburger, Western Bacon:			
Regular	7½-oz. serving	630	49.0
Double	10.4-oz. serving	890	61.0
Hot cakes, with margarine, excluding syrup	5½-oz. serving	360	59.0
Milk, 2% lowfat	10 fl. oz.	175	16.0
Muffins:			
Blueberry	3½-oz. muffin	256	40.0
Bran	4-oz. nuffin	220	34.0
English, with margarine	2-oz. muffin	180	28.0
Onion rings	3.2-oz. serving	310	38.0

Food and Description	Measure or Quantity	Calories	Carbo-hydrates (grams)
Orange juice, small	8 fl. oz.	94	21.0
Potato:			
Baked:			
Bacon & cheese	14.1-oz. serving	650	63.0
Broccoli & cheese	14-oz. serving	470	61.0
Cheese	14.2-oz. serving	550	72.0
Fiesta	15.2-oz. serving	550	60.0
Lite	9.8-oz. serving	250	54.0
Sour cream & chive	10.4-oz. serving	350	49.0
French fries, regular	6-oz. serving	360	43.0
Hash brown nuggets	3-oz. serving	170	20.0
Salad dressing:			
Regular:			
Blue cheese	2-oz. serving	150	3.0
House	2-oz. serving	186	6.0
1000 Island	2-oz. serving	231	7.0
Dietetic, Italian	2-oz. serving	80	0.
Sausage	1½-oz. patty	190	1.0
Shakes	1 regular size shake	353	61.0
Soft drink:			
Regular	1 regular size soft drink	243	62.0
Dietetic	1 regular size soft drink	2	0.
Soup:			
Broccoli, cream of	6 fl. oz.	140	14.0
Chicken & noodle	6 fl. oz.	80	11.0
Chowder, clam, Boston	6 fl. oz.	140	12.0
Vegetable, Lumber Jack mix	6 fl. oz.	70	10.0
Steak sandwich, *Country Fried*	7.2-oz. serving	610	54.0
Sunrise Sandwich:			
Bacon	4½-oz. serving	370	32.0
Sausage	6.1-oz. serving	500	31.0
Tea, iced	1 regular size drink	2	0.
Zucchini	4.3-oz. serving	300	33.0

Food and Description	Measure or Quantity	Calories	Carbo-hydrates (grams)
CARNATION DO-IT-YOURSELF DIET PLAN:			
Chocolate	2 scoops (1.1 oz.)	110	21.0
Vanilla	2 scoops (1.1 oz.)	110	22.0
CARNATION INSTANT BREAKFAST:			
Bar:			
Chocolate chip	1 bar (1.44 oz.)	200	20.0
Chocolate crunch	1 bar (1.34 oz.)	190	20.0
Honey nut	1 bar (1.35 oz.)	190	18.0
Peanut butter with chocolate chips	1 bar (1.4 oz.)	200	20.0
Peanut butter crunch	1 bar (1.35 oz.)	200	20.0
Drink packets:			
Chocolate or egg nog	1 packet	130	23.0
Chocolate malt	1 packet	130	22.0
Coffee, strawberry or vanilla	1 packet	130	24.0
CARROT:			
Raw (USDA):			
Whole	1 lb. (weighed with full tops)	112	26.0
Partially trimmed	1 lb. (weighed without tops, with skins)	156	36.1
Trimmed	5½" × 1" carrot (1.8 oz.)	21	4.8
Trimmed	25 thin strips (1.8 oz.)	21	4.8
Chunks	½ cup (2.4 oz.)	29	6.7
Diced	½ cup (1½ oz.)	30	7.0
Grated or shredded	½ cup (1.9 oz.)	23	5.3
Slices	½ cup (2.2 oz.)	27	6.2
Strips	½ cup (2 oz.)	24	5.6
Boiled, drained (USDA):			
Chunks	½ cup (2.9 oz.)	25	5.8
Diced	½ cup (2½ oz.)	24	5.2
Slices	½ cup (2.7 oz.)	24	5.4
Canned, regular pack, solids & liq.:			
(Comstock)	½ cup (4.2 oz.)	35	6.0
(Del Monte) diced, sliced or whole	½ cup (4 oz.)	30	7.0

Food and Description	Measure or Quantity	Calories	Carbo-hydrates (grams)
(Larsen) *Freshlike,* solids & liq.	½ cup	30	6.0
Canned, dietetic pack, solids & liq.:			
(Featherweight) sliced	½ cup	30	6.0
(Larsen) *Fresh-Lite,* sliced, low sodium	½ cup (4.4 oz.)	25	6.0
(S&W) *Nutradiet,* green label	½ cup	30	7.0
Frozen:			
(Birds Eye) whole, baby deluxe	⅓ of pkg. (3.3 oz.)	32	7.0
(Frosty Acres) cut or whole	3.3-oz. serving	40	9.0
(Green Giant) cuts, in butter sauce	½ cup	80	16.0
(McKenzie)	3.3-oz. serving	40	8.0
(Seabrook Farms) whole	⅓ pkg. (3.3 oz.)	39	8.1
CASABA MELON (USDA):			
Whole	1 lb. (weighed whole)	61	14.7
Flesh only, cubed or diced	4 oz.	31	7.4
CASHEW NUT:			
(USDA)	1 oz.	159	8.3
(USDA)	½ cup (2.5 oz.)	393	20.5
(USDA)	5 large or 8 med.	60	3.1
(Beer Nuts)	1 oz.	170	8.0
(Eagle Snacks):			
Honey Roast:			
Regular	1 oz.	170	9.0
With peanuts	1 oz.	170	8.0
Lightly salted	1 oz.	170	7.0
(Fisher):			
Dry roasted	¼ cup (1.2 oz.)	160	8.0
Honey roasted	1 oz.	150	7.0
Oil roasted	¼ cup (1.2 oz.)	170	8.0

(USDA): United States Department of Agriculture
(HEW/FAO):   Health, Education and Welfare/Food and Agriculture Organization
* Prepared as Package Directs

Food and Description	Measure or Quantity	Calories	Carbo-hydrates (grams)
(Planters):			
Dry roasted, salted or unsalted	1 oz.	160	9.0
Honey roasted:			
Plain	1 oz.	170	11.0
With peanuts	1 oz.	170	9.0
Oil roasted	1 oz.	170	8.0
(Tom's)	1 oz.	178	7.8
CATFISH, freshwater (USDA) raw fillet	4 oz.	117	0.
CATSUP:			
Regular:			
(Del Monte)	1 T. (.5 oz.)	17	3.9
(Del Monte)	¼ cup (2 oz.)	60	16.0
(Heinz)	1 T.	18	4.0
(Hunt's)	1 T. (.5 oz.)	16	4.0
(Smucker's)	1 T.	21	9.0
Dietetic or low calorie:			
(Del Monte) No Salt Added	1 T.	15	4.0
(Estee)	1 T. (.5 oz.)	6	0.
(Heinz) lite	1 T.	8	2.0
(Hunt's) no salt added	1 T.	20	5.0
CAULIFLOWER:			
Raw (USDA):			
Whole	1 lb. (weighed untrimmed)	49	9.2
Flowerbuds	½ cup (1.8 oz.)	14	2.6
Slices	½ cup (1.5 oz.)	11	2.2
Boiled (USDA) flowerbuds, drained	½ cup (2.2 oz.)	14	2.5
Frozen:			
(Birds Eye):			
Regular or florets, deluxe	⅓ of 10-oz. pkg.	23	5.0
With cheese sauce	½ of 10-oz. pkg.	130	12.0
(Frosty Acres)	3.3-oz. serving	25	5.0
(Green Giant):			
In cheese sauce, regular	3.3 oz.	50	7.5
Cuts, polybag	½ cup	12	3.0
(Larsen)	3.3 oz. serving	25	5.0
(McKenzie)	3.3-oz. serving	25	5.0
CAVATELLI, frozen (Celentano)	⅕ of 16-oz. pkg.	270	57.0

Food and Description	Measure or Quantity	Calories	Carbo-hydrates (grams)
CAVIAR, STURGEON (USDA):			
Pressed	1 oz.	90	1.4
Whole eggs	1 T. (.6 oz.)	42	.5
CELERIAC ROOT, raw (USDA):			
Whole	1 lb. (weighed unpared)	156	39.2
Pared	4 oz.	45	9.6
CELERY, all varieties (USDA): Fresh:			
Whole	1 lb. (weighed untrimmed)	58	13.3
1 large outer stalk	8″ × 1½ at root end (1.4 oz.)	7	1.6
Diced, chopped or cut in chunks	½ cup (2.1 oz.)	10	2.3
Slices	½ cup (1.9 oz.)	9	2.1
Boiled, drained solids:			
Diced or cut in chunks	½ cup (2.7 oz.)	10	2.4
Slices	½ cup (3 oz.)	12	2.6
Frozen (Larsen)	3½ oz. serving	14	3.0
CELERY SALT (French's)	1 tsp.	2	Tr.
CELERY SEED (French's)	1 tsp.	11	1.1
CERTS	1 piece	6	1.5
CERVELAT: (USDA):			
Dry	1 oz.	128	.5
Soft	1 oz.	87	.5
(Hormel) Viking	1-oz. serving	90	0.
CEREAL (See individual listings such as **BRAN BREAKFAST CEREAL,** *COCOA PUFFS,*			

(USDA): United States Department of Agriculture
(HEW/FAO): Health, Education and Welfare/Food and Agriculture Organization
* Prepared as Package Directs

Food and Description	Measure or Quantity	Calories	Carbo-hydrates (grams)
CORN FLAKES, NATURAL CEREAL, *NUTRI-GRAIN*, OATMEAL, etc.)			
CHABLIS WINE:			
(Almaden) light	3 fl. oz.	42	DNA
(Carlo Rossi)	3 fl. oz.	66	1.5
(Gallo):			
White	3 fl. oz.	60	.5
Pink	3 fl. oz.	60	3.0
(Louis M. Martini) 12½% alcohol	3 fl. oz.	59	.2
(Paul Masson):			
Regular, 11.8% alcohol	3 fl. oz.	71	2.7
Light, 7.1% alcohol	3 fl. oz.	45	2.7
CHAMPAGNE:			
(Great Western):			
Regular, 12% alcohol	3 fl. oz.	71	2.5
Brut, 12% alcohol	3 fl. oz.	74	3.4
Pink, 12% alcohol	3 fl. oz.	81	4.9
(Taylor) dry, 12½% alcohol	3 fl. oz.	78	3.9
CHARD, Swiss (USDA):			
Raw, whole	1 lb. (weighed untrimmed)	104	19.2
Raw, trimmed	4 oz.	29	5.2
Boiled, drained solids	½ cup (3.4 oz.)	17	3.2
CHARDONNAY WINE (Louis M. Martini) 12½% alcohol	3 fl. oz.	63	.2
CHARLOTTE RUSSE, homemade recipe (USDA)	4 oz.	324	38.0
CHEERIOS, cereal (General Mills):			
Regular	1¼ cups (1 oz.)	110	20.0
Honey & nut	¾ cup (1 oz.)	110	23.0
CHEESE:			
American or cheddar:			
(USDA):			
Regular	1 oz.	105	.5
Cube, natural	1″ cube (.6 oz.)	68	.3

Food and Description	Measure or Quantity	Calories	Carbo-hydrates (grams)
(Churny) cheddar, lite:			
Mild	1 oz.	80	1.0
Sharp	1 oz.	90	1.0
(Dorman's) *Chedda-De-Lite*			
or *Chedda Jack*	1 oz.	90	1.0
(Kraft):			
American Singles	1 oz.	90	2.0
Cheddar, regular or *Old*			
English	1 oz.	110	1.0
Laughing Cow, natural	1 oz.	100	Tr.
(Lite-Line) reduced sodium	1 oz.	·70	1.0
(Polly-O) cheddar, shredded	1 oz.	110	1.0
(Sargento):			
Midget, regular or sharp,			
sliced or sticks	1 oz.	114	1.0
Shredded, non-dairy	1 oz.	90	1.0
Wispride	1 oz.	115	1.0
Blue:			
(USDA) natural	1 oz.	104	.6
Laughing Cow	¾-oz. wedge	55	.5
(Sargento) cold pack or			
crumbled	1 oz.	100	1.0
Bonbino, *Laughing Cow*,			
natural	1 oz.	103	Tr.
Brick:			
(USDA) natural	1 oz.	105	.5
(Sargento) sliced	1 oz.	105	1.0
Brie (Sargento) *Danish Danko*	1 oz.	80	.1
Burgercheese (Sargento)			
Danish Danko	1 oz.	106	1.0
Camembert:			
(USDA) domestic	1 oz.	85	.5
(Sargento) *Danish Danko*	1 oz.	88	.1
Colby:			
(Churny) lite	1 oz.	80	1.0
(Featherweight) low sodium	1 oz.	100	0.
(Kraft)	1 oz.	110	1.0
(Pauly) low sodium	1 oz.	115	.6
(Sargento) shredded or sliced	1 oz.	112	1.0

(USDA): United States Department of Agriculture
(HEW/FAO): Health, Education and Welfare/Food and Agriculture
Organization
* Prepared as Package Directs

Food and Description	Measure or Quantity	Calories	Carbohydrates (grams)
Cottage:			
Unflavored:			
(USDA) creamed	½ cup (4.3 oz.)	130	3.5
(Breakstone):			
Low fat	4 oz.	90	4.0
Smooth & creamy or tangy	4 oz.	110	4.0
(Friendship) California			
style	1 oz.	30	1.0
(Light n' Lively)	4 oz.	80	4.0
(Sealtest)	4 oz.	120	4.0
Flavored (Friendship):			
Dutch apple	1 oz.	31	2.5
Garden salad	1 oz.	30	1.0
Pineapple	1 oz.	35	3.8
Cream, plain, unwhipped:			
(USDA)	1 oz.	106	.6
(Friendship)	1 oz.	103	.8
(Frigo)	1 oz.	100	1.0
(Kraft) *Philadelphia Brand*:			
Regular	1 oz.	100	1.0
With chive & onion	1 oz.	100	2.0
Light	1 oz.	60	2.0
Olive & pimento	1 oz.	90	2.0
Edam:			
(House of Gold)	1 oz.	100	1.0
(Kaukauna)	1 oz.	100	<1.0
Laughing Cow	1 oz.	100	Tr.
(Sargento)	1 oz.	101	1.0
Farmer:			
(Churny) *May-Bud*	1 oz.	90	1.0
Dutch Garden Brand	1 oz.	100	1.0
(Friendship) regular or			
no salt added	1 oz.	40	1.0
(Kaukauna)	1 oz.	100	<1.0
(Sargento)	1 oz.	72	1.0
Wispride	1 oz.	100	1.0
Feta (Sargento) Danish, cups	1 oz.	76	1.0
Gjetost (Sargento) Norwegian	1 oz.	118	13.0
Gouda:			
(Churny) *May-Bud*:			
Regular	1 oz.	100	1.0
Lite	1 oz.	81	1.0
(Kaukauna)	1 oz.	100	<1.0
Laughing Cow:			
Regular	1 oz.	110	Tr.

Food and Description	Measure or Quantity	Calories	Carbo-hydrates (grams)
Mini, waxed	¾ oz.	80	Tr.
(Sargento) baby, caraway, or smoked	1 oz.	101	1.0
Wispride	1 oz.	100	Tr.
Gruyère, *Swiss Knight*	1 oz.	100	Tr.
Havarti (Sargento):			
Creamy	1 oz.	90	.2
Creamy, 60% mild	1 oz.	177	.2
Hoop (Friendship) natural	1 oz.	21	.5
Hot pepper (Sargento) sliced	1 oz.	112	1.0
Jarlsberg (Sargento) Norwegian	1 oz.	100	1.0
Kettle Moraine (Sargento)	1 oz.	100	1.0
Limburger (Sargento) natural	1 oz.	93	14.0
Monterey Jack:			
(Churny) lite	1 oz.	80	0.
(Frigo)	1 oz.	100	1.0
(Kaukauna)	1 oz.	110	<1.0
(Kraft)	1 oz.	110	0.
(Sargento) midget, Longhorn, shredded or sliced	1 oz.	106	1.0
Mozzarella:			
(Dorman's)	1 oz.	80	1.0
(Frigo) part skim milk	1 oz.	90	1.0
(Kraft)	1 oz.	80	0.
(Polly-O):			
Fior di Latte	1 oz.	80	1.0
Lite	1 oz.	70	1.0
Part skim milk, regular or shredded	1 oz.	80	1.0
Smoked	1 oz.	85	1.0
Whole milk:			
Regular	1 oz.	90	1.0
Old fashioned, regular	1 oz.	70	1.0
(Sargento):			
Bar, rounds, shredded regular or with spices, sliced for pizza or square	1 oz.	79	1.0
Whole milk	1 oz.	100	1.0

(USDA): United States Department of Agriculture
(HEW/FAO):   Health, Education and Welfare/Food and Agriculture
            Organization
* Prepared as Package Directs

Food and Description	Measure or Quantity	Calories	Carbo-hydrates (grams)
Muenster:			
(Dorman's)	1 oz.	110	0.
(Kaukauna)	1 oz.	110	<1.0
(Sargento) red rind	1 oz.	104	1.0
Wispride	1 oz.	100	Tr.
Nibblin Curds (Sargento)	1 oz.	114	1.0
Parmesan:			
(USDA):			
Regular	1 oz.	111	.8
Grated	½ cup (not packed)	169	1.2
(Frigo):			
Grated	1 T.	23	Tr.
Whole	1 oz.	110	1.0
(Polly-O) grated	1 oz.	130	1.0
(Sargento):			
Grated, non-dairy	1 T.	27	2.3
Wedge	1 oz.	110	1.0
Pizza (Sargento) shredded or sliced, non-dairy	1 oz.	90	1.0
Pot (Sargento) regular, French onion or garlic	1 oz.	30	1.0
Provolone:			
(Frigo)	1 oz.	90	1.0
Laughing Cow:			
Cube	⅙ oz.	12	.1
Wedge	¾ oz.	55	.5
(Sargento) sliced	1 oz.	100	1.0
Ricotta:			
(Frigo) part skim milk	1 oz.	43	.9
(Polly-O):			
Lite	1 oz.	40	1.5
Old-fashioned	1 oz.	50	1.0
Part skim milk	1 oz.	45	1.0
Whole milk	1 oz.	50	1.0
(Sargento):			
Part skim milk	1 oz.	39	1.0
Whole milk	1 oz.	49	1.0
Romano (Polly-O) wedge	1 oz.	130	1.0
Roquefort, natural (USDA)	1 oz.	104	.6
Samsoe (Sargento) Danish	1 oz.	101	.2
Scamorze (Frigo)	1 oz.	79	.3
Semisoft:			
Bel Paese	1 oz.	90	.3

Food and Description	Measure or Quantity	Calories	Carbo-hydrates (grams)
Laughing Cow:			
Babybel:			
Regular	1 oz.	91	Tr.
Mini	¾ oz.	74	Tr.
Bonbel:			
Regular	1 oz.	100	Tr.
Mini	¾ oz.	74	Tr.
Reduced calorie	1 oz.	45	Tr.
Slim Jack (Dorman's)	1 oz.	90	1.0
Stirred curd (Frigo)	1 oz.	110	1.0
String (Sargento)	1 oz.	90	1.0
Swiss:			
(USDA) domestic, natural or process	1 oz.	105	.5
(Churny) lite	1 oz.	90	1.0
(Dorman's) light	1 oz.	100	1.0
(Fisher) natural	1 oz.	100	0.
(Frigo) domestic	1 oz.	100	0.
(Sargento) domestic or Finland, sliced	1 oz.	107	1.0
Taco (Sargento) shredded	1 oz.	105	1.0
Washed curd (Frigo)	1 oz.	110	1.0

CHEESE ENTREE (See MACARONI & CHEESE; SOUFFLE, Cheese; **WELSH RAREBIT)**

CHEESE FONDUE,
Swiss Knight

Swiss Knight	1 oz.	60	1.0

CHEESE FOOD:

American or cheddar:			
(USDA) process	1 oz.	92	2.0
(Borden) *Lite Line*	1 oz.	50	1.0
(Fisher) *Ched-O-Mate* or *Sandwich-Mate*	1 oz.	90	1.0
(Sargento)	1 oz.	94	2.0
(Weight Watchers) colored or white	1-oz. slice	50	1.0

(USDA): United States Department of Agriculture
(HEW/FAO): Health, Education and Welfare/Food and Agriculture Organization
* Prepared as Package Directs

Food and Description	Measure or Quantity	Calories	Carbo-hydrates (grams)
Wispride	1 oz.	100	3.0
Cheez-ola (Fisher)	1 oz.	90	1.0
Chef's Delight (Fisher)	1 oz.	70	4.0
Cracker snack (Sargento)	1 oz.	90	2.0
Garlic & Herb, *Wispride*	1 oz.	90	4.0
Jalapeño (Borden) *Lite Line*	1 oz.	50	1.0
Low sodium (Borden) *Lite Line*	1 oz.	70	2.0
Muenster (Borden) *Lite Line*	1 oz.	50	1.0
Mun-chee (Pauly)	1 oz.	100	2.0
Pimiento (Pauly)	.8-oz. slice	73	.8
Pizza-Mate (Fisher)	1 oz.	90	1.0
Swiss:			
(Borden) *Lite Line*	1 oz.	50	1.0
(Kraft) reduced fat	1 oz.	90	1.0
(Pauly)	.8-oz. slice	74	1.6
CHEESE SPREAD:			
American or cheddar:			
(USDA)	1 T. (.5 oz.)	40	1.1
(Fisher)	1 oz.	80	2.0
Laughing Cow	1 oz.	72	.7
(Nabisco) *Easy Cheese*	1 tsp.	16	.4
Blue, *Laughing Cow*	1 oz.	72	.7
Cheese 'n Bacon (Nabisco)			
Easy Cheese	1 tsp.	16	.4
Gruyère, *Laughing Cow,*			
La Vache Que Rit:			
Regular	1 oz.	72	.7
Reduced calorie	1 oz.	46	1.3
Nacho (Nabisco) *Easy Cheese*	1 tsp.	16	.4
Pimiento:			
(Nabisco) *Snack Mate*	1 tsp.	15	.3
(Price)	1 oz.	80	2.0
Provolone, *Laughing Cow*	1 oz.	72	.7
Velveeta (Kraft)	1 oz.	80	2.0
CHENIN BLANC WINE (Louis M. Martini) 12½% alcohol	3 fl. oz.	62	.2
CHERRY:			
Sour:			
Fresh (USDA):			
Whole	1 lb. (weighed with stems)	213	52.5

Food and Description	Measure or Quantity	Calories	Carbo-hydrates (grams)
Whole	1 lb. (weighed without stems)	242	59.7
Pitted	½ cup (2.7 oz.)	45	11.1
Canned, syrup pack, pitted: (USDA):			
Light syrup	4 oz. (with liq.)	84	21.2
Heavy syrup	½ cup (with liq.)	116	29.5
Extra heavy syrup	4 oz. (with liq.)	127	32.4
(Thank You Brand)	½ cup (4.5 oz.)	123	29.4
Canned, water pack, pitted, solid & liq.	½ cup (4.3 oz.)	52	13.1
Frozen, pitted:			
Sweetened	½ cup (4.6 oz.)	146	36.1
Unsweetened	4 oz.	62	15.2
Sweet:			
Fresh (USDA):			
Whole	1 lb. (weighed with stems)	286	71.0
Whole, with stems	½ cup (2.3 oz.)	41	10.2
Pitted	½ cup (2.9 oz.)	57	14.3
Canned, syrup pack: (USDA):			
Light syrup, pitted	4 oz. (with liq.)	74	18.7
Heavy syrup, pitted	½ cup (with liq., 4.2 oz.)	96	24.2
Extra heavy syrup, pitted	4 oz. (with liq.)	113	29.0
(Del Monte) solids & liq.:			
Dark	½ cup (4.3 oz.)	90	23.0
Light	½ cup (4.3 oz.)	100	26.0
(Stokely-Van Camp) pitted, solids & liq.	½ cup (4.2 oz.)	50	11.0
(Thank You Brand) heavy syrup	½ cup (4.5 oz.)	98	23.0
Canned, dietetic or water pack, solids & liq.:			
(Diet Delight)	½ cup (4.4 oz.)	70	17.0
(Featherweight):			
Dark	½ cup	60	13.0
Light	½ cup	50	11.0

(USDA): United States Department of Agriculture
(HEW/FAO): Health, Education and Welfare/Food and Agriculture
       Organization
* Prepared as Package Directs

Food and Description	Measure or Quantity	Calories	Carbohydrates (grams)
(Thank You Brand) water pack	½ cup (4.5 oz.)	61	14.1
CHERRY, CANDIED (USDA)	1 oz.	96	24.6
CHERRY DRINK:			
Canned:			
(Hi-C)	6 fl. oz.	100	24.7
(Johanna Farms) *Ssips*	8.45-fl.-oz. container	130	32.0
(Lincoln) cherry berry	6 fl. oz.	100	25.0
*Mix (Hi-C)	6 fl. oz.	72	18.0
CHERRY HEERING			
(Hiram Walker)	1 fl. oz.	80	10.0
CHERRY JELLY:			
Sweetened (Smucker's)	1 T. (.5 oz.)	53	13.5
Dietetic (Featherweight)	1 T.	16	4.0
CHERRY LIQUEUR			
(DeKuyper) 50 proof	1 fl. oz.	75	8.5
CHERRY, MARASCHINO			
(USDA)	1 oz. (with liq.)	33	8.3
CHERRY PRESERVES OR JAM:			
Sweetened (Smucker's)	1 T. (.7 oz.)	53	13.5
Dietetic:			
(Estee)	1 T. (.6 oz.)	6	0.
(Louis Sherry)	1 T. (.6 oz.)	6	0.
(S&W) *Nutradiet*, red label	1 T. (.6 oz.)	12	3.0
CHESTNUT (USDA):			
Fresh:			
In shell	1 lb. (weighed in shell)	713	154.7
Shelled	4 oz.	220	47.7
Dried:			
In shell	1 lb. (weighed in shell)	1402	292.4
Shelled	4 oz.	428	89.1

Food and Description	Measure or Quantity	Calories	Carbo-hydrates (grams)
CHEWING GUM:			
Sweetened:			
Bazooka, bubble	1 slice	18	4.5
Beechies	1 piece	6	2.0
Beech Nut; Beeman's, Big Red; Black Jack; Clove; Doublemint; Freedent; Fruit Punch; Juicy Fruit, Spearmint (Wrigley's); *Teaberry*	1 stick	10	2.3
Bubble Yum	1 piece	25	7.0
Dentyne	1 piece	4	1.2
Extra (Wrigley's)	1 piece	8	Tr.
Fruit Stripe:			
Regular	1 piece	9	2.0
Bubble	1 piece	10	2.0
Hubba Bubba (Wrigley's)	1 piece (8 grams)	23	5.8
Dietetic:			
Bubble Yum	1 piece	20	5.0
(*Care*Free*)	1 piece	8	2.0
(Estee) bubble or regular	1 piece	5	1.4
(Featherweight) bubble or regular	1 piece	4	1.0
Orbit (Wrigley's)	1 piece	8	Tr.
CHEX, cereal (Ralston Purina):			
Bran (See **BRAN BREAKFAST CEREAL**)			
Corn	1 cup (1 oz.)	110	25.0
Rice	1⅛ cups (1 oz.)	110	25.0
Wheat	⅔ cup (1 oz.)	110	23.0
Wheat & raisins	¾ cup (1.3 oz.)	130	31.0
CHIANTI WINE (Italian Swiss Colony) 13% alcohol	3 fl. oz.	64	1.5
CHICKEN (USDA):			
Broiler, cooked, meat only	4 oz.	154	0.

(USDA): United States Department of Agriculture
(HEW/FAO): Health, Education and Welfare/Food and Agriculture Organization
* Prepared as Package Directs

Food and Description	Measure or Quantity	Calories	Carbo-hydrates (grams)
Capon, raw, with bone	1 lb. (weighed ready-to-cook)	937	0.
Fryer:			
Raw:			
Ready-to-cook	1 lb. (weighed ready-to-cook)	382	0.
Breast	1 lb. (weighed with bone)	394	0.
Leg or drumstick	1 lb. (weighed with bone)	313	0.
Thigh	1 lb. (weighed with bone)	435	0.
Fried. A 2½-lb. chicken (weighed before cooking with bone) will give you:			
Back	1 back (2.2 oz.)	139	2.7
Breast	½ breast (3⅓ oz.)	154	1.1
Leg or drumstrick	1 leg (2 oz.)	87	.4
Neck	1 neck (2.1 oz.)	121	1.9
Rib	1 rib (.7 oz.)	42	.8
Thigh	1 thigh (2¼ oz.)	118	1.2
Wing	1 wing (1¾ oz.)	78	.8
Fried, Frozen (See **CHICKEN, Fried**, Frozen)			
Fried skin	1 oz.	199	2.6
Hen and cock:			
Raw	1 lb. (weighed ready-to-cook)	987	0.
Stewed:			
Meat only	4 oz.	236	0.
Chopped	½ cup (2.5 oz.)	150	0.
Diced	½ cup (2.4 oz.)	139	0.
Ground	½ cup (2 oz.)	116	0.
Roaster:			
Raw:	1 lb. (weighed ready-to-cook)	791	0.
Roasted:			
Dark meat without skin	4 oz.	209	0.
Light meat without skin	4 oz.	206	0.
CHICKEN A LA KING:			
Home recipe (USDA)	1 cup (8.6 oz.)	468	12.3
Canned (Swanson)	½ of 10½-oz. can	180	9.0
Frozen:			
(Banquet)	4-oz. pkg.	110	9.0

Food and Description	Measure or Quantity	Calories	Carbo-hydrates (grams)
(Blue Star) *Dining Lite*, with rice	9½-oz. meal	290	33.8
(Le Menu)	10¼-oz. dinner	320	29.0
(Morton) Light	8-oz. dinner	280	33.0
(Stouffer's) with rice	9½-oz. pkg.	290	34.0
(Weight Watchers)	9-oz. pkg.	230	15.0
CHICKEN BOUILLON:			
(Borden) *Lite-Line*, low sodium	1 tsp.	12	2.0
(Herb-Ox):			
Cube	1 cube	6	.6
Packet	1 packet	12	1.9
(Maggi) cube	1 cube	7	1.0
(Wyler's)	1 cube	8	1.0
Low sodium (Featherweight)	1 tsp.	18	2.0
CHICKEN, BONED, CANNED:			
Regular:			
(USDA)	1 cup (7.2 oz.)	406	0.
(Hormel) chunk:			
Breast	6¾-oz. serving	350	0.
Dark	6¾-oz. serving	327	0.
White & dark:			
Regular	6¾-oz. serving	340	0.
Low salt	6¾-oz. serving	330	0.
(Swanson) chunk:			
Regular	2½ oz.	100	0.
Mixin' chicken	2½ oz.	130	0.
White	2½ oz.	90	0.
Low sodium (Featherweight)	2½ oz.	154	0.
CHICKEN, CREAMED, frozen			
(Stouffer's)	6½ oz. pkg.	300	5.9
CHICKEN DINNER OR ENTREE:			
Canned:			
*(Hunt's) *Minute Gourmet*, microwave entree maker:			
Barbecued	6.8-oz. serving	320	37.0

(USDA): United States Department of Agriculture
(HEW/FAO):   Health, Education and Welfare/Food and Agriculture
                      Organization
* Prepared as Package Directs

Food and Description	Measure or Quantity	Calories	Carbo- hydrates (grams)
Cacciatore	8.3-oz. serving	280	20.0
Sweet & sour	7.8-oz. serving	300	32.0
(Swanson) & dumplings	7½-oz. serving	220	19.0
Frozen:			
(Armour):			
Classic Lites:			
Breast medallion marsala	11-oz. meal	250	28.0
Burgundy	10½-oz. meal	210	25.0
Cacciatore	11-oz. meal	250	30.0
Oriental	10-oz. meal	230	29.0
Sweet & sour	10½-oz. meal	240	37.0
Dinner Classics:			
BBQ	10-oz. meal	280	32.0
Fricassee	11¾-oz. meal	340	31.0
Hawaiian	10½-oz. meal	280	38.0
Milan	11½-oz. meal	320	33.0
With wine & mushroom sauce	10¾-oz. meal	350	27.0
(Banquet):			
American Favorites, fried	11-oz. dinner	359	46.0
Family Entrees, & dumplings	32-oz. pkg.	1720	124.0
Family Favorites, & dumplings	9-oz. dinner	286	28.0
Gourmet Entrees:			
Cacciatore	10-oz. entree	260	35.0
French	10-oz. entree	190	25.0
(Blue Star) *Dining Lite:*			
Glazed with vegetables & rice	8½-oz. meal	243	25.8
With vegetables & vermicelli	12¾-oz. meal	280	32.3
(Celentano):			
Parmigiana, cutlets	9-oz. pkg.	310	40.0
Primavera	11½-oz. pkg.	270	15.0
(Chun King):			
Imperial	13-oz. entree	294	53.0
Walnut, crunchy	13-oz. entree	117	2.0
(Conagra) *Light & Elegant*:			
Cheese	8¾-oz. entree	293	30.0
Glazed	8-oz. entree	240	23.0
Parmigiana	8-oz. entree	260	23.0
(La Choy) *Fresh & Lite:*			
Almond, with rice & vegetables	9¾-oz. meal	270	40.1
Imperial	11-oz. meal	260	45.0
Oriental, spicy	9¾-oz. meal	270	52.0

Food and Description	Measure or Quantity	Calories	Carbo- hydrates (grams)
Sweet & sour	10-oz. meal	260	50.1
(Le Menu):			
Cordon Bleu	11-oz. dinner	460	47.0
Florentine	12½-oz. dinner	480	40.0
Parmigiana	11½-oz. dinner	380	28.0
Sweet & sour	11½-oz. dinner	450	43.0
(Morton):			
Regular:			
Boneless	11-oz. dinner	329	44.7
Fried	11-oz. dinner	431	64.1
Light, boneless	11-oz. dinner	250	30.0
(Stouffer's):			
Regular:			
Cashew, in sauce with rice	9½-oz. meal	380	29.0
Creamed	6½-oz. meal	300	8.0
Divan	8½-oz. meal	320	11.0
Escalloped, & noodles	10-oz. meal	420	27.0
Lean Cuisine:			
a l'orange, with almond rice	8-oz. meal	260	30.0
Breast, in herbed cream sauce	9½-oz. meal	260	11.0
Breast, marsala, with vegetables	8⅛-oz. meal	190	11.0
Breast, Parmesan	10-oz. meal	260	19.0
Cacciatore, with vermicelli	10⅞-oz. meal	250	26.0
Fiesta	8½-oz. meal	250	29.0
Glazed, with vegetable rice	8½-oz. meal	270	23.0
Oriental	9⅜-oz. meal	230	23.0
& vegetables with vermicelli	11¾-oz. meal	270	29.0
Right Course:			
Italiano, with fettucini & vegetables	9⅝-oz. meal	280	29.0
Sesame	10-oz. meal	320	34.0
Tenderloins in barbecue sauce with rice pilaf	8¾-oz. meal	270	38.0

(USDA): United States Department of Agriculture
(HEW/FAO):   Health, Education and Welfare/Food and Agriculture
Organization
* Prepared as Package Directs

Food and Description	Measure or Quantity	Calories	Carbo-hydrates (grams)
Tenderloins in peanut sauce with linguini & vegetables	9¼-oz. meal	330	32.0
(Swanson):			
Regular, fried:			
Barbecue	9¼-oz. dinner	560	49.0
Breast portion	10¾-oz. dinner	650	63.0
Dark meat	10¼-oz. dinner	610	55.0
Hungry Man:			
Boneless	17½-oz. dinner	670	60.0
Fried:			
Breast	14-oz. dinner	860	75.0
Breast	11¾-oz. entree	670	51.0
Dark portion	14-oz. dinner	860	75.0
Dark portion	11-oz. entree	620	42.0
Parmigiana	20-oz. dinner	810	53.0
(Tyson):			
à l'orange	8¼-oz. meal	300	31.0
Fiesta	10½-oz. meal	420	27.0
Francais	8¾-oz. meal	350	12.0
Oriental	10¼-oz. meal	300	31.0
Parmigiana	11¾-oz. meal	450	38.0
Sweet & sour	11-oz. meal	440	42.0
(Weight Watchers):			
Cacciatore	10-oz. serving	290	30.1
Imperial	9¼-oz. meal	240	29.0
Parmigiana	8-oz. serving	290	14.0
Southern fried patty	6½-oz. serving	260	10.0
Sweet & sour with oriental style vegetables	9-oz. serving	210	26.1
CHICKEN FRICASEE (USDA) home recipe	1 cup (8.5 oz.)	386	7.7
CHICKEN, FRIED, frozen:			
(Banquet):			
Assorted	2-lb. pkg.	1625	100.0
Breast portion	22-oz. pkg.	1190	70.0
Drum snackers	12-oz. pkg.	808	56.0
Hot & spicy	32-oz. pkg.	1625	90.0
Thigh & drumstick	25-oz. pkg.	1385	80.0
Wings	12-oz. pkg.	808	56.0
(Country Pride) southern fried:			
Chunks	3 oz.	276	14.0

Food and Description	Measure or Quantity	Calories	Carbo-hydrates (grams)
Patties	3 oz.	232	12.0
(Swanson) *Plump & Juicy:*			
Assorted	3¼-oz. serving	270	13.0
Breast portion	4½-oz. serving	350	19.0
Nibbles	3¼-oz. serving	300	16.0
Take-out style	3¼-oz. serving	270	13.0
Thighs & drumsticks	3¼-oz. serving	280	11.0
CHICKEN GIZZARD (USDA):			
Raw	4 oz.	128	.8
Simmered	4 oz.	168	.8
***CHICKEN HELPER**			
(General Mills):			
& biscuits, crispy	⅕ of pkg.	710	45.0
& dumplings	⅕ of pkg.	530	41.0
& mushrooms	⅕ of pkg.	470	29.0
Potato & gravy	⅕ of pkg.	600	45.0
& seasoned rice, crispy	⅕ of pkg.	689	47.0
Stuffing	⅕ of pkg.	570	34.0
Teriyaki	⅕ of pkg.	480	35.0
Tetrazzini	⅕ of pkg.	340	38.0
CHICKEN & NOODLES, frozen:			
(Armour) *Dinner Classics*	12-oz. dinner	340	30.0
(Green Giant) twin pouch, with vegetables	9-oz. pkg.	390	38.0
(Stouffer's) homestyle	10-oz. meal	310	21.0
CHICKEN NUGGETS, frozen:			
(Banquet) breaded & fried:			
Regular	12-oz. pkg.	932	56.0
& cheddar	12-oz. pkg.	1100	44.0
Hot & spicy	12-oz. pkg.	940	52.0
(Empire Kosher)	12-oz. pkg.	708	56.0
CHICKEN, PACKAGED:			
(Carl Buddig) smoked, sliced	1 oz.	50	Tr.
(Eckrich) breast	1 slice	20	.5

(USDA): United States Department of Agriculture
(HEW/FAO):   Health, Education and Welfare/Food and Agriculture Organization
* Prepared as Package Directs

Food and Description	Measure or Quantity	Calories	Carbo-hydrates (grams)
(Louis Rich) breast, oven roasted	1-oz. slice	40	Tr.
CHICKEN PATTIES, frozen:			
(Banquet) breaded & fried	12-oz. pkg.	900	52.0
(County Pride)	12-oz. pkg.	1080	52.0
(Empire Kosher)	12-oz. pkg.	792	52.0
CHICKEN PIE, frozen:			
(Banquet):			
Regular	7-oz pie	540	38.0
Microwave, supreme	7-oz. pie	429	30.0
(Empire Kosher)	8-oz. pie	463	49.0
(Morton)	7-oz. pie	415	27.0
(Stouffer's)	10-oz. pie	530	35.0
(Swanson):			
Regular	8-oz. pie	420	39.0
Chunky	10-oz. pie	570	53.0
Hungry Man	16-oz. pie	700	64.0
CHICKEN, POTTED (USDA)	1 oz.	70	0.
CHICKEN SALAD (Carnation)	¼ of 7½-oz. can	120	3.8
CHICKEN SOUP (See **SOUP,** Chicken)			
CHICKEN SPREAD:			
(Hormel):			
Regular	1 oz.	60	0.
Lunch Loaf	1 oz.	65	0.
Sandwich Makins	1 oz.	50	2.0
(Swanson)	1 oz.	60	2.0
(Underwood) chunky	½ of 4¾-oz. can	150	2.7
CHICKEN STEW, canned:			
Regular:			
(Libby's) with dumplings	8 oz.	194	20.2
(Swanson)	7⅜-oz.	170	16.0
Dietetic:			
(Dia-Mel)	8-oz. serving	150	19.0
(Featherweight)	7½-oz. serving	170	21.0

Food and Description	Measure or Quantity	Calories	Carbo-hydrates (grams)
CHICKEN STICKS, frozen:			
(Banquet) breaded, fried	12-oz. pkg.	912	60.0
(County Pride)	12-oz. pkg.	932	64.0
CHICKEN STOCK BASE			
(French's)	1 tsp. (3.2 grams)	8	1.0
CHICK-FIL-A:			
Brownie, fudge, with nuts	2.8 oz.	369	45.0
Chicken, without bun	3.6 oz.	219	1.5
Chicken nuggets, 8 pack	4 oz.	287	12.5
Chicken salad:			
Regular, plate	11.8 oz.	475	60.2
Sandwich, regular wheat bread	5.7 oz.	449	35.2
Sandwich, deluxe, regular	7.45 oz.	368	29.8
Cole slaw	3.7 oz. cup	175	11.2
Icedream	4½ oz.	134	18.9
Pie, lemon	4.1-oz. slice	329	63.8
Potato, *Waffle Potato Fries*	3 oz.	270	33.0
Potato salad	3.8-oz. cup	198	13.9
Salad, tossed:			
Plain	4½ oz.	21	4.2
With dressing:			
Honey french	6 oz.	246	6.9
Italian, lite	6 oz.	46	6.3
Thousand Island	6 oz.	231	8.7
Soup, hearty, small	8½ oz.	152	11.1
CHICK'N QUICK, frozen (Tyson):			
Breast fillet	3 oz.	190	14.0
Breast pattie	3 oz.	240	10.0
Chick'N Cheddar	3 oz.	260	13.0
Chunks	1 piece (.5 oz.)	42	2.2
Cordon bleu	5 oz.	310	19.0
Italian Hoagies	3 oz.	250	12.0
Kiev	5 oz.	430	18.0
Sticks	1 piece (1 oz.)	80	4.7

(USDA): United States Department of Agriculture
(HEW/FAO):   Health, Education and Welfare/Food and Agriculture
                        Organization
* Prepared as Package Directs

Food and Description	Measure or Quantity	Calories	Carbo-hydrates (grams)
Swiss'N Bacon	3 oz.	280	14.0
Turkey patties	3 oz.	240	12.0
CHICK-PEAS OR GARBANZOS:			
Dry (USDA)	1 cup (7.1 oz.)	720	122.0
Canned, regular pack, solids & liq.:			
(Allen's)	½ cup	110	18.0
(Furman's)	⅓ cup (2.6 oz.)	237	13.5
(Goya)	½ cup (4 oz.)	110	17.0
(Old El Paso)	½ cup	77	12.4
Canned, dietetic pack, solids & liq.			
(S&W) *Nutradiet*	½ cup	105	19.0
CHILI or CHILI CON CARNE:			
Canned, regular pack:			
Beans only:			
(Comstock)	½ cup (4.4 oz.)	140	23.0
(Hormel) in sauce	5 oz.	130	19.0
(Hunt's)	½ cup (3.5 oz.)	91	15.8
With beans:			
(Gebhardt) hot	½ of 15-oz. can	470	46.0
(Hormel):			
Regular	7½-oz. serving	310	23.0
Hot	½-oz. serving	310	24.0
Short Orders	7½-oz. can	300	23.0
(Libby's)	7½-oz. serving	270	25.0
(Old El Paso)	1 cup	349	12.3
(Swanson)	7¾-oz. serving	310	28.0
Without beans:			
(Gebhardt)	½ of 15-oz. can	410	13.0
(Hormel):			
Regular or hot	7½-oz. serving	370	12.0
Short Orders	7½-oz. can	360	11.0
(Libby's)	7½ oz. serving	390	11.0
Canned, dietetic pack:			
(Estee) with beans	7½-oz. serving	370	27.0
(Featherweight) with beans	7½-oz.	270	25.0
Frozen, with beans			
(Stouffer's)	9¾-oz. pkg.	280	45.0
CHILI MAC (Hormel) *Short Orders*	7½-oz. can	200	16.0

Food and Description	Measure or Quantity	Calories	Carbo-hydrates (grams)
CHILI SAUCE:			
(USDA)	½ cup (4.8 oz.)	142	33.8
(Del Monte)	¼ cup (2 oz.)	70	17.0
(El Molino) green, mild	1 T.	5	1.0
(Heinz)	1 T.	17	3.0
(LaVictoria) green	1 T.	3	1.0
(Ortega) green:			
Hot1 oz.		9	1.9
Medium or mild	1 oz.	7	1.7
CHILI SEASONING MIX:			
*(Durkee)	1 cup	465	31.2
(French's) *Chili-O:*			
Plain	⅙ of pkg.	25	5.0
Onion	⅙ of pkg.	35	7.0
(Lawry's)	1.6-oz. pkg.	143	26.6
(McCormick)	1.2-oz. pkg.	106	36.1
CHIMICHANGA, frozen			
(Fred's) *Marquez:*			
Beef, shredded	5-oz. serving	351	35.0
Chicken	5-oz. serving	350	42.0
CHIPS (See CRACKERS, PUFFS & CHIPS)			
CHIVES (USDA) raw	1 T. (3 grams)	1	.2
CHOCOLATE, BAKING:			
(Baker's):			
Bitter or unsweetened	1-oz. square	180	8.6
Semi-sweet:			
Regular	1-oz. square	156	16.8
Chips	¼ cup (1½ oz.)	207	31.7
Sweetened, *German's*	1 oz. square	158	17.3
(Hershey's):			
Bitter or unsweetened	1 oz.	190	7.0
Sweetened:			
Dark chips, regular or mini	1 oz.	151	17.8
Milk, chips	1 oz.	150	18.0

(USDA): United States Department of Agriculture
(HEW/FAO):   Health, Education and Welfare/Food and Agriculture
Organization
* Prepared as Package Directs

Food and Description	Measure or Quantity	Calories	Carbo-hydrates (grams)
Semi-sweet, chips (Nestlé):	1 oz.	147	17.3
Bitter or unsweetened, *Choco-bake*	1-oz. packet	180	8.0
Sweet or semi-sweet, morsels	1 oz.	150	17.0

CHOCOLATE ICE CREAM
(See **ICE CREAM**, Chocolate)

CHOCOLATE SYRUP (See **SYRUP**, Chocolate)

CHOP SUEY:

Home recipe (USDA) with meat	1 cup (8.8 oz.)	300	12.8
Frozen:			
(Banquet):			
Buffet Supper	2-lb. pkg.	418	39.1
Dinner	12-oz. dinner	282	38.8
(Stouffer's) beef, with rice	12-oz. pkg.	340	43.0

*CHOP SUEY SEASONING MIX (Durkee)

	1¾ cups	557	21.0

CHOWDER (See **SOUP**, Chowder)

CHOW CHOW (USDA):

Sour	1 cup (8.5 oz.)	70	9.8
Sweet	1 cup (8.6 oz.)	284	66.2

CHOW MEIN:

Canned:			
(Chun King) Divider-pak:			
Beef	¼ of pkg.	91	11.6
Chicken	½ of 24-oz. pkg.	110	12.7
Pork	¼ of pkg.	116	11.2
Shrimp	¼ of pkg.	91	13.0
(Hormel) pork, *Short Orders*	7½-oz. can	140	13.0
(La Choy):			
Regular:			
Beef	7 oz.	60	6.0
Chicken	7 oz.	70	6.0
Meatless	¾ cup	35	6.0
Shrimp	¾ cup	45	4.0
*Bi-pack:			

Food and Description	Measure or Quantity	Calories	Carbo-hydrates (grams)
Beef	¾ cup	70	8.0
Beef pepper oriental or shrimp	¾ cup	80	10.0
Chicken	¾ cup	80	8.0
Pork	¾ cup	80	7.0
Vegetable	¾ cup	50	8.0
Frozen:			
(Blue Star) *Dining Lite*, chicken, and rice	11¼-oz. meal	233	37.5
*(Chun King) chicken	13-oz. entree	361	53.0
(Empire Kosher)	7½-oz. serving	97	12.0
(La Choy):			
Chicken:			
Dinner	12-oz. dinner	260	44.0
Entree	⅔ cup	90	11.0
Shrimp:			
Dinner	12-oz. dinner	220	47.0
Entree	¾ cup	70	11.0
(Morton) chicken, light:			
Dinner	11-oz. meal	260	43.0
Entree	8-oz. meal	210	35.0
(Stouffer's):			
Regular, chicken	8-oz. pkg.	130	11.0
Lean Cuisine, chicken, with rice	11¼-oz. serving	250	36.0
(Van de Kamp's) Mandarin:			
Beef	11-oz. serving	310	40.0
Chicken	11-oz. serving	340	40.0
CHOW MEIN SEASONING MIX (Kikkoman)	1⅛-oz. pkg.	98	13.8
CHURCH'S FRIED CHICKEN:			
Chicken:			
Breast	4.3-oz serving	278	9.4
Leg	2.9-oz. serving	147	4.5
Thigh	4.2-oz. servng	306	9.2
Wing-breast	4.8-oz. serving	303	8.9
Corn, with butter oil	1 ear	237	32.9

(USDA): United States Department of Agriculture
(HEW/FAO):   Health, Education and Welfare/Food and Agriculture
                        Organization
* Prepared as Package Directs

Food and Description	Measure or Quantity	Calories	Carbo- hydrates (grams)
French fries	1 regular order	138	20.1
CINNAMON, GROUND (French's)	1 tsp. (1.7 grams)	6	1.4
CINNAMON SUGAR (French's)	1 tsp. (4.3 grams)	16	4.0
CINNAMON TOAST CRUNCH, cereal (General Mills)	¾ cup (1 oz.)	120	23.0
CIRCUS FUN, cereal (General Mills)	1 cup (1 oz.)	110	24.0
***CITRUS BERRY BLEND,** mix (Sunkist) dietetic	8 fl. oz.	6	2.0
CITRUS COOLER DRINK, canned (Hi-C)	6 fl. oz.	95	23.0
CLAM:			
Raw (USDA):			
Hard or round:			
Meat & liq.	1 lb. (weighed in shell)	71	6.1
Meat only	1 cup (8 oz.)	182	13.4
Soft:			
Meat & liq.	1 lb. (weighed in shell)	142	5.3
Meat only	1 cup (8 oz.)	186	3.0
Canned:			
(Doxsee):			
Chopped or minced:			
Drained solids	½ cup	97	1.9
Solids & liq.	½ cup	59	3.2
Whole:			
Drained solids	½ cup	97	1.9
Solids & liq.	½ cup	58	3.1
(Gorton's) minced, drained solids	1 can	140	8.0
Frozen:			
(Gorton's) fried strips, crunchy	1 pkg.	480	40.0
(Howard Johnson's) fried	5-oz. pkg.	395	32.0
(Mrs. Paul's) fried, light	2½-oz. serving	230	20.0

Food and Description	Measure or Quantity	Calories	Carbo-hydrates (grams)
CLAMATO COCKTAIL			
(Mott's)	6 fl. oz.	80	19.0
CLAM JUICE (Snow)	½ cup	15	1.2
CLARET WINE:			
(Gold Seal) 12% alcohol	3 fl. oz.	82	.4
(Taylor) 12.5% alcohol	3 fl. oz.	72	2.4
CLORETS, gum or mint	1 piece	6	1.3
CLUSTERS, cereal			
(General Mills)	½ cup (1 oz.)	100	19.0
COCKTAIL (See individual listings)			
COCKTAIL MIX (See individual listings such as **PINA COLADA COCKTAIL** or **WHISKEY SOUR COCKTAIL**)			
COCOA:			
Dry, unsweetened:			
(USDA):			
Low fat	1 T. (5 grams)	10	3.1
High fat	1 T. (5 grams)	14	2.8
(Hershey's) American process	1 T. (5 grams)	29	2.3
Mix, regular:			
(Alba '66) instant, all flavors	1 envelope	60	11.0
(Carnation) all flavors	1-oz. pkg.	110	23.0
(Hershey's)	1 T.	27	6.0
(Nestlé)	1¼ oz.	150	26.0
(Ovaltine) hot'n rich	1 oz.	120	22.0
Swiss Miss:			
Regular:			
Double rich	1 envelope	110	19.1
Milk chocolate or with mini marshmallows	1 envelope or 3-4 heaping tsps.	110	20.0
European creme:			

(USDA): United States Department of Agriculture
(HEW/FAO):   Health, Education and Welfare/Food and Agriculture
                          Organization
* Prepared as Package Directs

Food and Description	Measure or Quantity	Calories	Carbo-hydrates (grams)
Amaretto or chocolate	1 envelope	150	29.0
Creme de menthe	1¼-oz. envelope	145	25.0
Mocha	1¼-oz. envelope	140	24.0
Mix, dietetic:			
(Carnation):			
70 Calorie	¾-oz. packet	70	15.0
Sugar free	.5-oz. envelope	50	8.0
*(Estee)	6 fl. oz.	50	9.0
*(Featherweight)	6 fl. oz.	50	8.0
(Ovaltine) reduced calorie	.45-oz. envelope	50	8.0
Swiss Miss:			
Lite	1 envelope	70	17.0
Milk chocolate	.5-oz. envelope	50	10.0
With sugar-free mini marshmallows	.5-oz. envelope	50	9.0
COCOA KRISPIES, cereal (Kellogg's)	¾ cup (1 oz.)	110	25.0
COCOA PUFFS, cereal (General Mills)	1 cup (1 oz.)	110	25.0
COCONUT:			
Fresh (USDA):			
Whole	1 lb. (weighed in shell)	816	22.2
Meat only	4 oz.	392	10.7
Grated or shredded, loosely packed	½ cup (1.4 oz.)	225	6.1
Dried, canned or packaged:			
(Baker's):			
Angel Flake:			
Packaged in bag	⅓ cup (.9 oz.)	118	10.6
Canned	⅓ cup (.9 oz.)	120	10.4
Cookie cut	⅓ cup (1.3 oz.)	186	17.1
Premium shred	⅓ cup (1 oz.)	138	12.4
Southern style	⅓ cup (.9 oz.)	118	10.3
(Durkee) shredded	¼ cup	69	2.0
COCONUT, CREAM OF, canned (Coco Lopez)	1 T.	60	10.0
COCO WHEATS, cereal (Little Crow)	1 T. (12 grams)	44	9.3
COD:			
(USDA):			

Food and Description	Measure or Quantity	Calories	Carbo-hydrates (grams)
Raw, meat only	4 oz.	88	0.
Broiled	4 oz.	193	0.
Dehydrated, lightly salted	4 oz.	425	0.
Frozen:			
(Frionor) *Norway Gourmet*	4-oz. fillet	70	0.
(Gorton's) *Fishmarket Fresh*	4 oz.	90	0.
(Van de Kamp's) *Today's Catch*	4 oz.	80	0.
COD DINNER OR ENTREE,			
Frozen:			
(Armour) *Dinner Classics*, almondine	12-oz. meal	360	33.0
(Blue Star) *Dining Lite*, fillet	10-oz. meal	189	12.1
(Frionor) *Norway Gourmet:*			
With dill sauce	4½-oz. fillet	80	1.0
With toasted bread crumbs	4½-oz. fillet	160	3.0
COFFEE:			
Regular:			
Max-Pax; Maxwell House Electra Perk; Yuban, Yuban Electra Matic	6 fl. oz.	2	0.
Mellow Roast	6 fl. oz.	8	2.0
Decaffeinated:			
Brim, regular or electric perk	6 fl. oz.	2	0.
Brim, freeze-dried; *Decaf; Nescafe*	6 fl. oz.	4	1.0
Sanka, regular or electric perk	6 fl. oz.	2	0.
Instant:			
(Maxwell House)	6 fl. oz.	4	1.0
Mellow Roast	6 fl. oz.	8	2.0
Sunrise	6 fl. oz.	6	1.0
*Mix (General Foods) International Coffee:			
Café Amaretto	6 fl. oz.	59	7.0
Café Français	6 fl. oz.	59	6.6
Café Vienna, Orange			

(USDA): United States Department of Agriculture
(HEW/FAO): Health, Education and Welfare/Food and Agriculture Organization
* Prepared as Package Directs

Food and Description	Measure or Quantity	Calories	Carbo-hydrates (grams)
Capuccino	6 fl. oz.	65	10.3
Irish Mocha Mint	6 fl. oz.	55	7.4
Suisse Mocha	6 fl. oz.	58	7.6
COFFEE CAKE (See **CAKE,** Coffee)			
COFFEE LIQUEUR (DeKuyper)	1 fl. oz.	93	12.4
COFFEE SOUTHERN	1 fl. oz.	79	8.8
COGNAC (See **DISTILLED LIQUOR**)			
COLA SOFT DRINK (See **SOFT DRINK,** Cola)			
COLD DUCK WINE (Great Western) pink, 12% alcohol	3 fl. oz.	92	7.7
COLESLAW, solids & liq. (USDA):			
Prepared with commercial French dressing	4-oz. serving	108	8.6
Prepared with homemade French dressing	4-oz. serving	146	5.8
Prepared with mayonnaise	4-oz. serving	163	5.4
Prepared with mayonnaise type salad dressing	1 cup (4.2 oz.)	119	8.5
***COLESLAW MIX** (Libby's) Super Slaw*	½ cup	240	11.0
COLLARDS:			
Raw (USDA):			
Leaves, including stems	1 lb.	181	32.7
Leaves only	½ lb.	70	11.6
Boiled (USDA) drained:			
Leaves, cooked in large amount of water	½ cup (3.4 oz.)	29	4.6
Leaves & stems, cooked in small amount of water	½ cup (3.4 oz.)	31	4.8
Canned (Allen's) chopped, solids & liq.	½ cup (4.1 oz.)	25	2.0
Frozen, chopped:			
(Birds Eye)	⅓ pkg. (3.3 oz.)	31	4.4

Food and Description	Measure or Quantity	Calories	Carbo-hydrates (grams)
(Frosty Acres)	3.3-oz. serving	25	4.0
(McKenzie)	⅓ pkg. (3.3 oz.)	25	4.0
(Southland) chopped	⅕ of 16-oz. pkg.	25	4.0
COMPLETE CEREAL (Elam's)	1 oz.	109	17.5
CONCORD WINE (Gold Seal) 13–14% alcohol	3 fl. oz.	125	9.8
COOKIE:			
Home recipe (USDA):			
Brownie with nuts	1¾″ × 1¾″ × ⅞″	97	10.2
Chocolate chip	1 oz.	146	17.0
Sugar, soft, thick	1 oz.	126	19.3
Packaged:			
Almond Supreme (Pepperidge Farm)	1 piece	70	6.5
Animal:			
(USDA)	1 piece (3 grams)	11	2.1
(Dixie Belle)	1 piece (.7 oz.)	8	1.5
(Gerber)	.2-oz. piece	30	5.0
(Nabisco) *Barnum's Animals*	1 piece	12	1.9
(Ralston)	1 piece (2 grams)	8	1.5
(Sunshine)	1 piece	8	1.4
(Tom's)	1.7 oz.	210	37.0
Apple Newtons (Nabisco)	1 piece	73	14.0
Apricot Raspberry (Pepperidge Farm)	1 piece (.4 oz.)	50	7.6
Assortment:			
(Nabisco) Famous:			
Baronet	1 piece	47	6.7
Butter flavor	1 piece	22	3.3
Biscos sugar wafer	1 piece	19	2.5
Cameo creme sandwich	1 piece	47	7.0
Kettle cookie	1 piece	32	5.0
Lorna Doone	1 piece	35	4.5
Oreo, chocolate	1 piece	47	6.7
(Pepperidge Farm):			
Butter	1 piece	55	7.0

(USDA): United States Department of Agriculture
(HEW/FAO):   Health, Education and Welfare/Food and Agriculture Organization
* Prepared as Package Directs

Food and Description	Measure or Quantity	Calories	Carbo-hydrates (grams)
Champagne	1 piece	32	4.0
Chocolate laced Pirouette	1 piece	37	7.0
Seville	1 piece	55	6.5
Southport	1 piece	75	9.0
Blueberry (Pepperidge Farm)	1 piece	57	7.7
Blueberry Newtons (Nabisco)	1 piece	73	14.0
Bordeaux (Pepperidge Farm)	1 piece (7.1 grams)	33	5.3
Brown edge wafer (Nabisco)	1 piece (.2 oz.)	28	4.0
Brownie:			
(Hostess):			
Large	2-oz. piece	251	38.6
Small	1¼-oz. piece	157	24.1
(Nabisco) *Almost Home,*			
fudge & nut	1 piece	160	23.0
(Pepperidge Farm):			
Chocolate nut	.4-oz. piece	57	6.3
Nut, large	.9-oz. piece	140	15.0
(Sara Lee) frozen	⅛ of 13-oz. pkg.	199	26.1
Brussles (Pepperidge Farm)	1 piece (10 grams)	53	6.6
Brussles Mint			
(Pepperidge Farm)	1 piece (.4 oz.)	67	8.3
Butter flavored:			
(Nabisco)	1 piece (.2 oz.)	22	3.3
(Sunshine)	1 piece (.2 oz.)	30	4.5
Cappucino (Pepperidge Farm)	(9 grams)	53	6.0
Capri (Pepperidge Farm)	1 piece (.5 oz.)	80	10.0
Carmel Patties (FFV)	1 piece	75	10.0
Cherry Newton (Nabisco)	1 piece	73	13.3
Chessman (Pepperidge Farm)	1 piece (.3 oz.)	43	6.0
Chocolate & chocolate-covered:			
(Keebler) fridge covered			
fudge strips	1 piece (.4 oz.)	50	7.0
(Nabisco):			
Famous wafer	1 piece (.2 oz.)	22	5.2
Pinwheel, cake	1 piece (1.1 oz.)	130	20.0
Snap	1 piece (.14 oz.)	19	3.0
(Sunshine) nuggets	1 piece	23	3.3
Chocolate chip:			
(Archway) & toffee	.1-oz. piece	150	21.0
(Keebler):			
Chips deluxe	1 piece (.5 oz.)	90	10.0
Rich 'n chips	1 piece (.5 oz.)	80	10.0

Food and Description	Measure or Quantity	Calories	Carbohydrates (grams)
(Nabisco):			
Almost Home, fudge or real	1 piece (.5 oz.)	65	10.0
Chips Ahoy!:			
Regular	1 piece (.3 oz.)	47	6.0
Chewy	1 piece (.5 oz.)	65	9.0
Chips 'n More:			
Coconut	1 piece (.5 oz.)	75	9.0
Fudge	1 piece (.3 oz.)	47	6.3
Original	1 piece (.5 oz.)	75	9.0
Snaps	1 piece (.2 oz.)	22	3.5
(Pepperidge Farm):			
Regular	1 piece (.3 oz.)	53	6.3
Chocolate	1 piece (.4 oz.)	53	6.3
Mocha	1 piece	40	5.3
Peanut butter	1 piece	47	5.3
(Sunshine):			
Chip-A-Roos:			
Regular	1 piece (.5 oz.)	60	8.0
Chocolate	1 piece (.5 oz.)	60	7.0
Chippy Chews	1 piece	50	8.0
(Tom's)	1.7-oz. serving	230	34.0
Chocolate peanut bar			
(Nabisco) Ideal	1 piece (.6 oz.)	75	8.5
Cinnamon Raisin (Nabisco)			
Almost Home	1 piece (.5 oz.)	70	8.0
Coconut Fudge (FFV)	1 piece	80	10.0
Creme sticks (Dutch Twin)			
chocolate coated	1 piece (.3 oz.)	39	5.0
Danish (Nabisco) imported	1 piece (.2 oz.)	30	3.6
Date Nut Granola (Pepperidge			
Farm) *Kitchen Hearth*	1 piece (.4 oz.)	53	6.7
Date Pecan (Pepperidge Farm)	1 piece (.4 oz.)	53	7.3
Devil's food cake (Nabisco)	1 piece	140	30.0
Dinosaurs (FFV)	1 oz.	130	20.0
Fig bar:			
(FFV)	1 piece	70	12.0
(Nabisco): *Fig Newtons*	1 piece (.5 oz.)	50	10.0
(Sunshine) chewies	1 piece (.5 oz.)	50	11.0
(Tom's) bar	1 oz.	100	21.0
Fruit Stick (Nabisco) *Almost*			

(USDA): United States Department of Agriculture
(HEW/FAO):   Health, Education and Welfare/Food and Agriculture
                      Organization
* Prepared as Package Directs

Food and Description	Measure or Quantity	Calories	Carbohydrates (grams)
Home	1 piece (.7 oz.)	70	14.0
Geneva (Pepperidge Farm)	1 piece (.4 oz.)	57	6.3
Gingerboys (FFV)	1 oz.	120	20.0
Gingersnap:			
(Archway)	1 piece (.5oz.)	25	4.0
(FFV)	1 oz.	130	22.0
(Nabisco)	1 piece	30	5.5
(Sunshine)	1 piece (.2 oz.)	20	3.0
Golden Fruit Raisin (Sunshine)	1 piece (smallest portion after breaking on scoreline) (.6 oz.)	70	14.0
Hazelnut (Pepperidge Farm)	1 piece (.4 oz.)	57	7.5
Heyday (Nabisco)	1 piece	140	15.0
Jelly Tart (FFV)	1 piece	60	11.0
Ladyfinger (USDA)	3¼″ × 1⅜″ × 1⅛″ (.4 oz.)	40	7.1
Lemon (Archway)	1 piece	155	23.0
Lemon Cooler (Sunshine)	1 piece (.2 oz.)	30	4.3
Lemon nut crunch (Pepperidge Farm)	1 piece (.4 oz.)	57	6.3
Lido (Pepperidge Farm)	1 piece (.6 oz.)	95	10.5
Macaroon (Nabisco) soft	1 piece	190	23.0
Mallo Puffs (Sunshine)	1 piece (.6 oz.)	70	12.0
Marshmallow:			
(Nabisco):			
Mallomars	1 piece (.5 oz.)	65	9.0
Puffs, cocoa covered	1 piece (.1 oz.)	120	20.0
Sandwich	1 piece (.3 oz.)	30	5.5
Twirls cakes	1 piece (1 oz.)	130	19.0
(Planters) banana pie	1 oz.	127	22.0
Milano (Pepperidge Farm)	1 piece (.4 oz.)	60	7.0
Mint fudge (FFV)	1 piece	80	11.0
Mint Milano (Pepperidge Farm)	1 piece (.5 oz.)	76	8.3
Molasses (Nabisco) *Pantry*	1 piece (.5 oz.)	65	10.5
Molasses Crisp (Pepperidge Farm)	1 piece (.2 oz.)	33	4.0
Nassau (Pepperidge Farm)	1 piece (.5 oz.)	85	9.0
Nilla wafer (Nabisco)	1 piece (.1 oz.)	19	3.0
Oatmeal:			
(Archway):			
Regular	1 piece	110	19.0
Apple bran	1 piece	107	18.0
Apple filled	1 piece	90	18.0

Food and Description	Measure or Quantity	Calories	Carbo-hydrates (grams)
Date filled, raisin or raisin bran	1 piece	100	18.0
Golden, *Ruth's*	1 piece	120	20.0
Iced	1 piece	140	22.0
(FFV):			
Regular	1 piece	26	4.0
Bar	1 piece	70	11.0
(Keebler) old fashioned	1 piece (18 grams)	80	12.0
(Nabisco) *Bakers Bonus*	1 piece (.5 oz.)	65	10.0
Cookie Little	1 piece (.1 oz.)	6	1.0
(Pepperidge Farm):			
Irish	1 piece (.3 oz.)	47	6.7
Raisin	1 piece (.4 oz.)	57	7.7
(Sunshine):			
Country style	1 piece	60	8.0
Peanut sandwich	1 piece	70	9.0
Orange Milano (Pepperidge Farm)	1 piece (.5 oz.)	76	8.3
Orbits (Sunshine):			
Butter flavored	1 piece	15	2.5
Chocolate	1 piece	15	2.3
Orleans (Pepperidge Farm)	1 piece (.2 oz.)	30	3.6
Peanut & peanut butter:			
(Nabisco):			
Almost Home	1 piece	70	8.0
Nutter Butter:			
Creme pattie	1 piece (.3 oz.)	37	4.3
Sandwich	1 piece (.5 oz.)	70	9.0
(Sunshine) wafer	1 piece	40	5.0
Pecan Sandies (Keebler)	1 piece (16 grams)	80	9.0
Praline Pecan (FFV)	1 piece	40	10.0
Raisin (USDA)	1 oz.	107	22.9
Raisin bran (Pepperidge Farm)	1 piece (.4 oz.)	53	6.7
Rocky road (Archway)	1 piece	130	20.0
Royal Dainty (FFV)	1 piece	60	7.0
Sandwich:			
(Keebler):			
Fudge creme	1 piece		

(USDA): United States Department of Agriculture
(HEW/FAO): Health, Education and Welfare/Food and Agriculture Organization
* Prepared as Package Directs

Food and Description	Measure or Quantity	Calories	Carbo-hydrates (grams)
	(12 grams)	60	8.0
(Sunshine) wafer	1 piece (.3 oz.)	40	5.0
Oatmeal cream	(.5 oz.)	80	11.0
Pitter Patter	1 piece		
	(17 grams)	90	11.0
(Nabisco):			
Almost Home	1 piece	140	20.0
Baronet	1 piece (.3 oz.)	47	6.7
Cameo	1 piece (.3 oz.)	47	7.0
Gaity, fudge chocolate	1 piece (.3 oz.)	50	6.3
Giggles	1 piece (.3 oz.)	70	8.5
I Screams	1 piece (.5 oz.)	75	10.0
Mystic Mint	1 piece (.5 oz.)	75	9.5
Oreo:			
Regular	1 piece (.3 oz.)	47	6.7
Double Stuf	1 piece (.5 oz.)	70	9.5
Mint	1 piece (.5 oz.)	70	10.0
Vanilla, *Cookie Break*	1 piece (.3 oz.)	47	6.7
(Sunshine):			
Regular:			
Chocolate fudge or cup custard	1 piece (.5 oz.)	70	9.0
Hydrox	1 piece (.4 oz.)	50	7.0
Vienna Fingers	1 piece	70	11.0
Chips 'n Middles:			
Fudge	1 piece (.5 oz.)	70	10.0
Peanut butter	1 piece (.5 oz.)	70	9.0
Tru Blue, any flavor	1 piece (.6 oz.)	80	11.0
Shortbread or shortcake:			
(FFV) country	1 piece	70	9.0
(Nabisco):			
Fudge striped	1 piece	50	6.3
Lorna Doone	1 piece (.3 oz.)	35	4.5
Pecan	1 piece (.5 oz.)	75	8.0
(Pepperidge Farm)	1 piece (.5 oz.)	75	8.5
Social Tea, biscuit (Nabisco)	1 piece	22	3.5
Sprinkles (Sunshine)	1 piece (.6 oz.)	70	12.0
Strawberry (Pepperidge Farm)	1 piece (.4 oz.)	50	7.6
Sugar:			
(Nabisco) rings, *Bakers Bonus*	1 piece (.5 oz.)	65	10.0
(Pepperidge Farm)	1 piece (.4 oz.)	50	6.7
Sugar wafer:			
(Dutch Twin) any flavor	1 piece (.3 oz.)	36	4.7
(Nabisco) *Biscos*	1 piece (.1 oz.)	19	2.5

Food and Description	Measure or Quantity	Calories	Carbo- hydrates (grams)
(Sunshine)	1 piece (.3 oz.)	45	6.0
Super Heroes (Nabisco)	1 piece (.1 oz.)	12	1.8
Tahiti (Pepperidge Farm)	1 piece (.5 oz.)	85	8.5
Tango (FFV)	1 piece	80	13.0
Toy (Sunshine)	1 piece (.1 oz.)	12	2.0
Vanilla wafer (Keebler)	1 piece (4 grams)	20	2.7
Waffle creme:			
(Dutch Twin)	1 piece (.3 oz.)	45	5.7
(Nabisco)	1 piece (.3 oz.)	50	6.7
Zanzibar (Pepperidge Farm)	1 piece (.3 oz.)	40	4.3
COOKIE CRISP, cereal,			
(Ralston Purina) any flavor	1 cup (1 oz.)	110	25.0
COOKIE, DIETETIC (Estee)	1 piece	30	4.0
***COOKIE DOUGH:**			
Refrigerated (Pillsbury):			
Brownie, fudge			
microwave	⅑ of pkg.	70	9.0
Chocolate chip or sugar	1 cookie	70	9.0
Peanut butter	1 cookie	70	8.0
Frozen (Rich's):			
Chocolate chip	1 cookie	138	20.3
Oatmeal	1 cookie	125	18.3
Oatmeal & raisins	1 cookie	122	19.1
Peanut butter	1 cookie	128	14.6
Sugar	1 cookie	118	17.4
COOKIE MIX:			
Regular:			
Brownie:			
*(Betty Crocker):			
Chocolate chip	¼ of pan	130	20.0
Frosted	¼ of pan	160	27.0
Fudge:			
Regular size	⅟₁₆ of pan	150	23.0
Family size	¼ of pan	130	21.0
Supreme	¼ of pan	120	21.0
German chocolate	¼ of pan	160	24.0

(USDA): United States Department of Agriculture
(HEW/FAO):   Health, Education and Welfare/Food and Agriculture
                        Organization
* Prepared as Package Directs

Food and Description	Measure or Quantity	Calories	Carbo-hydrates (grams)
Walnut	⅟₁₆ of pan	140	18.0
(Duncan Hines)	⅟₂₄ of pkg.	119	22.0
(Nestlé)	⅟₂₄ of pkg.	150	22.0
(Pillsbury) fudge:			
Regular size	2″ sq. (⅟₁₆ pkg.)	150	23.0
Family size	2″ sq. (⅟₂₄ pkg.)	150	22.0
Chocolate (Duncan Hines)			
double	⅟₃₆ of pkg.	67	9.2
Chocolate chip:			
*(Betty Crocker)			
Big Batch	1 cookie	60	8.0
(Duncan Hines)	⅟₃₆ of pkg.	72	9.1
*(Quaker)	1 cookie	75	8.5
Date bar (Betty Crocker)	⅟₂₄ of pkg.	60	8.0
Macaroon, coconut			
(Betty Crocker)	⅟₂₄ of pkg.	80	10.0
Oatmeal:			
(Duncan Hines)	⅟₃₆ of pkg.	68	9.1
*(Nestlé)	1 cookie	60	9.0
*(Quaker)	1 cookie	66	9.4
Peanut butter:			
(Duncan Hines)	⅟₃₆ pkg.	68	7.5
*(Nestlé)	1 cookie	65	7.5
*(Quaker)	1 cookie	75	8.0
Sugar:			
*(Betty Crocker)			
Big Batch	1 cookie	60	9.0
(Duncan Hines) golden	⅟₃₆ of pkg.	59	8.4
*(Nestlé)	1 cookie	65	8.5
*Vienna dream bar			
(Betty Crocker)	⅟₂₄ of pkg.	90	10.0
*Dietetic (Estee) brownie	2″ × 2″-sq. cookie	45	8.0
COOKING SPRAY, *Mazola No Stick*	2½-second spray	6	0.
CORIANDER SEED (French's)	1 tsp. (1.4 grams)	6	.8
CORN:			
Fresh, white or yellow (USDA):			
Raw:			
Untrimmed, on the cob	1 lb. (weighed in husk)	167	36.1
Trimmed, on cob	1 lb. (husk removed)	240	55.1

Food and Description	Measure or Quantity	Calories	Carbo-hydrates (grams)
Boiled:			
Kernels, cut from cob, drained	1 cup (5.8 oz.)	137	31.0
Whole	4.9-oz. ear (5" × 1¾")	70	16.2
Trimmed, on the cob	5" × 1¾" ear	70	16.2
Canned, regular pack:			
(USDA):			
Golden or yellow, whole kernel, solids & liq., vacuum pack	½ cup (3.7 oz.)	87	21.6
Golden or yellow, whole kernel, wet pack	½ cup (4.5 oz.)	84	20.1
Golden or yellow, whole kernel, drained solids, wet pack	½ cup (3 oz.)	72	16.4
White kernel, drained solids	½ cup (2.8 oz.)	70	16.4
White, whole kernel, drained liq., wet pack	4 oz.	29	7.8
Cream style	½ cup (4.4 oz.)	105	25.6
(Allen's) whole kernel, golden	½ cup (4.2 oz.)	80	3.0
(Comstock):			
Cream style	½ cup (4.4 oz.)	100	20.0
Whole kernel	½ cup (4.4 oz.)	90	20.0
(Del Monte) solids & liq.:			
Cream style, golden,	½ cup (4 oz.)	80	18.0
Cream style, white	½ cup (4 oz.)	90	21.0
Whole kernel, golden or white	½ cup	70	17.0
Whole kernel, vacuum pack	½ cup	90	22.0
(Green Giant) solids & liq.:			
Cream style	½ cup	100	24.0
Whole kernel or shoe peg, golden	4¼ oz.	90	18.0
Whole kernel, vacuum pack	½ cup	80	16.0

(USDA): United States Department of Agriculture
(HEW/FAO):   Health, Education and Welfare/Food and Agriculture
                 Organization
* Prepared as Package Directs

Food and Description	Measure or Quantity	Calories	Carbo-hydrates (grams)
Whole kernel, *Mexicorn*	3½ oz.	80	19.0
Whole kernel, white, vacuum pack	½ cup	80	20.0
(Larsen) *Freshlike:*			
Whole kernel, vacuum pack	½ cup (3.9 oz.)	100	22.0
Whole kernel, vacuum pack, with pepper	½ cup (4 oz.)	90	23.0
(Le Sueur) whole kernel, solids & liq.	4¼ oz.	80	18.0
(Libby's) cream style	½ cup (4.3 oz.)	100	21.2
(Stokely-Van Camp) solids & liq.:			
Cream style, golden	½ cup (4.5 oz.)	105	23.5
Cream style, white	½ cup (4.6 oz.)	110	24.5
Whole kernel, golden	½ cup	90	19.5
Canned, dietetic pack, solids & liq.:			
(Del Monte) No Salt Added:			
Cream style	½ cup	80	20.0
Whole kernel:			
Regular	½ cup (4.3 oz.)	70	17.0
Vacuum pack	½ cup (4 oz.)	90	22.0
(Diet Delight) whole kernel	½ cup	60	15.0
(Featherweight) whole kernel	½ cup (4 oz.)	80	16.0
(Larsen) *Fresh-Lite,* whole kernel, no salt added	½ cup (4.5 oz.)	80	19.0
(S&W) *Nutradiet,* whole kernel, green label	½ cup	100	21.0
Frozen:			
(Birds Eye):			
On the cob:			
Regular	4.4-oz. ear	120	28.7
Big Ears	5.7-oz. ear	156	37.0
Little Ears	4.6-oz. ear	126	30.0
Whole kernel:			
Cob corn, deluxe baby	⅓ of 8-oz. pkg.	23	4.0
Deluxe, petite	⅓ of 8-oz. pkg.	66	1.6
Sweet:			
Regular	¼ of 12-oz. pkg.	74	18.0
Butter sauce	⅓ of 10-oz. pkg.	85	17.0
Deluxe, tender	⅓ of 10-oz. pkg.	82	20.0
(Frosty Acres):			
On the cob	1 ear	120	29.0
Whole kernel	3.3-oz. serving	80	20.0

Food and Description	Measure or Quantity	Calories	Carbo-hydrates (grams)
(Green Giant):			
On the cob:			
Nibbler, regular	1 ear	60	13.0
Niblet Ear, regular	1 ear	120	26.0
Cream style	½ cup	110	25.0
Whole kernel, *Niblets:*			
In butter sauce, golden	½ cup	100	19.0
Harvest Fresh, golden	3 oz.	80	17.0
Polybag, white	½ cup	70	15.0
(Larsen):			
On the cob:			
3-inch piece	2.2-oz. piece	60	15.0
5-inch piece	4.4-oz. piece	120	29.0
Cut	3.3 oz.	80	20.0
(McKenzie):			
On the cob	5″ ear (4.4 oz.)	140	30.0
Whole kernel	3.3 oz.	90	20.0
(Seabrook Farms):			
On the cob	5″ ear	140	30.0
Whole kernel	⅓ of 10-oz. pkg.	97	19.9
CORN BREAD:			
Home recipe (USDA):			
Corn pone, prepared with white, whole-ground cornmeal	4 oz.	231	41.1
Johnnycake, prepared with yellow, degermed cornmeal	4 oz.	303	51.6
Southern style, prepared with degermed cornmeal	2½″ × 2½″ × 1⅝″ piece	186	28.8
Southern style, prepared with whole-ground cornmeal	4 oz.	235	33.0
Spoon bread, prepared with white, whole-ground cornmeal	4 oz.	221	19.2
*Mix:			
(Aunt Jemima)	⅙ of pkg.	220	34.0
(Dromedary)	2″ × 2″ piece (1/16 of pkg.)	130	20.0
(Pillsbury) *Ballard*	⅛ of recipe	140	25.0

(USDA): United States Department of Agriculture
(HEW/FAO): Health, Education and Welfare/Food and Agriculture Organization
* Prepared as Package Directs

Food and Description	Measure or Quantity	Calories	Carbo-hydrates (grams)
*CORN DOG, frozen:			
(Fred's) *Little Juan*	2¾-oz. serving	231	24.6
(Hormel)	1 piece	220	21.0
CORNED BEEF:			
Cooked (USDA), boneless, medium fat	4-oz. serving	422	0.
Canned, regular pack:			
Dinty Moore (Hormel)	2-oz. serving	130	0.
(Libby's)	⅓ of 7-oz. can	160	2.0
Canned, dietetic (Featherweight) loaf	2½-oz. serving	90	0.
Packaged:			
(Eckrich) sliced	1-oz. slice	40	1.0
(Carl Buddig) smoked, sliced	1 oz.	40	Tr.
(Eckrich) slender sliced	1 oz.	40	1.0
(Oscar Mayer)	.6-oz. slice	16	.1
CORNED BEEF HASH, canned:			
(Libby's)	⅓ of 24-oz. can	420	21.0
Mary Kitchen (Hormel):			
Regular	½ of 15-oz. can	360	19.0
Short Orders	7½-oz. can	360	17.0
CORNED BEEF HASH DINNER, frozen (Banquet)	10-oz. dinner	372	421.6
CORNED BEEF SPREAD, canned:			
(Hormel)	1 oz.	70	0.
(Underwood)	½ of 4½-oz. can	120	Tr.
CORN FLAKE CRUMBS (Kellogg's)	¼ cup (1 oz.)	110	25.0
CORN FLAKES, cereal:			
(General Mills) *Country*	1 cup (1 oz.)	110	25.0
(Kellogg's):			
Regular	1 cup (1 oz.)	110	25.0
Honey & Nut	¾ cup (1 oz.)	120	24.0
Sugar Frosted Flakes	¾ cup (1 oz.)	110	26.0
(Ralston Purina):			
Regular	1 cup (1 oz.)	110	25.0
Sugar Frosted	¾ cup (1 oz.)	110	26.0

Food and Description	Measure or Quantity	Calories	Carbo-hydrates (grams)
CORNMEAL, WHITE or YELLOW:			
Dry:			
Bolted:			
(USDA)	1 cup (4.3 oz.)	442	90.9
(Aunt Jemima/Quaker)	1 cup (4 oz.)	408	84.8
Degermed:			
(USDA)	1 cup (4.9 oz.)	502	108.2
(Aunt Jemima/Quaker)	1 cup (4 oz.)	404	88.8
Self-rising degermed:			
(USDA)	1 cup (5 oz.)	491	105.9
(Aunt Jemima)	1 cup (6 oz.)	582	126.0
Self-rising, whole ground			
(USDA)	1 cup (5 oz.)	489	101.4
Whole ground, unbolted			
(USDA)	1 cup (4.3 oz.)	433	90.0
Cooked:			
(USDA)	1 cup (8.5 oz.)	120	25.7
(Albers) degermed	1 cup	119	25.5
Mix (Aunt Jemima/Quaker)			
bolted	1 cup (4 oz.)	392	80.4
***CORN POPS**, cereal (Kellogg's)	1 cup (1 oz.)	110	26.0
CORN PUDDING, home recipe (USDA)	1 cup (8.6 oz.)	255	31.9
CORN PUREE, canned (Larsen) no salt added	½ cup	100	22.5
CORNSTARCH (Argo; Kingsford's)	1 tsp. (8 grams)	10	8.3
CORN SYRUP (See **SYRUP,** Corn)			
COTTAGE PUDDING, home recipe (USDA):			
Without sauce	2 oz.	180	30.8
With chocolate sauce	2 oz.	195	32.1
With strawberry sauce	2 oz.	166	27.4

(USDA): United States Department of Agriculture
(HEW/FAO):   Health, Education and Welfare/Food and Agriculture
                    Organization
* Prepared as Package Directs

Food and Description	Measure or Quantity	Calories	Carbo-hydrates (grams)
COUGH DROP:			
(Beech-Nut)	1 drop	10	2.5
(Pine Bros.)	1 drop	10	2.4
COUNT CHOCULA, cereal			
(General Mills)	1 oz. (1 cup)	110	24.0
COWPEA (USDA):			
Immature seeds:			
Raw, whole	1 lb. (weighed in pods)	317	54.4
Raw, shelled	½ cup (2.5 oz.)	92	15.8
Boiled, drained solids	½ cup (2.9 oz.)	89	15.0
Canned, solids & liq.	4 oz.	79	14.1
Frozen (See **BLACK-EYED PEAS,** frozen)			
Young pods with seeds:			
Raw, whole	1 lb. (weighed untrimmed)	182	39.2
Boiled, drained solids	4 oz.	39	7.9
Mature seeds, dry:			
Raw	1 lb.	1556	279.9
Raw	½ cup (3 oz.)	292	52.4
Boiled	½ cup (4.4 oz.)	95	17.2
CRAB:			
Fresh, steamed (USDA):			
Whole	½ lb. (weighed in shell)	202	1.1
Meat only	4 oz.	105	.6
Canned, drained (USDA)	4 oz.	115	1.2
Frozen (Wakefield's)	4 oz.	86	.7
CRAB APPLE, flesh only			
(USDA)	¼ lb.	71	20.2
CRAB APPLE JELLY			
(Smucker's)	1 T. (.7 oz.)	53	13.5
CRAB AU GRATIN, frozen			
(Gorton's) Light Recipe	1 pkg.	280	18.0
CRAB, DEVILED:			
Home recipe (USDA)	**4 oz.**	**213**	**15.1**
Frozen (Mrs. Paul's) breaded &			

Food and Description	Measure or Quantity	Calories	Carbo-hydrates (grams)
fried	½ of 6-oz. pkg.	170	20.0
CRAB, IMITATION:			
(Louis Kemp) *Crab Delights,* chunks, flakes or legs	2-oz. serving	60	7.0
CRAB IMPERIAL:			
Home recipe (USDA)	1 cup (7.8 oz.)	323	8.6
Frozen (Gorton's) Light Recipe, stuffed	1 pkg.	340	36.0
CRACKERS, PUFFS & CHIPS:			
Animal (FFV)	1 oz.	130	21.0
Arrowroot biscuit (Nabisco)	1 piece (.2 oz.)	22	3.5
Bacon-flavored thins (Nabisco)	1 piece (.1 oz.)	10	1.1
Bran wafer (Featherweight)	1 piece	13	2.0
Bravos (Wise)	1 oz.	150	18.0
Bugles (Tom's)	1 oz.	150	18.0
Butter (Pepperidge Farm) thin	1 piece	20	2.5
Cafe Cracker (Sunshine)	1 piece (smallest portion after breaking on scoreline	20	2.3
Cheese flavored:			
American Heritage (Sunshine):			
Cheddar	1 piece	16	1.6
Parmesan	1 piece	18	1.8
Better Blue Cheese (Nabisco)	1 piece	7	.8
Better Cheddar (Nabisco)	1 piece	6	.7
Better Nacho (Nabisco)	1 piece	8	.9
Better Swiss (Nabisco)	1 piece	7	.8
Cheddar Sticks (Flavor Tree)	1 oz.	160	12.0
Cheese Bites (Tom's)	1½ oz.	200	26.0
Cheese 'n Crunch (Nabisco)	1 piece	4	.4
Cheese Doodles (Wise):			
Crunchy	1 oz.	160	16.0
Fried	1 oz.	150	16.0
Chee-Tos, crunchy or puffy	1 oz.	160	15.0
Cheez Balls (Planters)	1 oz.	160	14.0
Cheez Curls (Planters)	1 oz.	160	14.0
Cheez-It (Sunshine)	1 piece	6	.6

(USDA): United States Department of Agriculture
(HEW/FAO):   Health, Education and Welfare/Food and Agriculture
Organization
* Prepared as Package Directs

Food and Description	Measure or Quantity	Calories	Carbo-hydrates (grams)
Corn cheese (Tom's):			
Crunchy	⅝ oz.	280	25.0
Puffed, baked	1⅛ oz.	180	18.0
Curl (Featherweight)	1 oz.	150	16.0
Dip In A Chip (Nabisco)	1 piece (.1 oz.)	9	1.0
(Dixie Belle)	1 piece	6	.7
Nacho cheese cracker			
(Old El Paso)	1 oz.	76	15.3
Nips (Nabisco)	1 piece (.04 oz.)	5	.7
(Planters) squares	1 oz.	140	15.0
(Ralston)	1 piece (1.1 grams)	6	.7
Sandwich (Nabisco)	1 piece	35	4.0
Tid-Bit (Nabisco)	1 piece	4	.5
Chicken in a Biskit (Nabisco)	1 piece (.1 oz.)	10	1.1
Chipsters (Nabisco)	1 piece	2	.3
Cinnamon Treats (Nabisco)	1 piece	30	5.5
Club cracker (Keebler)	1 piece (3.2 grams)	15	2.0
Corn chips:			
(Bachman) regular or BBQ	1 oz.	150	15.0
Dippy Doodle (Wise)	1 oz.	160	12.0
(Featherweight) low sodium	1 oz.	170	15.0
(Flavor Tree)	1 oz.	150	17.0
Fritos:			
Regular	1 oz.	160	16.0
Barbecue flavor	1 oz.	150	15.5
(Laura Scudder's)	1 oz.	160	15.0
(Old Dutch)	1 oz.	160	15.0
(Tom's) regular	1 oz.	105	17.0
Corn Stick (Flavor Tree)	1 oz.	160	15.0
Country Cracker (Nabisco)	1 piece	16	1.8
Crown Pilot (Nabisco)	1 piece (.6 oz.)	60	11.0
Diggers (Nabisco)	1 piece	4	.5
Dip In A Chip (Nabisco)	1 piece	9	1.0
Doo Dads (Nabisco)	1 oz.	140	18.0
English Water Biscuit (Pepperidge Farm)	1 piece (.1 oz.)	27	3.2
Escort (Nabisco)	1 piece (.1 oz.)	21	2.6
Goldfish (Pepperidge Farm)			
Tiny	1 piece (.02 oz.)	3	.4
Graham:			
(Dixie Belle) sugar-honey coated	1 piece	15	2.6
Flavor Kist (Schulze and			

Food and Description	Measure or Quantity	Calories	Carbohydrates (grams)
Burch) sugar-honey coated	1 double cracker	57	10.0
Honey Maid (Nabisco)	1 piece (.25 oz.)	30	5.5
(Keebler):			
Cinnamon Crisp	1 piece	17	2.7
Honey coated	1 piece	17	3.0
Party Graham (Nabisco)	1 piece	47	6.0
(Ralston) sugar-honey coated	1 piece	15	2.6
(Rokeach)	8 pieces	120	21.0
(Sunshine):			
Cinnamon	1 piece (.1 oz.)	17	2.8
Honey	1 piece	15	2.5
Graham, chocolate or cocoa-covered (Keebler) deluxe	1 piece (.3 oz.)	40	5.5
Great Crisps (Nabisco):			
Cheese & chive, real bacon, sesame or tomato & celery	1 piece	8	.9
French onion	1 piece	10	1.1
Nacho	1 piece	9	1.0
Savory garlic	1 piece	9	1.1
Hi Ho Crackers (Sunshine)	1 piece	20	2.0
Meal Mates (Nabisco)	1 piece	23	3.0
Melba Toast (see **MELBA TOAST**)			
Mucho Macho Nacho, Flavor Kist (Schulze and Burch)	1 oz.	121	18.0
Nachips (Old El Paso)	1 piece	17	1.7
Nacho Rings (Tom's)	1 oz.	160	15.0
Onion Crisp (FFV)	1 piece	60	10.0
Onion rings (Wise)	1 oz.	130	21.0
Oyster:			
(Dixie Belle)	1 piece (.03 oz.)	4	.6
(Keebler) *Zesta*	1 piece	2	.3
(Nabisco) *Dandy* or *Oysterettes*	1 piece (.03 oz.)	3	.5
(Ralston)	1 piece	4	.6
(Sunshine)	1 piece	4	.6
Party Mix (Flavor Tree)	1 oz.	160	11.0
Peanut butter sandwich (Planters) toasted	1 oz.	140	15.0

Food and Description	Measure or Quantity	Calories	Carbo-hydrates (grams)
Pizza Crunchies (Planters)	1 oz.	160	15.0
Potato chips (see **POTATO CHIPS**)			
Ritz (Nabisco)	1 piece (.1 oz.)	17	2.0
Rich & Crisp, (Dixie Bell; Ralston)	1 piece	14	1.9
Roman Meal Wafer, boxed	1 piece	11	1.3
Royal Lunch (Nabisco)	1 piece	60	10.0
Rusk, *Holland* (Nabisco)	1 piece (.35 oz.)	60	10.0
Rye toast (Keebler)	1 piece	16	2.0
RyKrisp (Ralston Purina):			
Natural	1 triple cracker	20	5.5
Seasoned	1 triple cracker	22	5.5
Saltine:			
(Dixie Belle) regular or unsalted	1 piece (.1 oz.)	12	2.0
Flavor Kist (Schulze and Burch)	1 piece	12	2.0
Krispy (Sunshine)	1 piece	12	2.2
Premium (Nabisco)	1 piece (.1 oz.)	12	2.0
(Ralston) regular or unsalted	1 piece	12	2.0
(Rokeach)	1 piece	12	2.0
Zesta (Keebler)	1 piece	13	2.1
Schooners (FFV):			
Regular	½ oz.	60	10.0
Wholewheat	½ oz.	70	8.0
Sea Rounds (Nabisco)	1 piece (.5 oz.)	50	10.0
Sesame:			
(Estee)	½ oz.	70	9.0
Flavor Kist, wheat snacks	1 oz.	134	18.0
(Flavor Tree):			
Chip	1 oz.	150	13.0
Crunch	1 oz.	150	10.0
Sticks:			
Plain	1 oz.	150	13.0
With bran	1 oz.	160	11.0
No salt added	1 oz.	160	12.0
(Keebler) toasted	1 piece	16	2.0
(Pepperidge Farm)	1 piece	20	3.4
(Sunshine) *American Heritage*	1 piece	17	2.0
Snack Cracker (Rokeach)	1 piece (.1 oz.)	14	2.1
Snackers (Dixie Bell; Ralston)	1 piece	17	2.2
Snackin' Crisp (Durkee) O & C	1 oz.	155	15.0
Snacks Sticks			

Food and Description	Measure or Quantity	Calories	Carbo-hydrates (grams)
(Pepperidge Farm):			
Cheese	1 piece	17	2.3
Original, pumpernickel,			
rye & sesame	1 piece	16	2.5
Parmesan pretzel	1 piece	15	2.6
Sociables (Nabisco)	1 piece	12	1.5
Sour cream & onion stick			
(Flavor Tree)	1 oz.	150	13.0
Spirals (Wise)	1 oz.	160	15.0
Table Water Cracker (Carr's):			
Small	1 piece (.12 oz.)	15	2.6
Large	1 piece (3 oz.)	32	5.9
Taco chips (Laura Scudder) mini	1 oz.	150	17.0
Tortilla chips:			
(Bachman) nacho, taco			
flavor or toasted	1 oz.	140	17.0
Doritos, nacho or taco:	1 oz.	140	18.0
Regular or *Salsa Rio*	1 oz.	140	19.0
Cool Ranch:			
Regular	1 oz.	140	18.0
Light	1 oz.	120	21.0
Nacho cheese:			
Regular	1 oz.	140	18.0
Light	1 oz.	120	21.0
Taco	1 oz.	140	18.0
(Laura Scudder's)	1 oz.	140	17.0
(Nabisco):			
Nacho	1 piece	12	1.3
Toasted corn	1 piece	11	1.4
(Old Dutch):			
Nacho	1 oz.	156	15.0
Taco	1 oz.	152	15.0
(Planters)	1 oz.	150	18.0
(Tom's) nacho	1 oz.	140	18.0
Tostitos:			
Jalapeno & cheese or sharp			
nacho	1 oz.	150	17.0
Traditional	1 oz.	140	18.0
Town House Cracker (Keebler)	1 piece (3.1 grams)	16	1.8

(USDA): United States Department of Agriculture
(HEW/FAO): Health, Education and Welfare/Food and Agriculture Organization
* Prepared as Package Directs

Food and Description	Measure or Quantity	Calories	Carbo-hydrates (grams)
Triscuit (Nabisco)	1 piece (.2 oz.)	20	3.3
Tuc (Keebler)	1 piece (.2 oz.)	23	2.7
Twiddle Sticks (Nabisco)	1 piece	53	7.0
Twigs (Nabisco)	1 piece (.1 oz.)	14	1.6
Uneeda Biscuit (Nabisco)	1 piece	20	3.3
Unsalted:			
(Estee)	1 piece (.1 oz.)	15	2.5
(Featherweight)	2 sections		
	(½ cracker)	30	5.0
Vegetable thins (Nabisco)	1 piece	10	1.1
Waverly (Nabisco)	1 piece	17	2.5
Wheat:			
(Dixie Belle) snack	1 piece	9	1.2
(Estee) *6 calorie*	1 piece	6	2.0
(Featherweight) wafer, unsalted	1 piece	13	2.3
Flavor Kist, (Schulze & Burch) snack:			
Natural	1 oz.	138	16.0
Rye	1 oz.	130	17.0
Wild onion	1 oz.	125	18.0
(Flavor Tree) nuts	1 oz.	200	5.0
(Keebler) toast	1 piece (.1 oz.)	16	2.0
(Nabisco):			
Wheat Thins:			
Regular or low salt	1 piece (.1 oz.)	9	1.1
Cheese	1 piece (.1 oz.)	8	1.0
Nutty	1 piece (.1 oz.)	11	1.1
Wheatsworth	1 piece	14	1.9
(Pepperidge Farm):			
Cracked	1 piece	28	3.5
Hearty	1 piece	25	3.8
Toasted, with onion	1 piece	20	3.0
(Ralston) snack	1 piece (.1 oz.)	9	1.2
(Sunshine):			
American Heritage	1 piece	15	2.0
Wafer	1 piece	10	1.2
CRACKER CRUMBS, graham:			
(Nabisco)	⅛ of 9″ pie shell		
	(2 T.)	60	11.0
(Sunshine)	½ cup	275	47.5
CRACKER MEAL (Nabisco)	2 T.	50	12.0

Food and Description	Measure or Quantity	Calories	Carbo-hydrates (grams)
CRANAPPLE JUICE (Ocean Spray) canned:			
Regular	6 fl. oz.	129	32.1
Dietetic	6 fl. oz.	32	7.4
CRANBERRY, fresh (Ocean Spray)	½ cup (2 oz.)	26	6.1
CRANBERRY-APPLE JUICE COCKTAIL, frozen (Welch's)	6 fl. oz.	120	30.0
CRANBERRY JUICE COCKTAIL: Canned (Ocean Spray):			
Regular	6 fl. oz. (6.5 oz.)	106	26.4
Dietetic	6 fl. oz. (6.3 oz.)	36	8.3
*Frozen (Sunkist)	6 fl. oz.	110	28.2
CRANBERRY-ORANGE RELISH (Ocean Spray)	2 oz.	104	25.8
CRANBERRY-RASPBERRY SAUCE (Ocean Spray) jellied	2 oz.	89	20.8
CRANBERRY SAUCE: Home recipe (USDA) sweetened, unstrained	4 oz.	202	51.6
Canned (Ocean Spray):			
Jellied	2 oz.	88	21.7
Whole berry	2 oz.	89	22.0
CRANGRAPE (Ocean Spray)	6 fl. oz.	108	26.2
CRANICOT (Ocean Spray)	6 fl. oz.	120	30.0
CRANRASPBERRY (Ocean Spray)	6 fl. oz.	110	27.0
CRANTASTIC JUICE DRINK, canned (Ocean Spray)	6 fl. oz.	110	27.0

(USDA): United States Department of Agriculture
(HEW/FAO): Health, Education and Welfare/Food and Agriculture Organization
* Prepared as Package Directs

Food and Description	Measure or Quantity	Calories	Carbo-hydrates (grams)
CRAZY COW, cereal (General Mills)	1 cup (1 oz.)	110	25.0
CREAM:			
Half & Half (Dairylea)	1 fl. oz.	40	1.0
Light, table or coffee (Sealtest) 16% fat	1 T.	26	.6
Light, whipping, 30% fat (Sealtest)	1 T. (.5 oz.)	45	1.0
Heavy whipping (Dairylea)	1 fl. oz.	60	1.0
Sour (Dairylea)	1 fl. oz.	60	1.0
Sour, imitation (Pet)	1 T. (.5 oz.)	25	1.0
Substitute (See **CREAM SUBSTITUTE**)			
CREAM PUFF, home recipe (USDA) custard filling	3½″ × 2″ piece	303	26.7
CREAMSICLE (Popsicle Industries)	2½-fl.-oz. piece	80	13.0
CREAM SUBSTITUTE:			
Coffee Mate (Carnation)	1 tsp.	11	1.1
Coffee Rich (Rich's)	½ oz.	22	2.2
Cremora (Borden)	1 tsp.	12	1.0
Dairy Light (Alba)	2.8-oz. envelope	10	1.0
Mocha Mix (Presto Food Products)	1 T. (.5 oz.)	19	1.2
N-Rich	1 tsp.	10	2.0
(Pet)	1 tsp.	10	1.0
CREAM OF RICE, cereal	1 oz.	100	23.0
CREAM OF WHEAT, cereal (Nabisco):			
Regular	1 T.	40	8.8
Instant	1 T.	40	8.8
Mix'n Eat:			
Regular	1-oz. packet	100	21.0
Baked apple & cinnamon	1.25-oz. packet	130	30.0
Brown sugar	1.25-oz. packet	130	30.0
Maple & brown sugar	1.25-oz. packet	130	30.0
Strawberry	1.25-oz. packet	140	29.0
Quick	1 T.	40	8.8

Food and Description	Measure or Quantity	Calories	Carbo-hydrates (grams)
CREME DE BANANA			
LIQUEUR (Mr. Boston):			
Regular, 27% alcohol	1 fl. oz.	93	12.1
Connoisseur, 21% alcohol	1 fl. oz.	82	11.4
CREME DE CACAO:			
(Hiram Walker) (54 proof)	1 fl. oz.	104	15.0
(Mr. Boston) 27% alcohol:			
Brown	1 fl. oz.	102	14.3
White	1 fl. oz.	93	12.0
CREME DE CASSIS			
(Mr. Boston) 17½% alcohol	1 fl. oz.	85	14.1
CREME DE MENTHE:			
(De Kuyper)	1 fl. oz.	94	11.3
(Mr. Boston) 27% alcohol:			
Green	1 fl. oz.	109	16.0
White	1 fl. oz.	97	13.0
CREME DE NOYAUX			
(Mr. Boston) 27% alcohol	1 fl. oz.	99	13.5
CREPE, frozen:			
(Mrs. Paul's):			
Crab	5½-oz. pkg.	248	24.6
Shrimp	5½-oz. pkg.	252	23.8
(Stouffer's):			
Chicken with mushroom			
sauce	8¼-oz. pkg.	390	19.0
Ham & asparagus	6¼-oz. pkg.	325	21.0
Ham & swiss cheese with			
cheddar cheese sauce	7½-oz. pkg.	410	23.0
Spinach with cheddar cheese			
sauce	9½-oz. pkg.	415	30.0
CRISP, cereal (General Mills):			
Bran muffin	⅔ cup (1.4 oz.)	130	30.0
Honey Buc*Wheat	¾ cup (1 oz.)	110	24.0
Oatmeal raisin	½ cup (1 oz.)	110	21.0

(USDA): United States Department of Agriculture
(HEW/FAO):   Health, Education and Welfare/Food and Agriculture
                         Organization
* Prepared as Package Directs

Food and Description	Measure or Quantity	Calories	Carbo- hydrates (grams)
CRISPIX, cereal (Kellogg's)	¾ cup (1 oz.)	110	25.0
CRISP RICE CEREAL:			
(Featherweight) low sodium	1 cup (1 oz.)	110	26.0
(Ralston Purina)	1 cup (1 oz.)	110	25.0
CRISPY WHEATS 'N RAISINS, cereal (General Mills)	¾ cup (1 oz.)	110	23.0
CROAKER (USDA):			
Atlantic:			
Raw, whole	1 lb. (weighed whole)	148	0.
Raw, meat only	4 oz.	109	0.
Baked	4 oz.	151	0.
White, raw meat only	4 oz.	95	0.
Yellowfin, raw, meat only	4 oz.	101	0.
CROUTON:			
(Arnold):			
Bavarian or English style	½ oz.	65	9.5
French, Italian or Mexican style	½ oz.	66	8.7
(Kellogg's) *Croutettes*	⅔ cup (.7 oz.)	70	14.0
(Mrs. Cubbison's):			
Cheese & garlic or seasoned	½ oz.	60	9.0
Onion & garlic	½ oz.	70	10.0
(Pepperidge Farm)	½ oz	70	9.0
C-3PO'S, cereal (Kellogg's)	¾ cup (1 oz.)	110	24.0
CUCUMBER (USDA):			
Eaten with skin	8-oz. cucumber (weighed whole)	32	7.4
Pared	7½″ × 2″ pared (7.3 oz.)	29	6.6
Pared	3 slices (.9 oz.)	4	.5
CUMIN SEED (French's)	1 tsp.	7	.7
CUPCAKE:			
Home recipe (USDA):			
Without icing	1.4-oz. cupcake	146	22.4
With chocolate icing	1.8-oz. cupcake	184	29.7

Food and Description	Measure or Quantity	Calories	Carbo-hydrates (grams)
With boiled white icing	1.8-oz. cupcake	176	30.9
With uncooked white icing	1.8-oz. cupcake	184	31.6
Regular:			
(Dolly Madison) Chocolate	1.6-oz. piece	170	29.0
(Hostess):			
Chocolate	1¾-oz. piece	166	29.8
Orange	1½-oz. piece	151	26.8
Frozen (Sara Lee) yellow	1 cupcake (1¾ oz.)	190	31.5
*CUPCAKE MIX (Flako)	1 cupcake	150	25.0
CUP O'NOODLES			
(Nissin Foods):			
Beef	2½-oz. serving	343	39.2
Beef, twin pack	1.2-oz. serving	151	18.2
Beef onion	2½-oz. serving	323	36.8
Beef onion, twin pack	1.2-oz. serving	158	19.4
Chicken	2½-oz. serving	343	40.0
Chicken, twin pack	1.2-oz. serving	155	18.6
Pork	2½-oz. serving	331	40.7
Shrimp	2½-oz. serving	336	40.0
CURACAO LIQUEUR:			
(Bols)	1 fl. oz.	105	10.3
(Hiram Walker)	1 fl. oz.	96	11.8
CURRANT:			
Fresh (USDA):			
Black European:			
Whole	1 lb. (weighed with stems)	240	58.2
Stems removed	4 oz.	61	14.9
Red and white:			
Whole	1 lb. (weighed with stems)	220	53.2
Stems removed	1 cup (3.9 oz.)	55	13.3
Dried:			
(Del Monte) Zante	½ cup (2.4 oz.)	200	53.0
(Sun-Maid)	½ cup	220	53.0

(USDA): United States Department of Agriculture
(HEW/FAO): Health, Education and Welfare/Food and Agriculture Organization
* Prepared as Package Directs

Food and Description	Measure or Quantity	Calories	Carbo-hydrates (grams)
CUSTARD:			
Home recipe (USDA)	½ cup (4.7 oz.)	152	14.7
Canned (Thank You Brand) egg	½ cup (4.6 oz.)	135	18.2
Chilled, *Swiss Miss*, chocolate			
or egg flavor	4-oz. container	150	22.0
*Mix, dietetic (Featherweight)	½ cup	80	15.0
*Mix, sweetened			
Jell-O Americana	½ cup	164	23.2
(Royal) regular	½ cup	150	22.0
C.W. POST, cereal:			
Plain	¼ cup (1 oz.)	131	20.3
With raisins	¼ cup	128	20.4

Food and Description	Measure or Quantity	Calories	Carbo-hydrates (grams)
DAIQUIRI MIX:			
(Bar-Tender's)	3½ fl. oz.	177	18.0
(Mr. Boston):			
Regular, 12% alcohol	3 fl. oz.	99	9.0
Strawberry, 12½% alcohol	3 fl. oz.	111	12.0
DAIRY CRISP, cereal (Pet) high calcium	¼ cup	120	19.0
DAIRY QUEEN/BRAZIER:			
Banana split	13.5-oz. serving	540	103.0
Brownie Delight, hot fudge	9.4-oz. serving	600	85.0
Buster Bar	5¼-oz. piece	460	41.0
Chicken sandwich	7.8-oz. sandwich	670	46.0
Cone:			
Plain, any flavor:			
Small	3-oz. cone	140	22.0
Regular	5-oz. cone	240	38.0
Large	7½-oz. cone	340	57.0
Dipped, chocolate:			
Small	3¼-oz. cone	190	25.0
Regular	5½-oz. cone	340	42.0
Large	8¼-oz. cone	510	64.0
Dilly Bar	3-oz. piece	210	21.0
Double Delight	9-oz. serving	490	69.0
DQ Sandwich	2.1-oz. sandwich	140	24.0
Fish sandwich:			
Plain	6-oz. sandwich	400	41.0
With cheese	6¼-oz. sandwich	440	39.0
Float	14-oz. serving	410	82.0
Freeze, vanilla	12-oz. serving	500	89.0

(USDA): United States Department of Agriculture
(HEW/FAO): Health, Education and Welfare/Food and Agriculture
Organization
* Prepared as Package Directs

Food and Description	Measure or Quantity	Calories	Carbo-hydrates (grams)
French fries:			
Regular	2½-oz. serving	200	25.0
Large	4-oz. serving	320	40.0
Hamburger:			
Plain:			
Single	5.2-oz. burger	360	33.0
Double	7.4-oz. burger	530	33.0
Triple	9.6-oz. burger	710	33.0
With cheese:			
Single	5.7-oz. burger	410	33.0
Double	8.4-oz. burger	650	34.0
Triple	10.63-oz. burger	820	34.0
Hot dog:			
Regular:			
Plain	3.5-oz. serving	280	21.0
With cheese	4-oz. serving	330	21.0
With chili	4½-oz. serving	320	23.0
Super:			
Plain	6.2-oz. serving	520	44.0
With cheese	6.9-oz. serving	580	45.0
With chili	7.7-oz. serving	570	47.0
Malt, chocolate:			
Small	10¼-oz. serving	520	91.0
Regular	14¾-oz. serving	760	134.0
Large	20¾-oz. serving	1060	187.0
Mr. Misty:			
Plain:			
Small	8¼-oz. serving	190	48.0
Regular	11.64-oz. serving	250	63.0
Large	15½-oz. serving	340	84.0
Kiss	3.14-oz. serving	70	17.0
Float	14.5-oz. serving	390	74.0
Freeze	14.5-oz. serving	500	94.0
Onion rings	3-oz. serving	280	31.0
Parfait	10-oz. serving	430	76.0
Peanut Butter Parfait	10¾-oz. serving	750	94.0
Shake, chocolate:			
Small	10¼-oz. serving	490	82.0
Regular	14¾-oz. serving	710	120.0
Large	20¾-oz. serving	990	168.0
Strawberry shortcake	11-oz. serving	540	100.0
Sundae, chocolate:			
Small	3¾-oz. serving	190	33.0
Regular	6¼-oz. serving	310	56.0
Large	8¾-oz. serving	440	78.0

Food and Description	Measure or Quantity	Calories	Carbo-hydrates (grams)
Tomato	½ oz.	4	1.0
DAMSON PLUM (See **PLUM**)			
DANDELION GREENS, raw (USDA):			
Trimmed	1 lb.	204	41.7
Boiled, drained	½ cup (3.2 oz.)	30	5.8
DANISH (See **ROLL OR BUN**)			
DATE, dry:			
Domestic:			
(USDA):			
With Pits	1 lb. (weighed with pits)	1081	287.7
Without pits	4 oz.	311	82.7
Without pits chopped	1 cup (6.1 oz.)	477	126.8
(Dromedary):			
Without pits	1 date	20	4.6
Without pits, chopped	¼ cup (1¼ oz.)	130	31.0
Imported (Bordo) Iraq:			
With pits	4 average dates (.9 oz.)	73	18.2
Without pits, chopped	½ cup (2 oz.)	159	39.8
DE CHAUNAC WINE (Great Western) 12% alcohol	3 fl. oz.	71	2.4
DELI'S, frozen			
(Pepperidge Farm):			
Beef with barbecue sauce	4-oz. piece	270	30.0
Mexican style	4-oz. piece	280	27.0
Pizza style	4-oz. piece	290	29.0
Reuben in rye pastry	4-oz. piece	360	25.0
Savory chicken salad	4-oz. piece	340	26.0
Scrambled eggs, bacon & cheese	3½-oz. piece	290	25.0
Sliced beef with brown sauce	4-oz. piece	270	27.0

(USDA): United States Department of Agriculture
(HEW/FAO): Health, Education and Welfare/Food and Agriculture Organization
* Prepared as Package Directs

Food and Description	Measure or Quantity	Calories	Carbo-hydrates (grams)
Turkey, ham & cheese	4-oz. piece	270	24.0
Western style omelet	4-oz. piece	290	27.0
DESSERT (See individual listings such as **APPLE BROWN BETTY, CAKE, FROZEN DESSERT, ICE CREAM, PRUNE WHIP, PUDDING, etc.)**			
DESSERT CUPS (Hostess)	¾-oz. piece	62	13.8
DILL SEED (French's)	1 tsp. (2.1 grams)	9	1.2
DING DONG (Hostess)	1 cake (1⅓ oz.)	172	21.5
DINNER, FROZEN (See individual listings such as **BEAN & FRANKFURTER, BEEF, CHICKEN, FISH, ITALIAN, MEATBALL, etc.)**			
DIP:			
Acapulco (Ortega):			
Plain	1 oz.	8	1.8
American cheese	1 oz.	60	1.1
Cheddar cheese	1 oz.	64	1.2
Monterey Jack cheese	1 oz.	59	1.4
Avocado (Nalley's)	1 oz.	114	.9
Barbecue (Nalley's)	1 oz.	114	1.1
Blue cheese:			
(Dean) tang	1 oz.	61	2.3
(Nalley's)	1 oz.	110	.9
Chili (La Victoria)	1 T.	6	1.0
Clam (Nalley's)	1 oz.	101	1.1
Enchilada, *Fritos*	1 oz.	37	3.9
Guacamole (Calavo)	1 oz.	55	3.5
Jalapeno:			
Fritos	1 oz.	34	3.7
(Hain) natural	1 oz.	40	2.5
(Wise)	1 T.	12	2.5
Onion (Thank You Brand)	1 T. (.8 oz.)	45	2.5
Onion bean (Hain) natural	1 oz.	41	3.6
Picante sauce (Wise)	1 T.	6	1.5
Taco (Thank You Brand)	1 T. (.8 oz.)	44	2.0

Food and Description	Measure or Quantity	Calories	Carbo-hydrates (grams)
DIP 'UM SAUCE, canned (French's):			
BBQ	1 T.	22	5.0
Creamy mustard	1 T.	40	6.0
Hot mustard	1 T.	35	7.0
Sweet 'n Sour	1 T.	40	10.0
DISTILLED LIQUOR. The values below would apply to unflavored bourbon whiskey, brandy, Canadian whiskey, gin, Irish whiskey, rum, rye whiskey, Scotch whisky, tequila and vodka. The caloric content of distilled liquors depends on the percentage of alcohol. The proof is twice the alcohol percent and the following values apply to all brands (USDA):			
80 proof	1 fl. oz.	65	Tr.
86 proof	1 fl. oz.	70	Tr.
90 proof	1 fl. oz.	74	Tr.
94 proof	1 fl. oz.	77	Tr.
100 proof	1 fl. oz.	83	Tr.
DONUTZ, cereal (General Mills):			
Chocolate flavor	1 cup (1 oz.)	120	23.0
Powdered sugar	1 cup (1 oz.)	120	22.0
DOUGHNUT (See also **WINCHELL'S**): (USDA):			
Cake type	1.1-oz. piece	125	16.4
Yeast leavened	2-oz. piece	235	21.4
(Dolly Madison): Regular:			
Plain	1¼-oz. piece	140	17.0

(USDA): United States Department of Agriculture
(HEW/FAO):   Health, Education and Welfare/Food and Agriculture
                      Organization
* Prepared as Package Directs

Food and Description	Measure or Quantity	Calories	Carbo-hydrates (grams)
Chocolate coated	1¼-oz. piece	150	18.0
Coconut crunch	1¼-oz. piece	140	20.0
Powdered sugar	1¼-oz. piece	140	19.0
Dunkin' Stix	1⅜-oz. piece	210	18.0
Gems:			
Chocolate coated	.5-oz. piece	65	7.0
Cinnamon sugar	.5-oz. piece	55	7.5
Coconut crunch	.5-oz. piece	60	8.0
Powdered sugar	.5-oz. piece	60	7.5
Jumbo:			
Plain	1.6-oz. piece	190	23.0
Cinnamon sugar	1.6-oz. piece	190	24.0
Sugar	1.7-oz. piece	210	27.0
Old fashioned:			
Cinnamon chip	2.2-oz. piece	280	32.0
Chocolate glazed	2.2-oz. piece	260	36.0
Chocolate iced	2.2-oz. piece	300	33.0
Glazed or orange crush	2.2-oz. piece	280	33.0
Powdered sugar	1.8-oz. piece	260	24.0
White iced	2.2-oz. piece	300	35.0
Frozen (Morton):			
Regular:			
Bavarian creme	2-oz. piece	180	22.0
Boston creme	2⅓-oz. piece	210	28.0
Chocolate iced	1.5-oz. piece	150	20.0
Glazed	1.5-oz. piece	150	19.0
Jelly	1.8-oz. piece	180	23.0
Mini	1.1-oz. piece	120	16.0
Donut Holes	⅕ of 7¾-oz. pkg.	160	21.0
Morning Light:			
Chocolate	2-oz. piece	200	26.0
Glazed	2-oz. piece	200	26.0
Jelly	2.6-oz. piece	250	33.0
DRAMBUIE (Hiram Walker) (80 proof)	1 fl. oz.	110	11.0
DRUMSTICK, frozen:			
Ice Cream, in a cone:			
Topped with peanuts	1 piece	181	22.7
Topped with peanuts & cone bisque	1 piece	168	23.6
Ice Milk, in a cone:			
Topped with peanuts	1 piece	163	24.3

Food and Description	Measure or Quantity	Calories	Carbo-hydrates (grams)
Topped with peanuts & cone bisque	1 piece	150	25.2
DUCK, raw (USDA):			
Domesticated:			
Ready-to-cook	1 lb. (weighed with bone)	1213	0.
Meat only	4 oz.	187	0.
Wild:			
Dressed	1 lb. (weighed dressed)	613	0.
Meat only	4 oz.	156	0.
DULCITO, frozen (Hormel):			
Apple	4-oz. serving	290	44.0
Cherry	4-oz. serving	300	48.0
DUMPLINGS, stuffed, canned, dietetic:			
(Estee Dia-Mel)	8 oz. serving	160	15.0
(Featherweight)	7½-oz. serving	160	18.0

Food and Description	Measure or Quantity	Calories	Carbo-hydrates (grams)

E

ECLAIR:
Home recipe (USDA), with custard filling and chocolate icing

Home recipe (USDA), with custard filling and chocolate icing	4-oz. piece	271	26.3
Frozen (Rich's) chocolate	1 piece (2 oz.)	196	25.5
EEL (USDA):			
Raw, meat only	4 oz.	264	0.
Smoked, meat only	4 oz.	374	0.
EGG (USDA) (See also **EGG SUBSTITUTE**):			
Chicken:			
Raw:			
White only	1 large egg (1.2 oz.)	17	.3
White only	1 cup (9 oz.)	130	2.0
Yolk only	1 large egg (.6 oz.)	59	.1
Yolk only	1 cup (8.5 oz.)	835	1.4
Whole, small	1 egg (1.3 oz.)	60	.3
Whole, medium	1 egg (1.5 oz.)	71	.4
Whole, large	1 egg (1.8 oz.)	81	.4
Whole	1 cup (8.8 oz.)	409	2.3
Whole, extra large	1 egg (2. oz.)	94	.5
Whole, jumbo	1 egg (2.3 oz.)	105	.6
Cooked:			
Boiled	1 large egg (1.8 oz.)	81	.4
Fried in butter	1 large egg	99	.1
Omelet, mixed with milk and cooked in fat	1 large egg	107	1.5
Poached	1 large egg	78	.4
Scrambled, mixed with milk & cooked in fat	1 large egg	111	1.5

Food and Description	Measure or Quantity	Calories	Carbohydrates (grams)
Scrambled, mixed with milk & cooked in fat	1 cup (7.8 oz.)	381	5.3
Dried:			
Whole	1 cup (3.8 oz.)	639	4.4
White, powder	1 oz.	105	1.6
Yolk	1 cup (3.4 oz.)	637	2.4
Duck, raw	1 egg (2.8 oz.)	153	.6
Goose, raw	1 egg (5.8 oz.)	303	2.1
Turkey, raw	1 egg (3.1 oz.)	150	1.5
EGG DINNER OR ENTREE, frozen (Swanson):			
Omelet:			
With cheese & ham	7-oz. meal	400	12.0
Spanish style	7¾-oz. meal	250	14.0
Scrambled & sausage	6¼-oz. meal	410	17.0
***EGG FOO YOUNG,** dinner, canned:			
(Chun King) stir fry	5-oz. serving	138	9.1
(La Choy)	1 patty + ¼ cup sauce	164	19.2
EGG MIX (Durkee):			
Omelet:			
*With bacon	½ of pkg.	310	10.0
*Puffy	½ of pkg.	302	10.5
Scrambled:			
Plain	.8-oz. pkg.	124	4.0
With bacon	1.3-oz. pkg.	181	6.0
EGG NOG, dairy:			
(Borden)	½ cup	160	16,0
(Johanna)	½ cup	195	22.4
(Meadow Gold) 6% fat	½ cup	164	25.5
EGG NOG COCKTAIL			
(Mr. Boston) 15% alcohol	3 fl. oz.	177	18.9
EGGPLANT:			
Raw (USDA) whole	1 lb. (weighed whole)	92	20.6

(USDA): United States Department of Agriculture
(HEW/FAO):   Health, Education and Welfare/Food and Agriculture Organization
* Prepared as Package Directs

Food and Description	Measure or Quantity	Calories	Carbo-hydrates (grams)
Boiled (USDA) drained, diced	1 cup (7.1 oz.)	38	8.2
Frozen:			
(Buitoni) parmigiana	5-oz. serving	168	17.6
(Celentano):			
Parmigiana	½ of 16-oz. pkg.	330	22.0
Rollettes	11-oz. pkg.	420	18.0
(Mrs. Paul's):			
Parmesan	5½-oz. serving	270	20.0
Sticks, breaded & fried	3½-oz. serving	240	29.0
(Weight Watchers)			
parmigiana	13-oz. pkg.	285	25.0
EGG ROLL, frozen:			
(Chun King):			
Regular:			
Chicken	3½ oz. piece	210	31.0
Meat & shrimp	3½-oz. piece	214	30.0
Shrimp	3½-oz. piece	189	30.0
Restaurant style, pork	3-oz. piece	172	23.0
(La Choy):			
Chicken	.5-oz. piece	30	4.0
Lobster	.5-oz. piece	27	4.3
Lobster	3-oz. piece	180	25.0
Meat & shrimp	.5-oz. piece	27	4.0
Shrimp	3-oz. piece	160	24.0
EGG ROLL DINNER OR ENTREE, frozen:			
(La Choy) entree:			
Almond chicken	2 pieces	450	43.0
Beef & broccoli	2 pieces	380	45.0
Spicy oriental chicken	2 pieces	300	32.0
Sweet & sour pork	2 pieces	430	56.0
(Van de Kamp's) Cantonese	10½-oz. serving	560	80.0
EGG SUBSTITUTE:			
Egg Magic (Featherweight)	½ of envelope	60	1.0
Egg Beaters (Fleischmann's):			
Regular	¼ cup	25	1.0
With cheese	½ cup	130	3.0
Scramblers (Morningstar Farms)	1 egg substitute	35	1.5
Second Nature (Avoset)	3 T.	42	2.0

Food and Description	Measure or Quantity	Calories	Carbohydrates (grams)
ELDERBERRY, fresh (USDA):			
Whole	1 lb. (weighed with stems)	307	69.9
Stems removed	4 oz.	82	18.6
EL POLLO LOCO **RESTAURANT:**			
Beans	3½-oz. serving	110	17.0
Chicken	2 pieces (4.8 oz. edible portion)	310	2.0
Cole slaw	2.8-oz. serving	80	5.0
Combo	16-oz. meal	720	70.0
Corn	3.3-oz. piece	110	20.0
Dole Whip	4½-oz. serving	90	19.0
Potato salad	4.3-oz. serving	140	15.0
Rice	2½-oz. serving	100	22.0
Salsa	1.8-oz. serving	10	1.0
Tortilla:			
Corn	3.3-oz. serving	210	42.0
Flour	3.3-oz. serving	280	45.0
ENCHANADA, frozen (Stouffer's) *Lean Cuisine:*			
Bean & beef	9¼-oz. meal	280	32.0
Chicken	9⅞-oz. meal	270	31.0
ENCHILADA OR ENCHILADA DINNER:			
Canned (Old El Paso) beef	1 enchilada	85	9.0
Frozen:			
Beef:			
(Banquet):			
Dinner, International Favorites	12-oz. dinner	497	72.0
Family Entree	2-lb. pkg.	1056	148.0
(Fred's Frozen Foods) *Marquez*	7½-oz. serving	304	23.5
(Hormel)	1 enchilada	140	17.0
(Morton)	11-oz. dinner	280	44.0
(Patio)	13¼-oz. dinner	514	59.0
(Swanson) *TV Brand*	15-oz. dinner	570	72.0

(USDA): United States Department of Agriculture
(HEW/FAO): Health, Education and Welfare/Food and Agriculture Organization
* Prepared as Package Directs

Food and Description	Measure or Quantity	Calories	Carbo-hydrates (grams)
(Van de Kamp's):			
Dinner:			
Regular	12-oz. meal	390	45.0
Shredded	14¾-oz. meal	490	60.0
Entree:			
Regular	7½-oz. meal	250	20.0
Shredded	5½-oz. serving	180	15.0
Cheese:			
(Banquet):			
Extra Helping	21¼-oz. dinner	777	105.0
International Favorites	12-oz. dinner	543	71.0
(Hormel)	1 enchilada	151	18.0
(Patio)	12¼-oz. dinner	378	60.0
(Van de Kamp's):			
Dinner	12-oz. dinner	390	45.0
Entree	7½-oz. pkg.	250	20.0
Chicken (Van de Kamp's):			
Regular	7½-oz. pkg.	250	25.0
Suiza	5½-oz. serving	220	20.0
ENCHILADA SAUCE:			
Canned:			
(Del Monte) hot or mild	½ cup (4 oz.)	45	11.0
(El Molino) hot	1 T.	8	1.0
(La Victoria)	1 T.	5	1.0
(Old El Paso):			
Green chili	½ cup	36	7.2
Hot	½ cup	54	7.6
Mild	½ cup	50	7.2
(Rosarita)	3 oz.	19	4.0
Mix:			
*(Durkee)	½ cup	29	6.2
(French's)	1⅜-oz. pkg.	120	20.0
ENCHILADA SEASONING			
MIX (Lawry's)	1.6-oz. pkg.	152	29.9
ENDIVE, CURLY raw (USDA):			
Untrimmed	1 lb. (weighed untrimmed)	80	16.4
Trimmed	½ lb.	45	9.3
Cut up or shredded	1 cup (2.5 oz.)	14	2.9
ESCAROLE, raw (USDA):			
Untrimmed	1 lb. (weighed untrimmed)	80	16.4

Food and Description	Measure or Quantity	Calories	Carbo-hydrates (grams)
Trimmed	½ lb.	46	9.2
Cut up or shredded	1 cup (2.5 oz.)	14	2.9
EULACHON or SMELT, raw			
(USDA) meat only	4 oz.	134	0.
EXPRESSO COFFEE			
LIQUEUR (Mr. Boston)			
26½% alcohol	1 fl. oz.	104	15.0

(USDA): United States Department of Agriculture
(HEW/FAO): Health, Education and Welfare/Food and Agriculture
            Organization
* Prepared as Package Directs

Food and Description	Measure or Quantity	Calories	Carbohydrates (grams)

F

FAJITA SEASONING
  MIX (Lawry's) | 1.3-oz. pkg. | 63 | 14.0

FARINA:
  (H-O) dry, regular | 1 T. (.4 oz.) | 40 | 8.5
  Malt-O-Meal, dry:
    Regular | 1 oz. | 96 | 21.0
    Quick cooking | 1 oz. | 100 | 22.2
  *(Pillsbury) made with water
    and salt | ⅔ cup | 80 | 17.0

FAT, COOKING:
  (USDA):
    Lard | 1 T. (.5 oz.) | 115 | 0.
    Vegetable oil | 1 T. (1.4 oz.) | 106 | 0.
  Crisco:
    Regular | 1 T. (.4 oz.) | 110 | 0.
    Butter flavor | 1 T. (.5 oz.) | 126 | 0.
  (Mrs. Tucker's) | 1 T. | 120 | 0.
  (Rokeach) neutral nyafat | 1 T. | 99 | 0.
  Spry | 1 T. (.4 oz.) | 94 | 0.

FENNEL SEED (French's) | 1 tsp. (2.1 grams) | 8 | 1.3

FETTUCINI ALFREDO, frozen
  (Stouffer's) | ½ of 10 oz. pkg. | 270 | 17.0

FETTUCINI PRIMAVERA,
  frozen (Green Giant) | 9½-oz. meal | 230 | 26.0

FIBER ONE, cereal
  (General Mills) | ½ cup (1 oz.) | 60 | 21.0

FIG:
  Fresh (USDA):
    Regular size | 1 lb. | 363 | 92.1
    Small | 1.3-oz. fig (1½" dia.) | 30 | 7.7

Food and Description	Measure or Quantity	Calories	Carbo-hydrates (grams)
Candied (Bama)	1 T. (.7 oz.)	37	9.6
Canned, regular pack, solids & liq.: (USDA):			
Light syrup	4 oz.	74	19.1
Heavy Syrup	3 figs & 2 T. syrup (4 oz.)	96	24.9
Heavy syrup	½ cup (4.4 oz.)	106	27.5
Extra heavy syrup	4 oz.	117	30.3
(Del Monte) whole	½ cup (4.3 oz.)	100	28.0
Canned, unsweetened or dietetic, solids & liq.:			
(USDA) water pack	4 oz.	54	14.1
(Diet Delight) Kadota	½ cup (4.4 oz.)	76	18.2
(Featherweight) Kadota water pack	½ cup	60	15.0
Dried (Sun-Maid):			
Calimyrna	½ cup (3.5 oz.)	250	58.0
Mission, regular or figlets	½ cup (3 oz.)	210	50.0
FIG JUICE (Sunsweet)	6 fl. oz.	120	30.0
FIGURINES (Pillsbury) all flavors	1 bar	138	10.5
FILBERT: (USDA):			
Whole	1 lb. (weighed in shell)	1323	34.9
Shelled	1 oz.	180	4.7
(Fisher) oil dipped, salted	½ cup (2 oz.)	360	5.4
FISH (See individual listings)			
FISH CAKE:			
Home recipe (USDA)	2 oz.	98	5.3
Frozen (Mrs. Paul's):			
Beach Haven	2-oz. piece	110	12.0
Thins, breaded & fried	½ of 10-oz. pkg.	150	12.5

(USDA): United States Department of Agriculture
(HEW/FAO):   Health, Education and Welfare/Food and Agriculture
                        Organization
* Prepared as Package Directs

Food and Description	Measure or Quantity	Calories	Carbo-hydrates (grams)
FISH & CHIPS, frozen:			
(Gorton's)	1 pkg.	1350	132.0
(Swanson):			
Entree	5½-oz. meal	320	32.0
4-compartment dinner	10½-oz. dinner	570	58.0
Hungry Man	14¾-oz. dinner	770	73.0
(Van de Kamp's) batter dipped, french fried	7-oz. pkg.	440	35.0
FISH DINNER OR ENTREE, frozen (See also individual listings such as **Cod Dinner**):			
(Banquet) platters	8¾-oz. dinner	445	33.0
(Morton)	10-oz. dinner	367	45.0
(Mrs. Paul's):			
Regular, parmesan	5-oz. meal	220	16.0
Light:			
Dijon	8½-oz. meal	250	7.0
Florentine	9-oz. meal	200	16.0
Mornay	10-oz. meal	230	11.0
(Stouffer's) *Lean Cuisine, filet:*			
Divan	12⅜-oz. pkg.	260	17.0
Florentine	9-oz. pkg.	230	13.0
(Weight Watchers):			
Au gratin	9¼-oz. meal	200	14.0
Oven fried	6¾-oz. meal	220	8.0
FISH FILLET, frozen:			
(Frionor) *Bunch O' Crunch,* breaded	1½-oz. piece	140	3.8
(Gorton's):			
Regular:			
Batter dipped, crispy	1 piece	250	18.0
Crunchy	1 piece	175	9.5
Potato crisp	1 piece	170	10.0
Light Recipe:			
Lightly breaded	1 piece	170	16.0
Tempura batter	1 piece	190	10.0
(Mrs. Paul's):			
Batter fried, light:			
Crunchy	2¼-oz. piece	155	13.5
Supreme	3⅝-oz. piece	220	19.0
Breaded & fried:			
Crispy, crunchy	2.1-oz. piece	145	11.0

Food and Description	Measure or Quantity	Calories	Carbo-hydrates (grams)
Light & natural	6-oz. serving	290	21.0
Buttered	2½-oz. serving	105	0.
(Van de Kamp's):			
Batter dipped, french fried:			
Regular	3-oz. piece	180	15.0
Country seasoned	2.4-oz. piece	200	10.0
Light & crispy	2-oz. piece	180	10.0
Today's Catch	4-oz. serving	90	0.
FISH KABOBS, frozen:			
(Mrs. Paul's) batter fried,			
supreme light	⅓ of 10-oz. pkg.	200	17.7
(Van de Kamp's) batter dipped,			
french fried	4-oz. piece	240	15.0
FISH LOAF, Home recipe			
(USDA)	4 oz.	141	8.3
FISH NUGGET, frozen			
(Frionor) *Bunch O' Crunch,*			
breaded	.5-oz. piece	40	2.2
FISH SANDWICH, frozen			
(Frionor) *Bunch O' Crunch,*			
microwave	5-oz. sandwich	320	31.0
FISH STICKS, frozen:			
(Frionor) *Bunch O' Crunch,*			
breaded	.7-oz. piece	58	3.5
(Gorton's):			
Batter dipped, crispy	1 piece	58	4.5
Breaded	1 piece	52	6.0
Crunchy	1 piece	55	3.7
Potato crisp	1 piece	60	4.2
Value pack	1 piece	52	4.5
(Mrs. Paul's):			
Batter fried, light & crunchy	1 piece (.9 oz.)	60	5.3
Breaded & fried, crispy	1 piece (¾ oz.)	50	4.2

(USDA): United States Department of Agriculture
(HEW/FAO):   Health, Education and Welfare/Food and Agriculture
              Organization
* Prepared as Package Directs

Food and Description	Measure or Quantity	Calories	Carbo-hydrates (grams)
(Van de Kamp's) batter dipped, french fried:			
Regular	1-oz. piece	55	3.7
Light & crispy	¾-oz. piece	67	3.8
FLOUNDER:			
Raw (USDA):			
Whole	1 lb. (weighed whole)	118	0.
Meat only	4 oz.	90	0.
Baked (USDA)	4 oz.	229	0.
Frozen:			
(Frionor) *Norway Gourmet*	4-oz. piece	60	0.
(Gorton's):			
Fishmarket Fresh	4 oz.	90	1.0
Light Recipe:			
Fillet entree	1 piece	260	23.0
Stuffed	1 pkg.	260	11.0
(Le Menu) fillet, with salmon mousse	10½-oz. meal	340	26.0
(Mrs. Paul's):			
Batter fried, crunchy light	2¼-oz. piece	155	13.0
Breaded & fried:			
Crispy crunchy	2-oz. piece	140	12.5
Light & natural	1-oz. piece	320	24.0
(Van de Kamp's) *Today's Catch*	4 oz.	90	0.
FLOUR:			
(USDA):			
Buckwheat, dark, sifted	1 cup (3.5 oz.)	326	70.6
Buckwheat, light sifted	1 cup (3.5 oz.)	340	77.9
Cake:			
Unsifted, dipped	1 cup (4.2 oz.)	433	94.5
Unsifted, spooned	1 cup (3.9 oz.)	404	88.1
Carob or St. John's bread	1 oz.	51	22.9
Chestnut	1 oz.	103	21.6
Corn	1 cup (3.9)	405	84.5
Cottonseed	1 oz.	101	9.4
Fish, from whole fish	1 oz.	95	0.
Lima bean	1 oz.	95	17.9
Potato	1 oz.	100	22.7
Rice, stirred spooned	1 cup (5.6 oz.)	574	125.6

Food and Description	Measure or Quantity	Calories	Carbo-hydrates (grams)
Rye:			
Light:			
Unsifted, spooned	1 cup (3.6 oz.)	361	78.7
Sifted, spooned	1 cup (3.1 oz.)	314	68.6
Medium	1 oz.	99	21.1
Dark:			
Unstirred	1 cup (4.5 oz.)	419	87.2
Stirred	1 cup (4.5 oz.)	415	86.5
Soybean, defatted, stirred	1 cup (3.6 oz.)	329	38.5
Soybean, high fat	1 oz.	108	9.4
Sunflower seed, partially defatted	1 oz.	96	10.7
Wheat:			
All-purpose:			
Unsifted, dipped	1 cup (5 oz.)	521	108.8
Unsifted, spooned	1 cup (4.4 oz.)	459	95.9
Sifted, spooned	1 cup (4.1 oz.)	422	88.3
Bread:			
Unsifted, dipped	1 cup (4.8 oz.)	496	101.6
Unsifted, spooned	1 cup (4.3 oz.)	449	91.9
Sifted, spooned	1 cup (4.1 oz.)	427	87.4
Gluten:			
Unsifted, dipped	1 cup (5 oz.)	537	67.0
Sifted, spooned	1 cup (4.8 oz.)	514	64.2
Self-rising:			
Unsifted, dipped	1 cup (4.6 oz.)	458	96.5
Sifted, spooned	1 cup (3.7 oz.)	373	78.7
Whole wheat	1 oz.	94	20.1
(Aunt Jemima) self-rising	¼ cup (1 oz.)	109	23.6
Ballard:			
Self-rising	¼ cup	91	23.6
All-purpose	¼ cup (1 oz.)	100	21.8
Bisquick (Betty Crocker)	¼ cup (1 oz.)	115	18.5
(Drifted Snow)	¼ cup	100	21.8
(Elam's):			
Brown rice, whole grain, sodium & gluten free	¼ cup (1.2 oz.)	125	.2
Buckwheat, pure	¼ cup (¼ oz.)	131	27.2
Pastry, whole wheat	¼ cup (1.2 oz.)	122	24.9
Rye, whole grain	¼ cup	118	24.2

(USDA): United States Department of Agriculture
(HEW/FAO):   Health, Education and Welfare/Food and Agriculture
                        Organization
* Prepared as Package Directs

Food and Description	Measure or Quantity	Calories	Carbo-hydrates (grams)
Soy, roasted, defatted	¼ cup (1.1 oz.)	108	9.8
3-in-1 mix	1 oz.	99	20.0
White, with wheat germ	¼ cup (1 oz.)	101	20.7
Whole wheat	¼ cup (1.1 oz.)	111	21.7
(Featherweight):			
Gluten	¼ cup	105	13.7
Soy	¼ cup	117	8.4
Gold Medal (Betty Crocker):			
All purpose or unbleached	¼ cup (1 oz.)	100	21.8
Better For Bread	¼ cup	100	20.7
Self-rising	¼ cup	95	20.8
Whole wheat	¼ cup	98	19.5
La Pina	¼ cup	100	21.8
Pillsbury's Best:			
All-purpose or rye and wheat Bohemian style	¼ cup	100	21.5
Bread or rye, medium	1.4 cup	100	20.8
Sauce & gravy	2 T.	50	11.0
Self-rising	¼ cup	95	21.0
Whole wheat	¼ cup	100	21.0
Presto, self-rising	¼ cup (1 oz.)	98	21.6
Red Band:			
All purpose or unbleached	¼ cup	97	21.2
Self-rising	¼ cup	95	20.8
Wondra	¼ cup	100	21.8
FOLLE BLANC WINE (Louis M. Martini) 12.5% alcohol	3 fl. oz.	63	.2
FOOD STICKS (Pillsbury) chocolate	1 piece	45	6.8
FRANKEN*BERRY, cereal (General Mills)	1 cup (1 oz.)	110	24.0
FRANKFURTER, raw or cooked: (USDA): Raw:			
All kinds	1 frankfurter (10 per lb.)	140	.8
Meat	1 frankfurter (10 per lb.)	134	1.1

Food and Description	Measure or Quantity	Calories	Carbo-hydrates (grams)
With cereal	1 frankfurter (10 per lb.)	112	<.1
Cooked, all kinds	1 frankfurter (10 per lb.)	136	.7
(Eckrich):			
Beef	1.2-oz. frankfurter	110	2.0
Beef	1.6-oz. frankfurter	150	3.0
Beef	2-oz. frankfurter	190	3.0
Cheese	2-oz. frankfurter	190	3.0
Meat	1.2-oz. frankfurter	120	2.0
Meat	1.6-oz. frankfurter	150	3.0
Meat	2.-oz. frankfurter	190	3.0
(Empire Kosher):			
Chicken	2-oz. frankfurter	106	1.0
Turkey	2-oz. frankfurter	107	1.0
Hebrew National:			
Beef	1.7-oz. frankfurter	149	<1.0
Collagen	2.3-oz. frankfurter	202	<1.0
Natural casing	2-oz. frankfurter	175	<1.0
(Hormel):			
Beef	1 frankfurter (12-oz. pkg.)	100	1.0
Beef	1 frankfurter (1 lb. pkg.)	140	1.0
Chili, *Frank 'n Stuff*	1 frankfurter	165	2.0
Meat	1 frankfurter (12-oz. pkg.)	110	1.0
Meat	1 frankfurter (1-lb. pkg.)	140	1.0
Range Brand	1 frankfurter	170	1.0
Wrangler, smoked:			
Beef	1 frankfurter	170	2.0
Cheese	1 frankfurter	180	1.0
(Hygrade) beef, *Ball Park*	2-oz. frankfurter	169	Tr.

(USDA): United States Department of Agriculture
(HEW/FAO): Health, Education and Welfare/Food and Agriculture Organization
* Prepared as Package Directs

Food and Description	Measure or Quantity	Calories	Carbo-hydrates (grams)
(Louis Rich):			
Turkey	1.5-oz. frankfurter	95	1.0
Turkey	1.6-oz. frankfurter	100	1.0
Turkey	2.-oz. frankfurter	125	1.0
(Ohse):			
Beef	1-oz. frankfurter	85	1.0
Wiener:			
Regular	1-oz. frankfurter	90	1.0
Chicken, beef & pork	1-oz. frankfurter	85	1.0
(Oscar Mayer):			
Bacon & cheddar	1.6-oz. frankfurter	139	1.0
Beef:			
Regular	1.6-oz. frankfurter	143	1.1
Jumbo	2-oz. frankfurter	179	1.4
Big One	4-oz. frankfurter	357	2.7
Cheese	1.6-oz. frankfurter	144	1.0
Little Wiener	2″ frankfurter	28	.2
Wiener	1.6-oz. frankfurter	144	1.1
Wiener	2-oz. frankfurter	180	1.4
(Swift)	1.6-oz. frankfurter	150	1.2
FRANKS-N-BLANKETS, frozen (Durkee)	1 piece	45	1.0
FRENCH TOAST, frozen:			
(Aunt Jemima):			
Regular	1 slice (1½ oz.)	85	13.2
Cinnamon swirl	1 slice (1½ oz.)	97	13.6
(Swanson) with sausage:			
Plain	6½-oz. meal	450	36.0
Cinnamon swirl	6½-oz. meal	480	39.0
FRITTERS:			
Home recipe (USDA):			
Clam	2″ × 1¾″ (1.4 oz.)	124	12.4

Food and Description	Measure or Quantity	Calories	Carbo-hydrates (grams)
Corn	2″ × 1½″ (1.2 oz.)	132	13.9
Frozen (Mrs. Paul's):			
Apple	2-oz. piece	140	16.5
Corn	2-oz. piece	125	15.0
FROG LEGS, raw (USDA):			
Bone-in	1 lb. (weighed with bone)	215	0.
Meat only	4 oz.	83	0.
FROOT LOOPS, cereal (Kellogg's)	1 cup (1 oz.)	110	25.0
FROSTED RICE, cereal (Ralston Purina)	1 cup (1 oz.)	110	26.0
FROSTING (See **CAKE ICING**)			
FROSTS (Libby's):			
Dry:			
Banana	.5 oz.	50	14.0
Orange, strawberry or pineapple	.5 oz.	60	16.0
Liquid:			
Banana	7 fl. oz.	120	25.0
Orange	8 fl. oz.	120	29.0
Pineapple	6 fl. oz.	110	22.0
Strawberry	8 fl. oz.	120	21.0
FROZEN DESSERT, dietetic (see also **TOFUTTI**):			
(Baskin-Robbins) chunky banana	½ cup	100	20.0
(Eskimo) bar, chocolate covered	2½-fl.-oz. bar	110	10.0

(USDA): United States Department of Agriculture
(HEW/FAO):   Health, Education and Welfare/Food and Agriculture
Organization
* Prepared as Package Directs

Food and Description	Measure or Quantity	Calories	Carbo-hydrates (grams)
Mocha Mix (Presto):			
Bar, vanilla, chocolate covered	4 oz.	230	20.0
Bulk:			
Dutch chocolate	½ cup	140	16.0
Heavenly hash	½ cup	160	18.0
Mocha almond fudge	½ cup	150	19.0
Neapolitan or vanilla	½ cup	140	17.0
Peach	½ cup	130	19.0
Strawberry swirl or very berry	½ cup	140	20.0
Toasted almond	½ cup	150	17.0
(SugarLo) ice cream or ice milk, all flavors	¼ pt. (2.6 fl. oz.)	135	14.0

FROZEN DINNER OR ENTREE (See individual listings such as **BEAN & FRANKFURTER, BEEF, CHICKEN, FISH, GERMAN STYLE, MACARONI & CHEESE, MEATBALL,** etc.)

FRUIT BARS (General Mills)
Fruit Corners:
Regular:

Cherry, grape or strawberry	1 bar	90	18.0
Orange pineapple or tropical	1 bar	90	17.0
Swirled	1 bar	90	18.0

FRUIT BITS, dried (Sun-Maid)

	1 oz.	90	21.0

FRUIT 'N APPLE JUICE (Tree Top):

Canned	6 fl. oz.	90	22.0
*Frozen	6 fl. oz.	90	23.0

FRUIT 'N CHERRY JUICE (Tree Top):

Canned	6 fl. oz.	80	21.0
*Frozen	6 fl. oz.	90	22.0

Food and Description	Measure or Quantity	Calories	Carbo-hydrates (grams)
FRUIT 'N CITRUS JUICE			
(Tree Top):			
Canned	6 fl. oz.	100	24.0
*Frozen	6 fl. oz.	90	22.0
FRUIT COCKTAIL:			
Canned, regular pack,			
solids & liq.:			
(USDA):			
Light syrup	4 oz.	68	17.8
Heavy syrup	½ cup (4.5 oz.)	97	25.2
Extra syrup	4 oz.	104	26.9
(Del Monte) regular or			
chunky	½ cup (4½ oz.)	80	23.0
(Libby's) heavy syrup	½ cup (4½ oz.)	101	24.7
(Stokely-Van Camp)	½ cup (4½ oz.)	95	23.0
Canned, dietetic or low calorie,			
solids & liq.:			
(Del Monte) Lite, syrup			
pack, regular or chunky	½ cup (4¼ oz.)	50	14.0
(Diet Delight):			
Juice pack	½ cup (4.4 oz.)	50	14.0
Water pack	½ cup (4.3 oz.)	40	10.0
(Featherweight):			
Juice pack	½ cup (4 oz.)	50	12.0
Water pack	½ cup (4 oz.)	40	10.0
(Libby's) Lite, water pack	½ cup (4.4 oz.)	50	13.0
(S&W) *Nutradiet,* white or			
blue label	½ cup	40	10.0
FRUIT COMPOTE, canned			
(Rokeach)	½ cup (4 oz.)	120	31.0
FRUIT COUNTRY			
(Comstock):			
Apple	¼ of pkg.	160	36.0
Blueberry	¼ of pkg.	160	33.0

(USDA): United States Department of Agriculture
(HEW/FAO): Health, Education and Welfare/Food and Agriculture
Organization
* Prepared as Package Directs

Food and Description	Measure or Quantity	Calories	Carbo-hydrates (grams)
Cherry	¼ of pkg.	180	38.0
Peach	¼ of pkg.	130	28.0
FRUIT CUP (Del Monte) solids & liq.:			
Mixed fruits	5-oz. container	110	26.7
Peach cling, diced	5-oz. container	116	27.8
FRUIT & FIBER CEREAL (Post)	½ cup (1 oz.)	103	22.3
FRUIT 'N GRAPE JUICE (Tree Top):			
Canned	6 fl. oz.	100	25.0
*Frozen	6 fl. oz.	110	27.0
FRUIT JUICE, canned (See also individual listings such as **CRANAPPLE JUICE, ORANGE-GRAPEFRUIT JUICE, PINEAPPLE JUICE,** etc.) (Sun-Maid):			
Golden	6 fl. oz.	100	23.0
Purple	6 fl. oz.	100	25.0
Red	6 fl. oz.	100	24.0
FRUIT 'N JUICE BAR (Dole):			
Pineapple	1 bar	70	17.0
Strawberry	1 bar	70	16.0
FRUIT & JUICE DRINK (Tree Top):			
Canned:			
Apple	6 fl. oz.	90	22.0
Berry	6 fl. oz.	80	21.0
Cherry	6 fl. oz.	100	24.0
Citrus	6 fl. oz.	90	22.0
Grape	6 fl. oz.	100	25.0
*Frozen:			
Apple	6 fl. oz.	90	23.0
Berry, cherry or citrus	6 fl. oz.	90	22.0
Grape	6 fl. oz.	110	27.0

Food and Description	Measure or Quantity	Calories	Carbo-hydrates (grams)
FRUIT, MIXED:			
Canned, solids & liq.:			
(Del Monte) Lite, chunky	½ cup	58	14.0
(Hunt's) *Snack Pack*	5-oz. container	120	31.0
Dried:			
(Del Monte)	2 oz.	130	34.0
(Sun-Maid/Sunsweet)	2 oz.	150	39.0
Frozen (Birds Eye) quick thaw	5-oz. serving	150	35.8
FRUIT & NUT MIX (Carnation):			
All fruit	.9-oz. pouch	80	18.0
Deluxe trail mix	.9-oz. pouch	130	9.0
Raisin & nuts	.9-oz. pouch	130	11.0
Tropical fruit & nuts	.9-oz. pouch	100	16.0
FRUIT PUNCH:			
Canned:			
Capri Sun, natural	6¾ fl. oz.	102	25.9
(Hi-C)	6 fl. oz.	96	23.7
(Lincoln) party	6 fl. oz.	90	23.0
Chilled:			
(Minute Maid)	6 fl. oz.	91	23.0
(Sunkist)	8.45 fl. oz.	140	34.0
*Mix:			
Regular (Hi-C)	6 fl. oz.	72	18.0
Dietetic:			
Crystal Light	6 fl. oz. (6.3 oz.)	2	.1
(Sunkist)	8 fl. oz.	6	2.0
FRUIT ROLLS:			
(Flavor Tree)	¾-oz. piece	80	18.0
Fruit Corners (General Mills):			
Apple, apricot, banana, cherry or grape	.5-oz. piece	50	12.0
Fruit punch	.5-oz. piece	60	12.0
(Sunkist)	.5-oz. piece	50	12.0

(USDA): United States Department of Agriculture
(HEW/FAO):   Health, Education and Welfare/Food and Agriculture
                        Organization
* Prepared as Package Directs

Food and Description	Measure or Quantity	Calories	Carbo-hydrates (grams)
FRUIT SALAD:			
Canned, regular pack, solids & liq.:			
(USDA):			
Light syrup	4 oz.	67	17.6
Heavy syrup	½ cup (4.3 oz.)	85	22.0
Extra heavy syrup	4 oz.	102	26.5
(Del Monte) fruits for salad:			
Regular	½ cup (4¼ oz.)	90	22.0
Tropical	½ cup (4 oz.)	90	26.0
(Libby's) heavy syrup	½ cup (4.4 oz.)	99	24.0
Canned, dietetic or low calorie, solids & liq.:			
(Diet Delight) juice pack	½ cup (4.4 oz.)	60	16.0
(S&W) *Nutradiet:*			
Juice pack, white label	½ cup	50	11.0
Water pack, blue label	½ cup	35	10.0
FRUIT SQUARES, frozen			
(Pepperidge Farm):			
Apple	2½-oz. piece	230	27.0
Blueberry or cherry	2½-oz. piece	230	29.0
FRUIT WRINKLES			
(General Mills) *Fruit Corners*	1 pouch	100	21.0

Food and Description	Measure or Quantity	Calories	Carbo-hydrates (grams)
GARLIC:			
Raw (USDA):			
Whole	2 oz. (weighed with skin)	68	15.4
Peeled	1 oz.	39	8.7
Flakes (Gilroy)	1 tsp.	13	2.6
Powder (French's)	1 tsp.	10	2.0
Salt (French's)	1 tsp.	4	1.0
Spread (Lawry's):			
Concentrate	1 T.	15	.2
Ready-to-use, bread spread	1 T.	94	2.0
GEFILTE FISH, canned:			
(Mother's):			
Jellied, old world	4-oz. serving	70	7.0
Jellied, white fish & pike	4-oz. serving	60	4.0
In liquid broth	4-oz. serving	70	7.0
(Rokeach):			
Natural Broth:			
12-oz. jar	2-oz. piece	46	3.0
24-oz. jar	2.6-oz. piece	60	4.0
Old Vienna:			
Regular:			
12-oz. jar	2-oz. piece	52	4.0
24-oz. jar	2.6-oz. piece	68	5.0
Jellied, Whitefish & Pike:			
12-oz. jar	2-oz. piece	54	4.0
24-oz. jar	2.6-oz. piece	70	5.0
Redi-Jell:			
12-oz. jar	2-oz. piece	46	3.0
24-oz. jar	2.6-oz. piece	60	4.0

(USDA): United States Department of Agriculture
(HEW/FAO): Health, Education and Welfare/Food and Agriculture Organization
* Prepared as Package Directs

Food and Description	Measure or Quantity	Calories	Carbo-hydrates (grams)
Whitefish & Pike, jellied broth:			
12-oz. jar	2-oz. piece	46	3.0
24-oz. jar	2.6-oz. piece	60	4.0
GELATIN, unflavored, dry:			
(USDA)	7-gram envelope	23	0.
Carmel Kosher	7-gram envelope	30	0.
(Knox)	1 envelope	25	0.
GELATIN DESSERT:			
Canned, dietetic (Dia-Mel; Louis Sherry)	4-oz. container	2	Tr.
*Powder:			
Regular:			
Carmel Kosher, all flavors	½ cup (4 oz.)	80	20.0
(Jell-O) all flavors	½ cup (4.9 oz.)	83	18.6
(Royal) all flavors	½ cup (4.9 oz.)	80	19.0
Dietetic:			
Carmel Kosher, all flavors	½ cup	8	0.
(D-Zerta) all flavors	½ cup (4.3 oz.)	7	.1
(Estee) all flavors	½ cup (4.2 oz.)	8	Tr.
(Featherweight):			
Regular	½ cup	10	1.0
Artificially sweetened	½ cup	10	0.
(Jell-O) sugar free:			
Cherry	½ cup (4.3 oz.)	12	.1
Lime	½ cup	9	.1
Orange, raspberry or strawberry	½ cup	8	.1
(Louis Sherry)	½ cup	8	Tr.
(Royal)	½ cup	12	0.
GELATIN, DRINKING			
(Knox) orange	1 envelope	39	4.0
GERMAN-STYLE DINNER, frozen (Swanson) *TV Brand*	11¾-oz. dinner	370	36.0
GIN, unflavored (See DISTILLED LIQUOR)			
GIN, SLOE:			
(DeKuyper)	1 fl. oz.	70	5.2
(Mr. Boston)	1 fl. oz.	68	4.7

Food and Description	Measure or Quantity	Calories	Carbo-hydrates (grams)
GINGER, powder (French's)	1 tsp.	6	1.2
GINGERBREAD:			
Home recipe (USDA)	1.9-oz piece (2″×2″×2″)	174	28.6
Mix:			
(Betty Crocker)	⅑ of cake	210	35.0
(Dromedary)	2″×2″square (¹⁄₁₆ of pkg.)	100	19.0
(Pillsbury)	3″ square (⅑ of cake)	190	36.0
GOLDEN GRAHAMS, cereal (General Mills)	¾ cup (1 oz.)	110	24.0
GOOBER GRAPE (Smucker's)	1 T.	90	9.0
GOOD HUMOR (See **ICE CREAM**)			
GOOD N' PUDDIN (Popsicle Industries) all flavors	2 ⅓-fl.-oz. bar	170	27.0
GOOSE, domesticated (USDA):			
Raw	1 lb. (weighed ready-to-cook)	1172	0.
Roasted:			
Meat & skin	4 oz.	500	0.
Meat only	4 oz.	264	0.
GOOSEBERRY (USDA):			
Fresh	1 lb.	177	44.0
Fresh	1 cup (5.3 oz.)	58	14.6
Canned, water pack, solids & liq.	4 oz.	29	7.5
GOOSE GIZZARD, raw (USDA)	4 oz.	158	0.

(USDA): United States Department of Agriculture
(HEW/FAO):   Health, Education and Welfare/Food and Agriculture Organization
* Prepared as Package Directs

Food and Description	Measure or Quantity	Calories	Carbohydrates (grams)
GRAHAM CRACKER (See **CRACKER, PUFFS & CHIPS,** Graham)			
GRAHAM CRACKOS, cereal (Kellogg's)	1 cup (1 oz.)	110	24.0
GRANOLA BAR:			
Nature Valley:			
Almond or oats 'n honey	1 bar	120	17.0
Chocolate chip	1 bar	110	16.0
Coconut	1 bar	130	15.0
Peanut	1 bar	120	16.0
Peanut butter	1 bar	120	15.0
New Trail (Hershey's) chocolate covered:			
Chocolate chip	1.3-oz. piece	200	22.0
Cocoa creme	1.3-oz. piece	190	24.0
Cookies & creme	1.3-oz. piece	200	23.0
Peanut butter	1.3-oz. piece	200	21.0
*GRANOLA BAR MIX, chewy, _Nature Valley, Bake-A-Bar:_			
Chocolate chip, oats & honey or raisins & spice	½₄ of pkg.	100	16.0
Peanut butter	½₄ of pkg.	100	15.0
GRANOLA CEREAL:			
Nature Valley:			
Cinnamon & raisin, fruit & nut or toasted oat	⅓ cup (1 oz.)	130	19.0
Coconut & honey	⅓ cup (1 oz.)	150	18.0
Sun Country (Kretschmer):			
With almonds	¼ cup (1 oz.)	138	19.3
Honey almond	1 oz.	130	19.0
With raisins	¼ cup (1 oz.)	133	19.9
With raisins & dates	¼ cup (1 oz.)	130	20.0
GRANOLA CLUSTERS, _Nature Valley:_			
Almond	1 piece (1.2 oz.)	140	27.0
Apple-cinnamon	1 piece (1.2 oz.)	140	25.0
Caramel or raisin	1 piece (1.2 oz.)	150	28.0
Chocolate chip	1 piece (1.2 oz.)	150	26.0

Food and Description	Measure or Quantity	Calories	Carbo-hydrates (grams)
GRANOLA & FRUIT BAR,			
Nature Valley	1 bar	150	25.0
GRANOLA SNACK:			
Nature Valley:			
Cinnamon or honey nut	1 pouch	140	19.0
Oats & honey	1 pouch	140	18.0
Peanut butter	1 pouch	140	17.0
Kudos (M&M/Mars):			
Chocolate chip	1.25-oz. pkg.	180	21.0
Nutty fudge	1.3-oz. pkg.	190	19.0
Peanut butter	1.3-oz. pkg.	190	17.0
GRAPE:			
Fresh:			
American type (slip skin),			
Concord, Delaware, Niagara,			
Catawba and Scuppernong:			
(USDA)	½ lb. (weighed with stem, skin & seeds)	98	22.4
(USDA)	½ cup (2.7 oz.)	33	7.5
(USDA)	3½″ × 3″ bunch (3.5 oz.)	43	9.9
European type (adherent skin,			
Malaga, Muscat, Tompson			
seedless, Emperor & Flame			
Tokay:			
(USDA)	½ lb. (weighed with stem & seeds)	139	34.9
(USDA) whole	20 grapes (¾″ dia.)	52	13.5
(USDA) whole	½ cup (.3 oz.)	56	14.5
(USDA) halves	½ cup (.3 oz.)	56	14.4
Canned, solids & liq., (USDA)			
Thompson, seedless, heavy syrup	4 oz.	87	22.7

(USDA): United States Department of Agriculture
(HEW/FAO): Health, Education and Welfare/Food and Agriculture Organization
* Prepared as Package Directs

Food and Description	Measure or Quantity	Calories	Carbo-hydrates (grams)
Canned, dietetic pack, solids & liq.:			
(USDA) Thompson, seedless, water pack	4 oz.	58	15.4
(Featherweight) water pack, seedless	½ cup	60	13.0
GRAPE DRINK:			
Canned:			
(Borden) *Bama*	8.45-fl.-oz. container	120	29.0
Capri Sun	6¾ fl. oz.	104	26.3
(Hi-C)	6 fl. oz.	96	23.7
(Johanna Farms) *Ssips*	8.45-fl-oz. container	130	32.0
(Lincoln)	6 fl. oz.	90	23.0
(Welchade)	6 fl. oz.	90	23.0
Chilled (Sunkist)	8.45 fl. oz.	140	33.0
*Mix:			
Regular (Hi-C)	6 fl. oz.	68	17.0
Dietetic (Sunkist)	8 fl. oz.	6	2.0
GRAPEFRUIT:			
Fresh (USDA):			
White:			
Seeded type	1 lb. (weighed with seeds & skin)	86	22.4
Seedless type	1 lb. (weighed with skin)	87	22.6
Seeded type	½ med. grapefruit (3¾" dia., 8.5 oz.)	54	14.1
Pink and red:			
Seeded type	1 lb. (weighed with seeds & skin)	87	22.6
Seedless type	1 lb. (weighed with skin)	93	24.1
Seeded type	½ med. grapefruit (3¾" dia., 8.5 oz.)	46	12.0
Canned, syrup pack (Del Monte) solids & liq.	½ cup	74	17.5

Food and Description	Measure or Quantity	Calories	Carbo-hydrates (grams)
Canned, unsweetened or dietetic pack, solids & liq.			
(USDA) water pack	½ cup (4.2 oz.)	36	9.1
(Del Monte) sections	½ cup	46	10.5
(Diet Delight) sections, juice pack	½ cup (4.3 oz.)	45	11.0
(Featherweight) sections, juice pack	½ of 8-oz. can	40	9.0
(S&W) *Nutradiet,* sections	½ cup	40	9.0
GRAPEFRUIT DRINK, canned (Lincoln)	6 fl. oz.	100	25.0
GRAPEFRUIT JUICE:			
Fresh (USDA) pink, red or white	½ cup (4.3 oz.)	46	11.3
Canned, sweetened:			
(Ardmore Farms)	6 fl. oz.	78	18.1
(Johanna Farms)	6 fl. oz.	76	18.0
(Texsun)	6 fl. oz.	77	18.0
Canned, unsweetened:			
(Del Monte)	6 fl. oz. (6.5 oz.)	70	17.0
(Libby's)	6 fl. oz.	75	18.0
(Ocean Spray)	6 fl. oz.	71	16.2
Chilled (Sunkist)	6 fl. oz.	72	17.0
*Frozen (Minute Maid)	6 fl. oz.	83	19.7
GRAPEFRUIT JUICE COCKTAIL, canned (Ocean Spray) pink	6 fl. oz.	80	20.0
GRAPEFRUIT-ORANGE JUICE COCKTAIL, canned, (Ardmore Farms)	6 fl. oz.	78	19.1
GRAPEFRUIT PEEL, CANDIED (USDA)	1 oz.	90	22.9
GRAPE JAM (Smucker's)	1 T. (.7 oz.)	53	13.7

(USDA): United States Department of Agriculture
(HEW/FAO):   Health, Education and Welfare/Food and Agriculture
                          Organization
* Prepared as Package Directs

Food and Description	Measure or Quantity	Calories	Carbo-hydrates (grams)
GRAPE JELLY:			
Sweetened:			
(Borden) *Bama*	1 T.	45	12.0
(Smucker's)	1 T. (.5 oz.)	53	13.5
(Welch's)	1 T.	52	13.5
Dietetic:			
(Diet Delight)	1 T. (.6 oz.)	12	3.0
(Estee)	1 T.	6	0.
(Featherweight) calorie			
reduced	1 T.	16	4.0
(S&W) *Nutradiet,* red label	1 T.	12	3.0
(Welch's) lite		30	6.2
GRAPE JUICE:			
Canned, unsweetened:			
(USDA)	½ cup (4.4 oz.)	83	20.9
(Ardmore Farms)	6 fl. oz.	99	24.9
(Borden) *Sippin' Pak*	8.45-fl.-oz. container	130	32.0
(Johanna Farms) *Tree Ripe*	8.45-fl.-oz. container	164	40.0
(Tree Top) sparkling	6 fl. oz.	120	29.0
(Welch's):			
Regular, red, sparkling white or white	6 fl. oz.	120	30.0
Sparkling red	6 fl. oz.	128	32.0
*Frozen:			
(Minute Maid)	6 fl. oz.	99	13.3
(Welch's)	6 fl. oz.	100	25.0
GRAPE JUICE DRINK, chilled:			
(Sunkist)	8.45 fl. oz.	140	33.0
(Welch's)	6 fl. oz.	110	27.0
GRAPE NUTS, cereal (Post):			
Regular	¼ cup (1 oz.)	108	23.3
Flakes	⅞ cup (1 oz.)	108	23.2
Raisin	¼ cup (1 oz.)	103	23.0
GRAPE PRESERVE OR JAM,			
sweetened (Welch's)	1 T.	52	13.5
GRAVY, canned:			
Regular:			
Au jus (Franco-American)	2-oz. serving	5	1.0

Food and Description	Measure or Quantity	Calories	Carbo-hydrates (grams)
Beef (Franco-American)	2-oz. serving	25	3.0
Brown:			
(Franco-American) with onion	2-oz. serving	25	4.0
(Howard Johnson's)	½ cup	51	4.9
Ready Gravy	¼ cup (2.2 oz.)	44	7.5
Chicken:			
(Franco-American):			
Regular	2-oz. serving	50	3.0
Giblet	2-oz. serving	30	3.0
Mushroom (Franco-American)	2-oz. serving	25	3.0
Pork (Franco-American)	2-oz. serving	40	3.0
Turkey:			
(Franco-American)	2-oz. serving	30	3.0
(Howard Johnson's) giblet	½ cup	55	5.5
Dietetic (Estee):			
Brown	¼ cup	14	3.0
Chicken & herb	¼ cup	20	4.0
GRAVYMASTER	1 tsp. (.2 oz.)	12	2.4
GRAVY MIX:			
Regular:			
Au jus:			
(Durkee):			
*Regular	½ cup	15	3.2
Roastin' Bag	1-oz. pkg.	64	14.0
*(French's) *Gravy Makins*	½ cup	20	4.0
*(Lawry's)	½ cup	42	5.5
Brown:			
*(Durkee):			
Regular	½ cup	29	5.0
With mushroom	½ cup	29	5.5
With onion	½ cup	33	6.5
*(French's) *Gravy Makins*	½ cup	40	8.0
*(Lawry's)	½ cup	47	18.2
(McCormick)	.85-oz. pkg.	87	12.8
*(Pillsbury)	½ cup	30	6.0
*(Spatini)	1 fl. oz.	8	2.0

(USDA): United States Department of Agriculture
(HEW/FAO):   Health, Education and Welfare/Food and Agriculture
            Organization
* Prepared as Package Directs

Food and Description	Measure or Quantity	Calories	Carbohydrates (grams)
Chicken:			
(Durkee):			
*Regular	½ cup	43	7.0
*Creamy	½ cup	78	7.0
Roastin' Bag:			
Regular	1.5-oz. pkg.	122	24.0
Creamy	2-oz. pkg.	242	22.0
Italian Style	1.5-oz. pkg.	144	31.0
*(French's) Gravy Makins	½ cup	50	8.0
(McCormick)	.85-oz. pkg.	82	13.4
*(Pillsbury)	½ cup	50	8.0
Homestyle:			
*(Durkee)	½ cup	35	5.5
*(French's) Gravy Makins	½ cup	40	8.0
*(Pillsbury)	½ cup	30	6.0
Meatloaf (Durkee) Roastin' Bag	1.5-oz. pkg.	129	18.0
Mushroom:			
*(Durkee)	½ cup	30	22.0
*(French's) Gravy Makins	½ cup	40	6.0
Onion:			
*(Durkee)	½ cup	42	7.5
*(French's) Gravy Makins	½ cup	50	8.0
*(McCormick)	.85-oz. pkg.	72	9.8
Pork:			
(Durkee):			
*Regular	½ cup	35	7.0
Roastin' Bag	1.5-oz. pkg.	130	26.0
*(French's) Gravy Makins	½ cup	40	8.0
Pot roast (Durkee) Roastin' Bag, regular or onion	1.5-oz. pkg.	125	25.0
*Swiss steak (Durkee)	½ cup	22	5.4
Turkey:			
*(Durkee)	½ cup	47	7.0
*(French's) Gravy Makins	½ cup	50	8.0
*Dietetic (Estee):			
Brown	½ cup	28	6.0
Chicken, & herbs	½ cup	40	8.0
GRAVY WITH MEAT OR TURKEY, frozen:			
(Banquet):			
Entrees for One:			
& sliced beef	4 oz.	90	4.0

Food and Description	Measure or Quantity	Calories	Carbo-hydrates (grams)
& sliced turkey	5 oz.	110	7.0
Family Entree:			
& sliced beef	2-lb. pkg.	640	36.0
& sliced turkey	2-lb. pkg.	640	32.0
(Morton) Light:			
& beef, sliced	8-oz. meal	280	30.0
& chicken, sliced	8-oz. meal	240	32.0
& salisbury steak	8-oz. meal	290	34.0
& turkey	8-oz. meal	270	45.0
(Swanson) & sliced beef	8-oz. meal	200	18.0
GREAT BEGINNINGS			
(Hormel):			
With chunky beef	5 oz.	136	7.0
With chunky chicken	5 oz.	147	7.0
With chunky pork	5 oz.	140	5.0
With chunky turkey	5 oz.	138	7.0
GREENS, MIXED, canned,			
solids & liq.:			
(Allen's)	½ cup (4 oz.)	25	3.0
(Sunshine)	½ cup (4.1 oz.)	20	2.7
GRENADINE (Garnier)			
non-alcoholic	1 fl. oz.	103	26.0
GROUPER, raw (USDA):			
Whole	1 lb. (weighed whole)	170	0.
Meat only	4 oz.	99	0.
GUACAMOLE SEASONING MIX (Lawry's)	.7-oz. pkg.	60	12.6
GUAVA, COMMON, fresh (USDA):			
Whole	1 lb. (weighed untrimmed)	273	66.0
Whole	1 guava (2.8 oz.)	48	11.7
Flesh only	4 oz.	70	17.0

(USDA): United States Department of Agriculture
(HEW/FAO):   Health, Education and Welfare/Food and Agriculture
            Organization
* Prepared as Package Directs

Food and Description	Measure or Quantity	Calories	Carbo-hydrates (grams)
GUAVA JAM (Smucker's)	1 T.	53	13.5
GUAVA JELLY (Smucker's)	1 T.	53	13.5
GUAVA NECTAR (Libby's)	6 fl. oz.	70	17.0
GUAVA, STRAWBERRY, fresh (USDA):			
Whole	1 lb. (weighed untrimmed)	289	70.2
Flesh only	4 oz.	74	17.9
GUINEA HEN, raw (USDA):			
Ready-to-cook	1 lb. (weighed ready-to-cook)	594	0.
Meat & skin	4 oz.	179	0.

Food and Description	Measure or Quantity	Calories	Carbo-hydrates (grams)

H

HADDOCK:

Food and Description	Measure or Quantity	Calories	Carbo-hydrates (grams)
Raw (USDA) meat only	4 oz.	90	0.
Fried, breaded (USDA)	4″ × 3″ × ½″ fillet (3.5 oz.)	165	5.8
Smoked (USDA)	4-oz. serving	117	0.
Frozen:			
(Frionor) *Norway Gourmet*	4-oz. fillet	70	0.
(Gorton's):			
Fishmarket Fresh	4 oz.	90	0.
Light Recipe, fillet, entree size	1 piece	260	33.0
(Mrs. Paul's):			
Batter dipped	2¼-oz. fillet	160	14.0
Breaded & fried	2-oz. fillet	140	12.5
Bread & fried, light	6-oz. serving	320	23.0
(Van de Kamp's) batter dipped, french fried	2-oz. piece	120	10.0
(Weight Watchers) with stuffing, 2-compartment meal	7-oz. pkg.	205	14.1

HALIBUT:

Food and Description	Measure or Quantity	Calories	Carbo-hydrates (grams)
Raw (USDA):			
Whole	1 lb. (weighed whole)	144	0.
Meat only	4 oz.	84	0.
Broiled (USDA)	4″ × 3″ × ½″ steak (4.4 oz.)	214	0.
Smoked (USDA)	4 oz.	254	0.
Frozen (Van de Kamp's) batter dipped, french fried	½ of 8-oz. pkg.	260	15.0

(USDA): United States Department of Agriculture
(HEW/FAO): Health, Education and Welfare/Food and Agriculture Organization
* Prepared as Package Directs

Food and Description	Measure or Quantity	Calories	Carbo-hydrates (grams)
HAM (See also **PORK**):			
Canned:			
(Hormel):			
Black Label (3- or 5-lb. size)	4 oz.	140	0.
Chopped	3 oz. (8-lb. ham)	240	1.0
Chunk	6¾-oz. serving	310	0.
Curemaster, smoked	4 oz.	140	1.0
EXL	4 oz.	120	0.
Holiday Glaze	4 oz. (3-lb. ham)	140	2.9
Patties	1 patty	180	0.
(Oscar Mayer) *Jubilee,* extra lean, cooked	1-oz. serving	31	.1
(Swift) *Premium*	1¾-oz. slice	111	.3
Deviled:			
(Hormel)	1 T.	35	0.
(Libby's)	1 T. (.5 oz.)	43	0.
(Underwood)	1 T. (.5 oz.)	49	Tr.
Packaged:			
(Carl Buddig) smoked	1-oz. slice	50	Tr.
(Eckrich):			
Chopped	1 oz.	45	1.0
Loaf	1 oz.	70	1.0
Cooked or imported, danish	1.2-oz. slice	30	1.2
(Hormel):			
Black peppered, *Light & Lean*	1 slice	25	0.
Chopped	1 slice	44	0.
Cooked, *Light & Lean*	1 slice	25	0.
Glazed, *Light & Lean*	1 slice	25	0.
Red peppered, *Light & Lean*	1 slice	25	0.
Smoked, cooked, *Light & Lean*	1 slice	25	0.
(Oscar Mayer):			
Chopped	1-oz. slice	64	.9
Cooked, smoked	1-oz. slice	34	0.
Jubilee boneless:			
Sliced	8-oz. slice	232	0.
Steak	2-oz. steak	59	0.1
HAM & ASPARAGUS BAKE, frozen (Stouffer's)	9½-oz. meal	510	31.0

Food and Description	Measure or Quantity	Calories	Carbo-hydrates (grams)
HAMBURGER (See **BEEF**, Ground; see also *MCDONALD'S, BURGER KING, DAIRY QUEEN, WHITE CASTLE*, etc.)			
HAMBURGER MIX:			
Hamburger Helper (General Mills):			
Beef noodle	⅓ of pkg.	320	26.0
Beef romanoff	⅓ of pkg.	350	30.0
Cheeseburger macaroni	⅓ of pkg.	360	28.0
Chili:			
With beans	¼ of pkg.	350	25.0
Without beans, hot	¼ of pkg.	350	26.0
Chili tomato	⅓ of pkg.	330	31.0
Hash	⅓ of pkg.	320	27.0
Lasagna	⅓ of pkg.	340	33.0
Pizza dish	⅓ of pkg.	360	37.0
Potatoes au gratin	⅓ of pkg.	320	28.0
Potato Stroganoff	⅓ of pkg.	320	28.0
Rice oriental	⅓ of pkg.	340	38.0
Spaghetti	⅓ of pkg.	340	32.0
Stew	⅓ of pkg.	300	25.0
Tamale bake	⅓ of pkg.	380	39.0
Make a Better Burger (Lipton) mildly seasoned or onion	⅓ of pkg.	30	5.0
HAMBURGER SEASONING MIX:			
*(Durkee)	1 cup	663	7.5
(French's)	1-oz. pkg.	100	20.0
HAM & CHEESE:			
Canned (Hormel):			
Loaf	3 oz.	260	1.0
Patty	1 patty	190	0.
Packaged:			
(Eckrich) loaf	1-oz. serving	60	1.0
(Hormel) loaf	1-oz. slice	65	0.

(USDA): United States Department of Agriculture
(HEW/FAO):   Health, Education and Welfare/Food and Agriculture
                        Organization
* Prepared as Package Directs

Food and Description	Measure or Quantity	Calories	Carbo-hydrates (grams)
(Ohse) loaf	1 oz.	65	2.0
(Oscar Mayer) spread	1 oz.	66	.6
HAM DINNER, frozen:			
(Armour) *Dinner Classics*	11-oz. dinner	350	39.0
(Banquet) **American Favorites**	10-oz. dinner	532	61.0
(Morton)	10-oz. dinner	286	49.0
HAM SALAD, canned			
(Carnation)	¼ of 7½-oz. can (1.9 oz.)	110	4.0
HAM SALAD SPREAD (Oscar Mayer)	1 oz.	59	3.6
HARDEE'S:			
Apple turnover	3.2-oz. piece	270	38.0
Big Cookie	1.7-oz. piece	260	31.0
Big Country Breakfast:			
Bacon	7.65-oz. meal	660	51.0
Country ham	8.96-oz. meal	670	52.0
Ham	8.85-oz. meal	620	51.0
Sausage	9.7-oz. meal	850	51.0
Biscuit:			
Bacon	3.3-oz. serving	360	34.0
Bacon & egg	4.4-oz. serving	410	35.0
Bacon, egg & cheese	4.8-oz. serving	460	35.0
Chicken	5.1-oz. serving	430	42.0
Country ham:			
Plain	3.8-oz. serving	350	35.0
& egg	4.9-oz. serving	400	35.0
'n gravy	7.8-oz. serving	440	45.0
Ham:			
Plain	3.7-oz. serving	320	34.0
With egg	4.9-oz. serving	370	35.0
With egg & cheese	5.3-oz. serving	420	35.0
Rise 'N Shine:			
Plain	2.9-oz. serving	320	34.0
Canadian bacon	5.7-oz. serving	470	35.0
Sausage:			
Plain	4.2-oz. serving	440	34.0
With egg	5.3-oz. serving	490	35.0
Steak:			
Plain	5.2-oz. serving	500	46.0
With egg	6.3-oz. serving	550	47.0

Food and Description	Measure or Quantity	Calories	Carbo-hydrates (grams)
Cheeseburger:			
Plain	4.3-oz. serving	320	33.0
Bacon	7.7-oz. serving	610	31.0
Quarter-pound	6.4-oz. serving	500	34.0
Chicken fillet sandwich	6.1-oz. sandwich	370	44.0
Chicken, grilled, sandwich	6.8-oz. sandwich	310	34.0
Chicken Stix:			
6-piece	3 ½-oz. serving	210	13.0
9-piece	5.3-oz. serving	310	20.0
Cool Twist:			
Cone:			
Chocolate:	4.2-oz. serving	200	31.0
Vanilla	4.2-oz. serving	190	28.0
Vanilla/chocolate	4.2-oz. serving	190	29.0
Sundae:			
Caramel	6-oz. serving	330	54.0
Hot fudge	5.9-oz. serving	320	45.0
Strawberry	5.9-oz. serving	260	43.0
Fisherman's Fillet, sandwich	7.3-oz. sandwich	500	49.0
Hamburger:			
Plain	3.9-oz. serving	270	33.0
Big Deluxe	7.6-oz. serving	500	32.0
Mushroom 'N Swiss	6.6-oz. serving	490	33.0
Hot dog, all beef	4.2-oz. serving	300	25.0
Hot ham 'n cheese	4.2-oz. sandwich	330	32.0
Margarine/butter blend	.2-oz. serving	35	0.
Pancakes, three:			
Plain	4.8-oz. serving	280	56.0
With sausage pattie	6.2-oz. serving	430	56.0
With bacon strips	5.3-oz. serving	350	56.0
Potato:			
French fries:			
Regular	2 ½-oz. order	230	30.0
Large	4-oz. order	360	48.0
Hash Rounds	2.8-oz. serving	230	24.0
Roast beef sandwich:			
Regular	4-oz. serving	260	31.0
Big Roast Beef	4.7-oz. serving	300	32.0
Salads:			
Chef	10.4-oz. serving	240	5.0

(USDA): United States Department of Agriculture
(HEW/FAO):   Health, Education and Welfare/Food and Agriculture
　　　　　　　　Organization
* Prepared as Package Directs

Food and Description	Measure or Quantity	Calories	Carbo-hydrates (grams)
Chicken & pasta	14.6-oz. serving	230	23.0
Garden	8.5-oz. serving	210	3.0
Side	3.9-oz. serving	20	1.0
Shake:			
Chocolate	12 fl. oz.	460	85.0
Strawberry	12 fl. oz.	440	82.0
Vanilla	12 fl. oz.	400	66.0
Syrup, pancake	1 ½-oz. serving	120	31.0
Turkey club sandwich	7.3-oz. serving	390	32.0
HAWAIIAN PUNCH, canned:			
Regular:			
Apple, fruit juicy red, island fruit cocktail, tropical fruit or very berry	6 fl. oz.	90	22.0
Cherry, grape or wild fruit	6 fl. oz.	90	23.0
Orange	6 fl. oz.	100	24.0
Dietetic:	6 fl. oz.	30	8.0
HAWS, SCARLET, raw (USDA):			
Whole	1 lb. (weighed with core)	316	75.5
Flesh & skin	4 oz.	99	23.6
HEADCHEESE:			
(USDA)	1 oz.	76	.3
(Oscar Mayer)	1 oz.	55	0.
HERRING:			
Raw (USDA):			
Atlantic:			
Whole	1 lb. (weighed whole)	407	0.
Meat only	4 oz.	200	0.
Pacific, meat only	4 oz.	111	0.
Canned:			
(USDA) in tomato sauce, solids & liq.	4-oz. serving	200	4.2
(Vita):			
Bismarck, drained	5-oz. jar	273	6.9
In cream sauce, drained	8-oz. jar	397	18.1
Matjis, drained	8-oz. jar	304	26.2
In wine sauce, drained	8-oz. jar	401	16.6

Food and Description	Measure or Quantity	Calories	Carbo-hydrates (grams)
Pickled (USDA) Bismarck type	4-oz. serving	253	0.
Salted or brined (USDA)	4-oz. serving	247	0.
Smoked (USDA):			
Bloaters	4-oz. serving	222	0.
Hard	4-oz. serving	340	0.
Kippered	4-oz. serving	239	0.
HICKORY NUT (USDA):			
Whole	1 lb. (weighed in shell)	1068	20.3
Shelled	4 oz.	763	14.5
HO-HO (Hostess)	1-oz. piece	126	17.0
HOMINY, canned, solids & liq.			
(Allen's) golden or white	½ cup	80	16.0
HOMINY GRITS:			
Dry:			
(USDA):			
Degermed	1 oz.	103	22.1
Degermed	½ cup (2.8 oz.)	282	60.9
(Albers) quick, degermed	1½ oz.	150	33.0
(Aunt Jemima)	3 T. (1 oz.)	101	22.4
(Pocono) creamy	1 oz.	101	23.6
(Quaker):			
Regular or quick	1 T. (.33 oz.)	34	7.5
Instant:			
Regular	.8-oz. packet	79	17.7
With imitation bacon bits	1-oz. packet	101	21.6
With artificial cheese flavor	1-oz. packet	104	21.6
With imitation ham bits	1-oz. packet	99	21.3
(3-Minute Brand) quick, enriched	⅙ cup (1 oz.)	98	22.2
Cooked (USDA) degermed	⅔ cup (5.6 oz.)	84	18.0

(USDA): United States Department of Agriculture
(HEW/FAO):   Health, Education and Welfare/Food and Agriculture Organization
* Prepared as Package Directs

Food and Description	Measure or Quantity	Calories	Carbo-hydrates (grams)
HONEY, strained:			
(USDA)	½ cup (5.7 oz.)	494	134.1
(USDA)	1 T. (.7 oz.)	61	16.5
HONEYCOMB, cereal (Post)			
regular	1⅓ cups (1 oz.)	117	24.5
HONEYDEW, fresh (USDA):			
Whole	1 lb. (weighed whole)	94	22.0
Wedge	2″ × 7″ wedge (5.3 oz.)	31	7.2
Flesh only	4 oz.	37	8.7
Flesh only, diced	1 cup (5.9 oz.)	55	12.9
HONEY SMACKS, cereal			
(Kellogg's)	¾ cup (1 oz.)	110	25.0
HORSERADISH:			
Raw, pared (USDA)	1 oz.	25	5.6
Prepared (Gold's)	1 tsp.	4	Tr.
HOT DOG (see **FRANKFURTER**)			
HYACINTH BEAN (USDA):			
Young bean, raw:			
Whole	1 lb. (weighed untrimmed)	140	29.1
Trimmed	4 oz.	40	8.3
Dry seeds	4 oz.	383	69.2

Food and Description	Measure or Quantity	Calories	Carbo-hydrates (grams)

I

ICE CREAM (Listed below by flavor or by type, such as Cookie sandwich or *Whammy*. See also **FROZEN DESSERT**):

Food and Description	Measure or Quantity	Calories	Carbo-hydrates (grams)
Almond (Good Humor)	4 fl. oz.	350	29.4
Almond amaretto (Baskin-Robbins)	4 fl. oz.	280	26.0
Blueberry & cream (Häagen-Dazs)	4 fl. oz.	190	25.0
Bon Bon, nuggets (Carnation):			
Chocolate	1 piece	34	3.1
Vanilla	1 piece	33	2.8
Bubble O Bill bar (Good Humor)	3 ½-fl.-oz. bar	149	17.0
Butter almond (Breyer's)	½ cup	170	15.0
Butter pecan:			
(Breyer's)	½ cup	180	15.0
(Good Humor)	4 fl. oz.	150	14.0
(Häagen-Dazs)	4 fl. oz.	312	19.2
(Lady Borden)	½ cup	180	16.0
Calippo (Good Humor):			
Cherry	4 ½ fl. oz.	140	34.9
Lemon	4 ½ fl. oz.	112	27.6
Orange	4 ½ fl. oz.	110	27.2
Cappuccino chip (Baskin-Robbins)	4 fl. oz.	310	31.0
Cherry vanilla (Breyer's)	4 fl. oz.	140	17.0
Chip crunch bar (Good Humor)	3-fl.-oz. bar	255	21.2

(USDA): United States Department of Agriculture
(HEW/FAO): Health, Education and Welfare/Food and Agriculture Organization
* Prepared as Package Directs

Food and Description	Measure or Quantity	Calories	Carbo-hydrates (grams)
Chocolate:			
(Baskin-Robbins):			
Regular	4 fl. oz.	264	32.6
Chip	4 fl. oz.	260	27.0
Deluxe	4 fl. oz.	270	32.0
Mousse Royale	4 fl. oz.	293	36.3
World Class	4 fl. oz.	280	35.0
(Borden) Old Fashioned			
Recipe, dutch	½ cup	130	16.0
(Breyer's)	½ cup	160	19.0
(Häagen-Dazs):			
Regular	4 fl. oz.	270	24.0
Mint	4 fl. oz.	290	28.0
(Meadow Gold)	½ cup	140	18.0
Chocolate bar (Häagen-Dazs) dark chocolate coating	1 bar	360	35.0
Chocolate chip (Häagen-Dazs)	4 fl. oz.	290	28.0
Chocolate eclair (Good Humor)	3-fl.-oz. bar	187	22.6
Chocolate malt bar (Good Humor)	3-fl.-oz. bar	190	16.0
Chocolate raspberry truffle (Baskin-Robbins)	4 fl. oz.	310	35.0
Chocolate swirl (Borden)	½ cup	130	18.0
Coffee:			
(Breyer's)	½ cup	140	15.0
(Häagen-Dazs)	4 fl. oz.	270	23.0
Cookies & cream (Breyers)	4 fl. oz.	170	19.0
Cookie sandwich (Good Humor)	2.7-fl.-oz. piece	290	42.0
Eskimo Pie:			
Chocolate fudge bar	1¾-fl.-oz. bar	60	14.0
Chocolate fudge bar	2½-fl.-oz. bar	90	20.0
Chocolate fudge bar	3-fl.-oz. bar	110	24.0
Dietary dairy bar, chocolate covered	2½-fl.-oz. bar	110	10.0
Old fashioned:			
Crispy	1 bar	290	24.0
Double chocolate	1 bar	280	25.0
Vanilla	1 bar	280	23.0
Original:			
Double chocolate	1 bar	140	12.0
Vanilla	1 bar	140	11.0
Pie:			

Food and Description	Measure or Quantity	Calories	Carbo-hydrates (grams)
Regular:			
Chocolate	3-fl.-oz. bar	170	16.0
Crunch	3-fl.-oz. bar	170	15.0
Vanilla	3-fl.-oz. bar	170	14.0
Junior:			
Chocolate	1¾-fl.-oz. bar	100	10.0
Crunch	1¾-fl.-oz. bar	100	9.0
Vanilla	1¾-fl.-oz. bar	100	9.0
Thin mints	2-fl.-oz. bar	130	10.0
Twin pops	1¾-fl.-oz. bar	40	10.0
Twin pops	3-fl.-oz. bar	70	17.0
Fat Frog (Good Humor)	3-fl.-oz. bar	154	16.0
Fudge Royal (Sealtest)	½ cup	140	19.0
Grand Marnier (Baskin-Robbins)	4 fl. oz.	240	31.0
Halo bar (Good Humor)	2 ½-fl.-oz. bar	230	22.8
Honey (Häagen-Dazs)	4 fl. oz.	250	22.0
Honey vanilla (Häagen-Dazs)	4 fl. oz.	240	8.0
Jamocha (Baskin-Robbins)	2½-fl.-oz. scoop	146	15.8
Jumbo Jet Star (Good Humor)	4½ fl. oz.	84	19.5
Keylime & cream (Häagen-Dazs)	4 fl. oz.	200	34.0
King cone (Good Humor):			
Regular	5½ fl. oz.	290	40.9
Boysenberry	5 fl. oz.	340	51.6
Laser Blazer (Good Humor):	3 fl. oz.	131	23.1
Macadamia brittle (Häagen-Dazs)	4 fl. oz.	280	25.2
Macadamia Nut (Häagen-Dazs)	4 fl. oz.	330	24.0
Maple Walnut (Häagen-Dazs)	4 fl. oz.	310	18.0
Milky pop (Good Humor)	1½-fl.-oz. pop	46	8.4
Mint chocolate chip (Breyer's)	½ cup	170	18.0
Mocha double nut (Häagen-Dazs)	4 fl. oz.	290	22.0
Orange & cream (Häagen-Dazs)	4 fl. oz.	200	30.0
Oreo, cookies & cream:			

(USDA): United States Department of Agriculture
(HEW/FAO):   Health, Education and Welfare/Food and Agriculture
              Organization
* Prepared as Package Directs

Food and Description	Measure or Quantity	Calories	Carbo- hydrates (grams)
Chocolate, mint or vanilla	3 fl. oz.	140	16.0
Sandwich	1 sandwich	240	31.0
Stick	1 bar	220	19.0
Peach:			
(Breyer's)	½ cup	140	19.0
(Häagen-Dazs)	4 fl. oz.	210	15.0
Peanut vanilla			
(Häagen-Dazs)	4 fl. oz.	280	19.0
Pralines & Cream: (Baskin-Robbins)	4-fl. oz.	280	35.0
Raspberry & cream (Häagen-Dazs)	4 fl. oz.	180	26.0
Rocky Road (Baskin-Robbins)	4 fl. oz.	300	39.0
Rum Raisin (Häagen-Dazs)	4 fl. oz.	250	21.0
Shark (Good Humor)	3-fl. oz. pop	68	17.0
Strawberry:			
(Baskin-Robbins) very berry	4 fl. oz.	220	30.0
(Borden)	½ cup	130	18.0
(Breyer's) natural	½ cup	130	17.0
(Häagen-Dazs)	4 fl.oz.	250	23.0
(Meadow Gold)	½ cup	146	19.0
Strawberry fudge bar (Good Humor)	2 ½-fl.-oz. bar	49	12.2
Strawberry shortcake (Good Humor)	3-fl.-oz. bar	176	23.8
Toasted almond bar (Good Humor)	3-fl.-oz. pop	212	24.3
Vanilla:			
(Baskin-Robbins):			
Regular	4 fl.-oz. scoop	235	25.0
French	4 fl.-oz. scoop	280	25.0
(Borden) Old Fashioned Recipe	½ cup	130	15.0
(Eagle Brand)	½ cup	150	16.0
(Häagen-Dazs)	4 fl. oz.	260	23.0
(Sealtest)	½ cup	140	16.0
Vanilla bar (Häagen-Dazs) with milk chocolate coating	1 bar	320	24.0
Vanilla sandwich (Good Humor)	3-fl.-oz. piece	191	31.1
Vanilla Swiss Almond (Häagen-Dazs)	4 fl. oz.	290	24.0

Food and Description	Measure or Quantity	Calories	Carbo-hydrates (grams)
Whammy (Good Humor) assorted	1.6-fl.-oz. piece	95	6.6
ICE CREAM CONE, cone only: (Baskin-Robbins):			
Sugar	1 piece	60	11.0
Waffle	1 piece	140	28.0
(Comet) sugar	1 piece (.35 oz.)	40	9.0
ICE CREAM CONES, cereal (General Mills)	¾ cup (1-oz.)	110	23.0
ICE CREAM CUP, cup only (Comet):			
Regular	1 cup	20	4.0
Chocolate	1 cup	25	5.0
*****ICE CREAM MIX** (Salada) any flavor	1 cup	310	31.0
ICE MILK: (USDA):			
Hardened	1 cup (4.6 oz.)	199	29.3
Soft-serve	1 cup (6.3 oz.)	266	39.2
(Borden):			
Chocolate	½ cup	100	18.0
Strawberry or vanilla	½ cup	90	17.0
(Dean):			
Count Calorie, 2.1% fat	1 cup (4.8 oz.)	155	17.1
5% fat	1 cup (4.9 oz.)	227	35.0
Light n' Lively, coffee	½ cup	100	17.0
(Meadow Gold):			
Chocolate, Viva	1 cup	200	36.0
Vanilla, Viva	1 cup	200	34.0
ICING (See **CAKE ICING**)			
INSTANT BREAKFAST (See individual brand name or company listings)			
IRISH WHISKEY (See **DISTILLED LIQUOR**)			

(USDA): United States Department of Agriculture
(HEW/FAO): Health, Education and Welfare/Food and Agriculture
           Organization
* Prepared as Package Directs

Food and Description	Measure or Quantity	Calories	Carbo-hydrates (grams)

J

JACKFRUIT, fresh (USDA):

Food and Description	Measure or Quantity	Calories	Carbo-hydrates (grams)
Whole	1 lb. (weighed with seeds & skin)	124	32.5
Flesh only	4 oz.	111	28.8
JACK-IN-THE-BOX RESTAURANT:			
Breakfast Jack	4.4-oz. serving	307	30.0
Breadstick, sesame	.6-oz. serving	70	12.0
Burger:			
Regular	3.6-oz. serving	267	28.0
Cheeseburger:			
Regular	4-oz. serving	315	33.0
Bacon	8.1-oz. serving	705	48.0
Double	5¼-oz. serving	467	33.0
Ultimate	9.9-oz. serving	942	33.0
Jumbo Jack:			
Regular	7.8-oz. serving	584	42.0
With cheese	8.5-oz. serving	677	46.0
Monterey Burger	9.9-oz. serving	865	72.0
Swiss & bacon	6.6-oz. serving	678	34.0
Cheesecake	3.5-oz. serving	309	29.0
Chicken fajita pita sandwich	6.7-oz. serving	292	29.0
Chicken fillet sandwich, grilled	7.2-oz. serving	408	33.0
Chicken strips	1 piece	87	7.0
Chicken supreme sandwich	8.1-oz. serving	575	34.0
Coffee, black	8 fl. oz.	2	.5
Egg, scrambled, platter	8.8-oz. serving	662	52.0
Egg roll	1 piece	135	14.0
Fish supreme sandwich	8-oz. sandwich	554	47.0
French fries:			
Regular	2.4-oz. order	221	27.0
Large	3.8-oz. order	353	43.0
Jumbo	4.8-oz. order	442	54.0
Jelly, grape	.5-oz. serving	38	9.0

Food and Description	Measure or Quantity	Calories	Carbo- hydrates (grams)
Ketchup	1 serving	10	2.0
Mayonnaise	1 serving	152	.5
Milk, low fat	8 fl. oz.	122	12.0
Milk shake:			
Chocolate	10-oz. serving	320	55.0
Strawberry	10-oz. serving	320	55.0
Vanilla	10-oz. serving	320	57.0
Mustard	1 serving	8	.7
Onion rings	3.8-oz. serving	382	39.0
Orange juice	6.5-oz. serving	80	20.0
Pancake platter	8.1-oz. serving	612	87.0
Salad:			
Chef	11.7-oz. salad	325	10.0
Mexican chicken	15.2-oz. salad	443	31.0
Side	3.9-oz. salad	51	Tr.
Taco	14.8-oz. salad	641	34.0
Salad dressing:			
Regular:			
Blue cheese	1.2-oz. serving	131	7.0
Buttermilk	1.2-oz. serving	181	4.0
Thousand Island	1.2-oz. serving	156	6.0
Dietetic or low calorie, French	1.2-oz. serving	80	13.0
Sauce:			
A-1	1.8-oz. serving	35	9.0
BBQ	.9-oz. serving	39	9.4
Guacamole	.9-oz. serving	55	1.8
Mayo-mustard	.8-oz. serving	124	2.0
Mayo-onion	.8-oz. serving	143	1.0
Salsa	.9-oz. serving	8	2.0
Seafood cocktail	1-oz. serving	32	6.8
Sweet & sour	1-oz. serving	40	11.0
Sausage crescent	5.5-oz. serving	585	28.0
Shrimp	1 piece (.3 oz.)	27	2.2
Soft drink:			
Sweetened:			
Coca-Cola Classic	12 fl. oz.	144	36.0
Dr. Pepper	12 fl. oz.	144	37.0
Root beer, *Ramblin'*	12 fl. oz.	176	46.0
Sprite	12 fl. oz.	144	36.0
Dietetic, *Coca-Cola*	12 fl. oz.	Tr.	.3

(USDA): United States Department of Agriculture
(HEW/FAO): Health, Education and Welfare/Food and Agriculture
        Organization
* Prepared as Package Directs

Food and Description	Measure or Quantity	Calories	Carbo-hydrates (grams)
Supreme crescent	5.1-oz. serving	547	27.0
Syrup, pancake	1.5-oz. serving	121	30.0
Taco:			
Regular	2.9-oz. serving	191	16.0
Super	4.8-oz. serving	288	21.0
Taquito	1-oz. piece	73	8.0
Tea, iced, plain	12 fl. oz.	3	.8
Tortilla chips	1 oz.	139	18.0
Turnover, hot apple	4.2-oz. piece	410	45.0
JACK MACKERAL, raw			
(USDA) meat only	4 oz.	162	0.
JAM, sweetened (See also individual listings by flavor)			
(USDA)	1 T. (.7 oz.)	54	14.0
JELL-O FRUIT BARS	1 bar	45	11.0
JELL-O GELATIN POPS:			
Cherry, grape, orange, or			
strawberry	1.7-oz. pop	37	8.5
Raspberry	1.7-oz. pop	34	7.7
JELL-O PUDDING POPS:			
Chocolate, chocolate-caramel swirl, chocolate with chocolate chips & vanilla with chocolate chips	1 bar	80	13.0
Chocolate covered chocolate & vanilla	1 bar	130	14.0
Chocolate-vanilla swirl & vanilla	1 bar	70	12.0
JELLY, sweetened (See also individual flavors) (Crosse & Blackwell) all flavors	1 T.	51	12.8
JERUSALEM ARTICHOKE (USDA):			
Unpared	1 lb. (weighed with skin)	207	52.3
Pared	4 oz.	75	18.9
JOHANNISBERG RIESLING WINE (Louis M. Martini)	3 fl. oz.	68	1.3

Food and Description	Measure or Quantity	Calories	Carbo-hydrates (grams)
JUICE (See individual listings)			
JUJUBE OR CHINESE DATE (USDA):			
Fresh, whole	1 lb. (weighed with seeds)	443	116.4
Fresh, flesh only	4 oz.	119	31.3
Dried, whole	1 lb. (weighed with seeds)	1159	297.1
Dried, flesh only	4 oz.	325	83.5
JUST RIGHT, cereal (Kellogg's):			
Fruit, nut & flake	¾ cup (1.3 oz.)	140	30.0
Nugget & flake	⅔ cup (1 oz.)	100	23.0

(USDA): United States Department of Agriculture
(HEW/FAO):   Health, Education and Welfare/Food and Agriculture
            Organization
* Prepared as Package Directs

Food and Description	Measure or Quantity	Calories	Carbo-hydrates (grams)

K

KABOOM, cereal (General Mills) | 1 cup (1 oz.) | 110 | 23.0

KALE:
Raw (USDA) leaves only	1 lb. (weighed untrimmed)	154	26.1
Boiled, leaves only (USDA)	4 oz.	44	6.9
Canned (Allen's) chopped, solids & liq.	½ cup (4.1 oz.)	25	2.0
Frozen, chopped:			
(Birds Eye)	⅓ of 10-oz. pkg.	31	4.6
(Frosty Acres)	3.3-oz. serving	25	5.0
(McKenzie)	⅓ of 10-oz. pkg.	30	5.0
(Southland)	⅕ of 16-oz. pkg.	25	5.0

KARO SYRUP (See **SYRUP**)

KENTUCKY FRIED CHICKEN:
Biscuit, buttermilk	2.3-oz. serving	232	27.1
Chicken:			
Original recipe:			
Breast:			
Center	1 piece	283	8.8
Side	1 piece	267	10.8
Drumstick	1 piece	146	4.2
Thigh	1 piece	294	11.1
Wing	1 piece	178	6.0
Extra crispy:			
Breast:			
Center	1 piece	353	14.4
Side	1 piece	354	17.3
Drumstick	1 piece	173	5.9
Thigh	1 piece	371	13.8
Wing	1 piece	218	7.8
Chicken Littles	1.7-oz. sandwich	169	13.8

Food and Description	Measure or Quantity	Calories	Carbo-hydrates (grams)
Chicken nugget	1 piece	46	2.2
Cole slaw	3.2-oz. serving	119	13.2
Corn on the cob	5-oz. serving	176	31.9
Potatoes:			
French fries	2.7-oz. regular order	244	41.0
Mashed, & gravy	3½-oz. serving	71	11.9
Salad:			
Chicken topper	8.4-oz. serving	158	6.2
Garden:			
Large	6.5-oz. serving	76	6.5
Mini	4.6-oz. serving	28	4.2
Salad dressing:			
Regular:			
Blue cheese	1 T.	72	.6
Buttermilk	1 T.	74	1.0
French	1 T.	54	2.0
Thousand Island	1 T.	57	2.0
Dietetic, vinaigrette	1 T.	18	1.7
Sauce:			
Barbecue	1-oz. serving	35	7.1
Honey	.5-oz. serving	49	12.1
Mustard	1-oz. serving	36	6.0
Sweet & sour	1-oz. serving	58	13.0

KETCHUP (See **CATSUP**)

KIDNEY (USDA):

Beef, braised	4 oz.	286	.9
Calf, raw	4 oz.	128	.1
Lamb, raw	4 oz.	119	1.0

KIELBASA (See **SAUSAGE**, Polish-style)

KINGFISH, raw (USDA):

Whole	1 lb. (weighed whole)	210	0.
Meat only	4 oz.	119	0.

(USDA): United States Department of Agriculture
(HEW/FAO): Health, Education and Welfare/Food and Agriculture Organization
* Prepared as Package Directs

Food and Description	Measure or Quantity	Calories	Carbo-hydrates (grams)
KIPPER SNACKS (King David Brand) Norwegian	3¼-oz. can	195	0.
KIWIFRUIT (Calavo)	1 fruit (5-oz. edible portion)	45	9.0
KIX, cereal (General Mills)	1½ cups (1 oz.)	110	24.0
KNOCKWURST (See SAUSAGE)			
KOHLRABI (USDA):			
Raw:			
Whole	1 lb. (weighed with skin, without leaves)	96	21.9
Diced	1 cup (4.8 oz.)	40	9.1
Boiled:			
Drained	4 oz.	27	6.0
Drained	1 cup (5.5 oz.)	37	8.2
KOO KOOS (Dolly Madison)	1½-oz. piece	190	25.0
KOOL-AID (General Foods):			
Unsweetened (sugar to be added)	8 fl. oz.	98	25.0
Pre-sweetened:			
Regular, sugar sweetened:			
Apple or sunshine punch	8 fl. oz.	96	24.5
Cherry or grape	8 fl. oz.	89	22.8
Orange, raspberry or strawberry	8 fl. oz.	88	22.5
Tropical punch	8 fl. oz.	99	25.2
Dietetic, sugar-free:			
Cherry or grape	8 fl. oz.	2	.1
Sunshine punch	8 fl. oz.	4	.3
Tropical punch	8 fl. oz.	3	.3

Food and Description	Measure or Quantity	Calories	Carbo-hydrates (grams)
KUMQUAT, fresh (USDA):			
Whole	1 lb. (weighed with seeds)	274	72.1
Flesh & skin	4 oz.	74	19.4

(USDA): United States Department of Agriculture
(HEW/FAO): Health, Education and Welfare/Food and Agriculture
Organization
* Prepared as Package Directs

Food and Description	Measure or Quantity	Calories	Carbo-hydrates (grams)

L

LAKE HERRING, raw
(USDA):

Whole	1 lb.	226	0.
Meat only	4 oz.	109	0.

LAKE TROUT, raw (USDA):

Drawn	1 lb. (weighed with head, fins & bones)	282	0.
Meat only	4 oz.	191	0.

LAKE TROUT or SISCOWET,
raw (USDA):
Less than 6.5 lb.:

Whole	1 lb. (weighed whole)	404	0.
Meat only	4 oz.	273	0.

More than 6.5 lb.:

Whole	1 lb. (weighed whole)	856	0.
Meat only	4 oz.	594	0.

LAMB, choice grade (USDA):
Chop, broiled:
Loin. One 5-oz. chop
(weighed before cooking
with bone) will give you:

Lean & fat	2.8 oz.	280	0.
Lean only	2.3 oz.	122	0.

Rib. One 5-oz. chop
(weighed before cooking
with bone) with give you:

Lean & fat	2.9 oz.	334	0.
Lean only	2 oz.	118	0.
Fat, separable, cooked	1 oz.	201	0.

Food and Description	Measure or Quantity	Calories	Carbo-hydrates (grams)
Leg:			
Raw, lean & fat	1 lb. (weighed with bone)	845	0.
Roasted, lean & fat	4 oz.	316	0.
Roasted, lean only	4 oz.	211	0.
Shoulder:			
Raw, lean & fat	1 lb. (weighed with bone)	1092	0.
Roasted, lean & fat	4 oz.	383	0.
Roasted, lean only	4 oz.	232	0.
LAMB'S QUARTERS (USDA):			
Raw, trimmed	1 lb.	195	33.1
Boiled, drained	4 oz.	36	5.7
LARD:			
(USDA)	1 cup (6.2 oz.)	1849	0.
(USDA)	1 T. (.5 oz.)	117	0.
LASAGNA:			
Dry:			
(Buitoni) pre-cooked	1 sheet	48	8.9
(Mueller's)	2 oz.	210	42.0
Canned (Hormel) *Short Orders*	7½-oz. can	260	25.0
Frozen:			
(Armour) *Dinner Classics*	10-oz. meal	380	42.0
(Banquet) *Family Entree* with meat sauce	32-oz. pkg.	1980	234.0
(Blue Star) *Dining Lite:*			
Vegetable	11-oz. meal	284	37.6
Zucchini	11-oz. meal	278	32.6
(Buitoni):			
Alforno	8-oz. meal	327	31.8
Cheese, sorrentino	8-oz. serving	286	37.4
Individual portion	9-oz. serving	342	30.9
With meat sauce	5-oz. serving	212	23.4
(Celentano):			
Regular	½ of 16-oz. pkg.	320	30.0
Regular	¼ of 25-oz. pkg.	250	58.0
Primavera	11-oz. pkg.	300	36.0

(USDA): United States Department of Agriculture
(HEW/FAO):   Health, Education and Welfare/Food and Agriculture Organization
* Prepared as Package Directs

Food and Description	Measure or Quantity	Calories	Carbo-hydrates (grams)
(Conagra) *Light & Elegant*, Florentine	11¼-oz. entree	280	35.0
(Le Menu) vegetable	11-oz. dinner	360	32.0
(Stouffer's):			
Regular:			
Plain	10 ½-oz. meal	360	33.0
Vegetable	10 ½-oz. meal	420	23.0
Lean Cuisine:			
With meat sauce	10 ¼-oz. meal	270	24.0
Tuna, with spinach noodles & vegetables	9¾-oz. meal	270	29.0
Zucchini	11-oz. meal	260	28.0
(Swanson):			
4-compartment meal	13-oz. dinner	410	55.0
Hungry Man, with meat	18¾-oz. dinner	730	99.0
Main course entree, with meat	13¼-oz. entree	450	50.0
(Van de Kamp's):			
Beef & mushroom	11-oz. meal	430	30.0
Italian sausage	11-oz. meal	440	35.0
(Weight Watchers):			
Regular	12-oz. meal	360	40.0
Italian cheese	11-oz. serving	360	35.0
Mix (Golden Grain) Stir-N-Serv	⅓ of pkg.	150	28.0
LATKES, frozen (Empire Kosher):			
Mini	3 oz.	190	20.0
Rounds	2 ½ oz.	120	20.0
Triangles	3 oz.	140	12.0
LEEKS, raw (USDA):			
Whole	1 lb. (weighed untrimmed)	123	26.4
Trimmed	4 oz.	59	12.7
LEMON fresh (USDA):			
Whole	2⅛″ lemon (109 grams)	22	11.7
Peeled	2⅛″ lemon (74 grams)	20	6.1
LEMONADE:			
Canned:			
(Ardmore Farms)	6 fl. oz.	89	22.5
Country Time	6 fl. oz.	69	17.2

Food and Description	Measure or Quantity	Calories	Carbo-hydrates (grams)
(Johanna Farms) *Ssips*	8.45-fl.-oz. container	85	21.0
Chilled (Minute Maid) regular or pink	6 fl. oz.	79	18.0
*Frozen:			
Country Time, regular or pink	6 fl. oz.	68	18.0
Minute Maid,	6 fl. oz.	74	19.6
(Sunkist)	6 fl. oz.	92	24.2
*Mix:			
Regular:			
Country Time, regular or pink	6 fl. oz.	68	20.6
Kool-Aid, regular or pink:			
Sugar to be added	6 fl. oz.	73	18.8
Pre-sweetened with sugar	6 fl. oz.	65	16.3
Lemon Tree (Lipton)	6 fl. oz.	68	16.5
(Minute Maid)	6 fl. oz.	80	20.0
Dietetic:			
Crystal Light	6 fl. oz.	4	.2
Kool-Aid	6 fl. oz.	3	.2
LEMONADE BAR (Sunkist)	3 fl. oz. bar	68	17.6
LEMON JUICE:			
Fresh (USDA)	1 T. (.5 oz.)	4	1.2
Plastic container, *ReaLemon*	1 T. (.5 oz.)	3	.5
*Frozen (Sunkist) unsweetened	1 fl. oz.	7	2.2
*LEMON-LIMEADE DRINK, MIX:			
Regular:			
(Minute Maid)	6 fl. oz.	80	20.0
Country Time	6 fl. oz.	65	16.2
Dietetic, *Crystal Light*	6 fl. oz.	3	.1
LEMON PEEL, CANDIED (USDA)	1 oz.	90	22.9

(USDA): United States Department of Agriculture
(HEW/FAO):   Health, Education and Welfare/Food and Agriculture
            Organization
* Prepared as Package Directs

Food and Description	Measure or Quantity	Calories	Carbo-hydrates (grams)
LEMON & PEPPER			
SEASONING:			
(Lawry's)	1 tsp.	6	1.2
(McCormick)	1 tsp.	7	.8
LENTIL:			
Whole:			
Dry:			
(USDA)	½ lb.	771	136.3
(USDA)	1 cup (6.7 oz.)	649	114.8
(Sinsheimer)	1 oz.	95	17.0
Cooked (USDA) drained	½ cup (3.6 oz.)	107	19.5
Split (USDA) dry	½ lb.	782	140.2
LETTUCE (USDA):			
Bibb, untrimmed	1 lb.	47	8.4
Bibb, untrimmed	7.8-oz. head (4″ dia.)	23	4.1
Boston, untrimmed	1 lb.	47	8.4
Boston, untrimmed	7.8-oz. head (4″ dia.)	23	4.1
Butterhead varieties (See Bibb & Boston)			
Cos (See Romaine)			
Dark green (See Romaine)			
Grand Rapids	1 lb. (weighed untrimmed)	52	10.2
Great Lakes	1 lb. (weighed untrimmed)	56	12.5
Great Lakes, trimmed	1 lb. head (4¾″ dia.)	59	13.2
Iceberg:			
Untrimmed	1 lb.	56	12.5
Trimmed	1 lb. head (4¾″ dia.)	59	13.2
Leaves	1 cup (2.3 oz.)	9	1.9
Chopped	1 cup (2 oz.)	8	1.7
Chunks	1 cup (2.6 oz.)	10	2.1
Looseleaf varieties (See Salad Bowl)			
New York	1 lb. (weighed untrimmed)	56	12.5
New York	1 lb. head (4¾″ dia.)	59	13.2
Romaine:			
Untrimmed	1 lb.	52	10.2

Food and Description	Measure or Quantity	Calories	Carbo-hydrates (grams)
Trimmed, shredded & broken into pieces	½ cup	4	.8
Salad Bowl	1 lb. (weighed untrimmed)	52	10.2
Salad Bowl	2 large leaves (1.8 oz.)	9	1.8
Simpson	1 lb. (weighed untrimmed)	52	10.2
Simpson	2 large leaves (1.8 oz.)	9	1.8
White Paris (See Romaine)			
LIFE, cereal (Quaker) regular or cinnamon	⅔ cup (1 oz.)	105	19.7
LIL' ANGELS (Hostess)	1-oz. piece	78	14.2
LIME, fresh (USDA) peeled fruit	2″ dia. lime (1.8 oz.)	15	4.9
*LIMEADE, frozen (Minute Maid)	6 fl. oz.	75	20.1
LIME JUICE, *ReaLime*	1 T.	2	.5
LINGCOD, raw (USDA): Whole	1 lb. (weighed whole)	130	0.
Meat only	34 oz.	95	0.
LINGUINI WITH CLAM SAUCE, frozen (Stouffer's)	10½-oz. pkg.	285	36.0
LIQUEUR (See individual kinds such as **CREME DE BANANA, PEACH LIQUEUR,** etc.)			
LIQUOR (See **DISTILLED LIQUOR**)			

(USDA): United States Department of Agriculture
(HEW/FAO): Health, Education and Welfare/Food and Agriculture Organization
* Prepared as Package Directs

Food and Description	Measure or Quantity	Calories	Carbo-hydrates (grams)
LITCHI NUT (USDA):			
Fresh:			
Whole	4 oz. (weighed in shell with seeds)	44	11.2
Flesh only	4 oz.	73	18.6
Dried:			
Whole	4 oz. (weighed in shell with seeds)	145	36.9
Flesh	2 oz.	157	40.1
LIVER:			
Beef:			
(USDA):			
Raw	1 lb.	635	24.0
Fried	4 oz.	260	6.0
(Swift) packaged, True-Tender, sliced, cooked	⅓ of 1-lb. pkg.	141	3.1
Calf (USDA):			
Raw	1 lb.	635	18.6
Fried	4 oz.	296	4.5
Chicken:			
Raw	1 lb.	585	13.2
Simmered	4 oz.	187	3.5
Goose, raw (USDA)	1 lb.	826	24.5
Hog (USDA):			
Raw	1 lb.	594	11.8
Fried	4 oz.	273	2.8
Lamb (USDA):			
Raw	1 lb.	617	13
LIVERWURST SPREAD,			
canned:			
(Hormel)	1 oz.	70	0.
(Underwood)	2.4 oz.	220	3.0
LOBSTER:			
Raw (USDA):			
Whole	1 lb. (weighed whole	107	.6
Meat only	4-oz.	103	.6
Cooked, meat only (USDA)	4-oz.	108	.3
Canned (USDA) meat only	4-oz.	108	.3
Frozen, South African rock lobster	2-oz. tail	65	.1

Food and Description	Measure or Quantity	Calories	Carbo- hydrates (grams)
LOBSTER NEWBURG:			
Home recipe (USDA)	4 oz.	220	5.8
Frozen (Stouffer's)	6½ oz.	380	9.0
LOBSTER PASTE, canned			
(USDA)	1 oz.	51	.4
LOBSTER SALAD, home			
recipe (USDA)	4 oz.	125	2.6
LOGANBERRY (USDA):			
Fresh:			
Untrimmed	1 lb. (weighed with caps)	267	64.2
Trimmed	1 cup (5.1 oz.)	89	21.5
Canned, solids & liq.:			
Extra heavy syrup	4 oz.	101	25.2
Heavy syrup	4 oz.	101	25.2
Juice pack	4 oz.	61	14.4
Light syrup	4 oz.	79	19.5
Water pack	4 oz.	45	10.7
LONGAN (USDA):			
Fresh:			
Whole	1 lb. (weighed with shell & seeds)	147	38.0
Flesh only	4 oz.	69	17.9
Dried:			
Whole	1 lb. (weighed with shell & seeds)	467	120.8
Flesh only	4 oz.	324	83.9
LONG ISLAND TEA COCKTAIL (Mr. Boston)			
12½% alcohol	3 fl. oz.	93	9.0
LONG JOHN SILVER'S:			
Catfish:			
Dinner	13.2-oz. serving	860	90.0

(USDA): United States Department of Agriculture
(HEW/FAO):   Health, Education and Welfare/Food and Agriculture
Organization
* Prepared as Package Directs

Food and Description	Measure or Quantity	Calories	Carbo-hydrates (grams)
Fillet	2½-oz. piece	180	10.0
Catsup	.4-oz. packet	15	3.0
Chicken plank:			
Dinner:			
3-piece	13-oz. serving	830	88.0
4-piece	14.6-oz. serving	940	94.0
Single piece	1.6-oz. piece	110	6.0
Children's meals:			
Chicken planks	7.1-oz. serving	510	52.0
Fish	6½-oz. serving	440	49.0
Fish & chicken planks	8.1-oz. serving	550	55.0
Chowder, clam, with cod	7-oz. serving	140	10.0
Clam:			
Breaded	2.3-oz. serving	240	26.0
Dinner	12.8-oz. serving	980	122.0
Cod, entree, broiled	5.4-oz. serving	160	2.0
Cole slaw, drained on fork	3.4-oz. serving	140	20.0
Corn on the cob, with whirl	6.6-oz. ear	270	38.0
Cracker, *Club*	.2-oz. package	35	5.0
Fish, battered	2.6-oz. piece	150	9.0
Fish dinner, 3-piece	16.1-oz. serving	960	97.0
Fish dinner, home-style:			
3-piece	13.1-oz. serving	880	97.0
4-piece	14.8-oz. serving	1,010	106.0
6-piece	18.1-oz. serving	1,260	124.0
Fish & fryes, entree:			
2-piece	10-oz. serving	660	68.0
3-piece	12.6-oz. serving	810	77.0
Fish, homestyle	1.6-oz. piece	125	9.0
Fish & more	13.4-oz. entree	800	88.0
Fish sandwich, homestyle	6.9-oz. serving	510	58.0
Fish sandwich platter, homestyle	13.4-oz. serving	870	108.0
Flounder, broiled	5.1-oz. piece	180	0.
Gumbo, with cod & shrimp bobs	7-oz. serving	110	4.0
Halibut steak, broiled	4.1-oz. serving	140	0.
Hushpuppie	.8-oz. piece	70	10.0
Pie:			
Lemon meringue	4.2-oz. slice	260	47.0
Pecan	4.4-oz. slice	530	70.0
Potato:			
Baked, without topping	7.1-oz. serving	150	33.0
Fryes	3-oz. serving	220	30.0
Rice pilaf	3-oz. serving	150	32.0
Roll, dinner, plain	.9-oz. piece	70	12.0

Food and Description	Measure or Quantity	Calories	Carbo-hydrates (grams)
Salad:			
Garden	8.7-oz. serving	170	13.0
Ocean chef	11.3-oz. serving	250	19.0
Seafood, entree	11.9-oz. serving	270	36.0
Side	4.3-oz. serving	20	5.0
Salad dressing:			
Regular:			
Bleu cheese	1.5-oz. packet	120	22.0
Ranch	1.5-oz. packet	140	27.0
Sea salad	1.6-oz. packet	140	20.0
Dietetic, Italian	1.6-oz. packet	18	2.0
Salmon, broiled	4.4-oz. piece	180	0.
Sauce:			
Honey mustard	1.2-oz. packet	60	13.0
Seafood	1.2-oz. packet	45	8.0
Sweet & sour	1.2-oz. packet	60	13.0
Tartar	1-oz. packet	80	13.0
Seafood platter	14.1-oz. entree	970	109.0
Shrimp, battered	.5-oz. piece	40	2.0
Shrimp, breaded	2.2-oz. serving	190	20.0
Shrimp dinner, battered:			
6-piece	11.1-oz. serving	740	82.0
9-piece	12.6-oz. serving	860	88.0
Shrimp feast, breaded:			
13-piece	12.6-oz. serving	880	110.0
21-piece	14.8-oz. serving	1070	130.0
Shrimp, fish & chicken dinner	13.4-oz. dinner	840	89.0
Shrimp & fish dinner	12.3-oz. dinner	770	85.0
Vegetables, mixed	4-oz. serving	60	9.0
Vinegar, malt	.4-oz. packet	2	0.
LOQUAT, fresh, flesh only (USDA)	2 oz.	27	7.0
LUCKY CHARMS, cereal (General Mills)	1 cup (1 oz.)	110	24.0
LUNCHEON MEAT (See also individual listings such as **BOLOGNA, HAM,** etc.):			

(USDA): United States Department of Agriculture
(HEW/FAO):   Health, Education and Welfare/Food and Agriculture
                       Organization
* Prepared as Package Directs

Food and Description	Measure or Quantity	Calories	Carbo-hydrates (grams)
All meat (Oscar Mayer)	1-oz. slice	95	.7
Banquet loaf (Eckrich)	¾-oz. slice	50	1.0
Bar-B-Que Loaf:			
(Eckrich)	1-oz. slice	35	1.0
(Oscar Mayer)	1-oz. slice	46	1.7
Beef, jellied (Hormel) loaf	1 slice	45	0.
Gourmet loaf (Eckrich):			
Regular	1-oz. slice	35	2.0
Smorgas Pac	¾-oz. slice	25	2.0
Ham & cheese (See **HAM & CHEESE**)			
Honey loaf:			
(Eckrich):			
Regular	1-oz. slice	40	3.0
Smorgas Pac	¾-oz. slice	30	2.0
Smorgas Pac	1-oz. slice	35	3.0
(Hormel)	1 slice	45	.5
(Oscar Mayer)	1-oz. slice	34	1.1
Iowa Brand (Hormel)	1 slice	45	0.
Liver cheese (Oscar Mayer)	1.3-oz. slice	114	.5
Liver loaf (Hormel)	1 slice	80	6.5
Macaroni-cheese loaf (Eckrich)	1-oz. slice	70	3.0
Meat loaf (USDA)	1-oz. serving	57	.9
New England Brand sliced sausage:			
(Eckrich)	1-oz. slice	35	1.0
(Hormel) *Light & Lean*	1 slice	45	0.
(Oscar Mayer)	.8-oz. slice	29	.4
Old fashioned loaf:			
(Eckrich):			
Regular	1-oz. slice	70	3.0
Smorgas Pac	¾-oz. slice	50	2.0
(Oscar Mayer)	1-oz. slice	62	2.3
Olive loaf:			
(Eckrich)	1-oz. slice	80	2.0
(Hormel)	1 slice	55	2.5
(Oscar Mayer)	1-oz. slice	60	3.1
Peppered loaf:			
(Eckrich)	1-oz. slice	40	1.0
(Oscar Mayer)	1-oz. slice	39	1.3
Pickle loaf:			
(Eckrich):			
Regular	1-oz. slice	80	2.0
Smorgas Pac	¾-oz. slice	50	1.0
(Hormel) *Light & Lean*	1 slice	50	1.5

Food and Description	Measure or Quantity	Calories	Carbo-hydrates (grams)
(Ohse)	1 oz.	60	2.0
Pickle & pimiento loaf (Oscar Mayer)	1-oz. slice	62	3.7
Picnic loaf (Oscar Mayer)	1-oz. slice	60	1.2
Spiced (Hormel)	1 slice	75	.5
LUNG, raw (USDA):			
Beef	1 lb.	435	0.
Calf	1 lb.	481	0.
Lamb	1 lb.	467	0.

(USDA): United States Department of Agriculture
(HEW/FAO):   Health, Education and Welfare/Food and Agriculture
Organization
* Prepared as Package Directs

Food and Description	Measure or Quantity	Calories	Carbo-hydrates (grams)

M

MACADAMIA NUT (Royal
Hawaiian)   1 oz.   197   4.5

MACARONI:
Dry:
  (USDA)   1 oz.   105   21.3
  Spinach (Creamette) ribbons 1 oz.   105   21.0
  Whole wheat (Pritikin)   1 oz.   110   18.0
Cooked (USDA):
  8-10 minutes, firm   4 oz.   168   34.1
  14-20 minutes, tender   4 oz.   126   26.1
Canned (Franco-American)
PizzOs, in pizza sauce   7½-oz. can   170   35.0

MACARONI & BEEF:
Canned (Franco-American)
BeefyO's, in tomato sauce   7½-oz. can   220   30.0
Frozen:
  (Morton)   10-oz. meal   245   30.4
  (Stouffer's) & tomatoes   11½-oz. meal   340   30.0
  (Swanson) 3-compartment   12-oz. dinner   360   46.0

MACARONI & CHEESE:
Frozen:
  (Banquet):
    Casserole   8-oz. pkg.   344   36.0
    Family Entree 2-lb. pkg.   920   124.0
    Family Favorites 9-oz. meal   334   37.0
  (Birds Eye):
    Classics   ½ of 10-oz. pkg.   236   24.0
    For One   5¾-oz. pkg.   304   27.0
  (Celentano) baked   ½ of 12-oz. pkg.   290   29.0
  (Conagra) *Light & Elegant* 9-oz. entree   300   38.0
  (Morton):
    Casserole   20-oz. casserole   648   91.2
    Dinner   11-oz. dinner   278   45.8

Food and Description	Measure or Quantity	Calories	Carbo-hydrates (grams)
Family Meal	2-lb. pkg.	1043	143.7
(Stouffer's)	6-oz. serving	250	22.0
(Swanson):			
Dinner, 3-compartment	12¼-oz. dinner	380	46.0
Entree	12-oz. entree	380	45.0
Mix:			
(Golden Grain) deluxe	¼ of 7¼-oz. pkg.	190	35.0
*(Kraft):			
Regular, plain or spiral	¼ of box	190	36.0
Velveeta	¼ of pkg.	270	32.0
MACARONI & CHEESE LOAF, packaged (Ohse)	1 oz.	60	4.0
MACARONI & CHEESE PIE, frozen (Swanson)	7-oz. pie	210	26.0
***MACARONI SALAD,** mix (Betty Crocker) creamy	⅙ of pkg.	200	20.0
MACE (French's)	1 tsp.	10	.8
MACKEREL (USDA):			
Atlantic:			
Raw:			
Whole	1 lb. (weighed whole)	468	0.
Meat only	4 oz.	217	0.
Broiled with butter	4 oz.	268	0.
Canned, solids & liq.		208	0.
Pacific:			
Raw:			
Dressed	1 lb. (weighed with bones & skin)	519	0.
Meat only	4 oz.	180	0.
Canned, solids & liq.	4 oz.	204	0.
Salted	4 oz.	346	0.
Smoked	4 oz.	248	0.

(USDA): United States Department of Agriculture
(HEW/FAO): Health, Education and Welfare/Food and Agriculture Organization
* Prepared as Package Directs

Food and Description	Measure or Quantity	Calories	Carbo-hydrates (grams)
MADEIRA WINE (Leacock) 19% alcohol	3 fl. oz.	120	6.3
MAGIC SHELL (Smucker's)	1 T. (17 grams)	95	8.0
MALT, dry (USDA)	1 oz.	104	21.9
MALTED MILK MIX (Carnation):			
Chocolate	3 heaping tsps. (.7 oz.)	85	18.0
Natural	3 heaping tsps. (.7 oz.)	88	15.8
MALT LIQUOR:			
Colt 45	12 fl. oz.	156	11.1
Kingsbury, no alcohol	12 fl. oz.	60	12.8
Mickey's	12 fl. oz.	156	11.1
Schlitz	12 fl. oz.	88	7.2
MALT-O-MEAL, cereal:			
Regular	1 T. (.3 oz.)	33	7.3
Chocolate flavored	1 T. (.3 oz.)	33	7.0
MAMEY or MAMMEE APPLE, fresh (USDA)	1 lb. (weighed with skin & seeds)	143	35.2
MANDARIN ORANGE (See TANGERINE)			
MANGO, fresh (USDA):			
Whole	1 lb. (weighed with seeds & skin)	201	51.1
Flesh only, diced or sliced	½ cup	54	13.8
MANHATTAN COCKTAIL (Mr. Boston) 20% alcohol	3 fl. oz.	123	12.3
MANICOTTI, frozen: (Buitoni):			
Plain	5½-oz. serving	310	26.0
Florentine	1 piece (2½ oz.)	142	14.3

Food and Description	Measure or Quantity	Calories	Carbo- hydrates (grams)
(Celentano):			
Plain	2 pieces (7 oz.)	380	34.0
With sauce	2 pieces (8 oz.)	300	22.0
MANWICH, sauce			
(Hunt's):			
Original	2½ oz.	40	10.0
Mexican	2½ oz.	35	9.0
MAPLE SYRUP (See **SYRUP**, Maple)			
MARGARINE, salted or unsalted:			
Regular:			
(USDA)	1 lb.	3266	1.8
(USDA)	1 cup (8 oz.)	1633	.9
(Autumn) soft or stick	1 T.	80	0.
(Blue Bonnet) soft or stick	1 T. (.5 oz.)	90	0.
(Chiffon):			
Soft	1 T.	90	0.
Stick	1 T.	100	0.
(Fleischmann's) soft or stick	1 T. (.5 oz.)	100	0.
(Golden Mist)	1 T.	100	0.
(Holiday)	1 T. (.5 oz.)	102	0.
(Imperial) soft or stick	1 T. (.5 oz.)		
(Mazola)	1 T.	100	0.
(Parkay)	1 T.	100	0.
(Promise) soft or stick	1 T.	90	Tr.
Whipped:			
(Blue Bonnet)	1 T. (9 grams)	70	0.
(Chiffon)	1 T.	70	0.
(Fleischmann's)	1 T.	70	0.
(Imperial)	1 T. (9 grams)	45	0.
(Parkay) cup	1 T.	67	Tr.
MARGARITA COCKTAIL,			
(Mr. Boston) 12½% alcohol:			
Regular	3 fl. oz.	105	10.8
Strawberry	3 fl. oz.	138	18.9

Food and Description	Measure or Quantity	Calories	Carbo-hydrates (grams)
MARINADE MIX:			
Chicken (Adolph's)	1-oz. packet	64	14.4
Meat:			
(Adolph's)	.8-oz. pkg.	38	8.5
(Durkee)	1-oz. pkg.	47	9.0
(French's)	1-oz. pkg.	80	16.0
(Kikkoman)	1-oz. pkg.	64	12.5
MARJORAM (French's)	1 tsp. (1.2 grams)	4	.8
MARMALADE:			
Sweetened:			
(USDA)	1 T. (.7 oz.)	51	14.0
(Keiller)	1 T.	60	15.0
(Smucker's)	1 T. (.7 oz.)	53	13.5
Dietetic:			
(Estee; Louis Sherry)	1 T. (.6 oz.)	6	0.
(Featherweight)	1 T.	16	4.0
(S&W) *Nutradiet*, red label	1 T.	12	3.0
MARSHMALLOW (See **CANDY, GENERIC, REGULAR**)			
MARSHMALLOW FLUFF	1 heaping tsp.	59	14.4
MARSHMALLOW KRISPIES, cereal (Kellogg's)	1¼ cups (1.3 oz.)	140	32.0
MARTINI COCKTAIL (Mr. Boston) 20% alcohol:			
Gin, extra dry	3 fl. oz.	99	Tr.
Vodka	3 fl. oz.	102	Tr.
MASA HARINA (Quaker)	⅓ cup (1.3 oz.)	237	27.4
MASA TRIGO (Quaker)	⅓ cup (1.3 oz.)	149	24.7
MATZO:			
(Goodman's):			
Diet-10s	1 sq.	109	23.0
Unsalted	1 matzo (1 oz.)	109	23.0
(Horowitz-Margareten) unsalted	1 matzo	135	28.2
(Manischewitz):			

Food and Description	Measure or Quantity	Calories	Carbo-hydrates (grams)
Regular:			
Plain	1 piece	110	24.0
American	1-oz. piece	115	22.0
Egg	1 piece	108	26.6
Egg & onion	1 piece	112	23.0
Miniature	1 piece	9	20.0
Tam Tams	1 piece	15	DNA
Wheat	1 piece	9	1.8
Dietetic:			
Tam Tams	1 piece	14	DNA
Thins	1 piece	91	19.0
MATZO MEAL (Manischewitz)	½ cup	267	DNA
MAYONNAISE:			
Real:			
(Bama)	1 T.	100	0.
(Bennett's)	1 T.	110	1.0
Blue Plate (Luzianne)	1 T.	100	1.0
Hellmann's (Best Foods)	1 T. (.5 oz.)	103	.1
(Kraft)	1 T.	100	0.
(Rokeach)	1 T.	100	0.
Imitation or dietetic:			
Hellmann's Lite (Best Foods)	1 T.	50	1.0
Blue Plate (Luzianne)	1 T.	50	1.0
(Estee)	1 T. (.5 oz.)	45	0.
(Kraft)	1 T.	45	1.0
MAYPO, cereal:			
30-second	¼ cup (.8 oz.)	89	16.4
Vermont style	¼ cup (1.1 oz.)	121	22.0
McDONALD'S:			
Apple pie	2.9-oz. serving	260	30.0
Bacon bits	.1 oz.	16	.1
Big Mac	1 hamburger	560	42.5
Biscuit:			
Plain, with spread	2.6-oz. piece	260	31.9
With bacon, egg & cheese	5.5-oz. piece	440	33.3
With sausage	4.3-oz. piece	440	31.9
With sausage & egg	6.2-oz. piece	520	32.6

(USDA): United States Department of Agriculture
(HEW/FAO):   Health, Education and Welfare/Food and Agriculture
              Organization
* Prepared as Package Directs

Food and Description	Measure or Quantity	Calories	Carbo-hydrates (grams)
Cheeseburger	1 cheeseburger	310	31.2
Chicken McNuggets	1 serving (4 oz.)	290	16.5
Chicken McNuggets Sauce:			
Barbecue	1.1-oz. serving	50	12.1
Honey	.5-oz. serving	45	11.5
Hot mustard	1-oz. serving	70	8.2
Sweet & sour	1.1-oz. serving	60	13.8
Cookies:			
Chocolate chip	1 package	330	41.9
McDonaldland	1 package	290	47.1
Danish:			
Apple	4-oz. piece	390	51.2
Cheese, iced	3.9-oz. piece	390	42.3
Cinnamon raisin	3.9-oz. piece	440	57.5
Raspberry	4.1-oz. piece	410	61.5
Egg McMuffin	1 serving	290	28.1
Egg, scrambled	1 serving	140	1.2
English muffin, with butter	1 muffin	170	26.7
Filet-O-Fish	1 sandwich	440	37.9
Grapefruit juice	6 fl. oz.	80	17.9
Hamburger	1 hamburger	260	30.6
Hot cakes with butter & syrup	1 serving	410	74.4
McD.L.T. sandwich	8¼-oz. serving	580	36.0
Milk shake:			
Chocolate	10.7 fl. oz.	390	62.6
Strawberry	10.7 fl. oz.	350	55.7
Vanilla	10.7 fl. oz.	380	63.2
Orange juice	6 fl. oz.	80	18.5
Potato:			
Fried	1 reg. order	220	26.6
Hash browns	1.9-oz. piece	130	14.9
Quarter Pounder:			
Plain	5.8-oz. serving	410	34.1
With cheese	6.8-oz. serving	520	35.1
Salad:			
Chef	10-oz. serving	230	7.5
Chicken, chunky	8.6-oz. serving	140	5.0
Garden	7.5-oz. serving	110	6.2
Side	4.1-oz. serving	60	3.3
Salad dressing:			
Regular:			
Bleu cheese	.5-oz. serving	70	1.2
Caesar	.5-oz. serving	60	.6
French	.5-oz. serving	58	2.7
Peppercorn	.5-oz. serving	80	.5

Food and Description	Measure or Quantity	Calories	Carbo-hydrates (grams)
Ranch	.5-oz. serving	83	1.3
1000 Island	.5-oz. serving	78	2.4
Dietetic:			
Ranch	.5-oz. serving	40	5.2
Vinaigrette	.5-oz. serving	15	2.0
Sausage	1.9-oz. piece	180	0.
Sausage McMuffin:			
Plain	4.1-oz. piece	370	27.3
With egg	5.8-oz. piece	440	27.9
Soft Drink:			
Sweetened:			
*Coca-Cola,*classic	12 fl. oz.	144	38.0
*Coca-Cola,*classic	16 fl. oz.	190	50.0
*Coca-Cola,*classic	22 fl. oz.	264	70.0
Orange drink	12 fl. oz.	133	33.0
Orange drink	16 fl. oz.	177	44.0
Orange drink	22 fl. oz.	243	60.0
Sprite	12 fl. oz.	144	36.0
Sprite	16 fl. oz.	190	48.0
Sprite	22 fl. oz.	264	66.0
Dietetic, *Coke*	12 fl. oz.	1	.3
Sundae:			
Caramel	6.1-oz. sundae	340	58.4
Hot fudge	6-oz. sundae	310	49.6
Strawberry	6-oz. sundae	280	48.3
Vanilla soft-serve, with cone	3 fl. oz.	140	21.9
MEATBALL DINNER OR ENTREE, frozen: (Green Giant) twin pouch, sweet & sour, with rice & vegetables	9.4-oz. entree	370	57.0
(Swanson) with brown gravy	8½-oz. meal	290	19.0
MEATBALL SEASONING MIX:			
*(Durkee) Italian	1 cup	619	4.5
(French's)	¼ of 1.5-oz. pkg.	35	7.0
MEATBALL STEW:			
Canned (Hormel) *Dinty Moore*	⅓ of 24-oz. can	240	15.0

(USDA): United States Department of Agriculture
(HEW/FAO):   Health, Education and Welfare/Food and Agriculture
              Organization
* Prepared as Package Directs

Food and Description	Measure or Quantity	Calories	Carbo-hydrates (grams)
Frozen (Stouffer's) *Lean Cuisine*	10-oz. meal	250	20.0
MEATBALL, SWEDISH, frozen:			
(Armour) *Dinner Classics*	11½-oz. meal	480	33.0
(Stouffer's) with parsley noodles	11-oz. meal	480	37.0
MEAT LOAF DINNER, frozen:			
(Banquet):			
Dinner, American Favorites	11-oz. dinner	395	24.0
Entree For One	5-oz. pkg.	240	12.0
(Morton)	10-oz. dinner	306	26.0
(Swanson)			
Dinner, 4-compartment	11-oz. dinner	500	48.0
Entree, with tomato sauce	9-oz. entree	310	28.0
MEAT LOAF SEASONING MIX:			
(Bell's)	4½-oz. serving	300	14.0
(Contadina)	3¾-oz. pkg.	360	72.4
(French's)	1.5-oz. pkg.	160	40.0
MEAT, POTTED:			
(Hormel)	1 T.	30	0.
(Libby's)	1-oz. serving	55	0.
MEAT TENDERIZER:			
Regular (Adolph's; McCormick)	1 tsp.	2	.5
Seasoned (McCormick)	1 tsp.	5	.8
MELBA TOAST, salted (Old London):			
Garlic, onion or white rounds	1 piece	10	1.8
Pumpernickel, rye, wheat or white	1 piece	17	3.4
Sesame, flat	1 piece	18	3.0
MELON (See individual kinds)			
MELON BALLS, in syrup, frozen (USDA)	½ cup (4.1 oz.)	72	18.2

Food and Description	Measure or Quantity	Calories	Carbo-hydrates (grams)
MENHADEN, Atlantic, canned			
(USDA) solids & liq.	4 oz.	195	0.
MENUDO, canned (Hormel)			
Casa Grande	7½-oz. can	90	10.0
MERLOT WINE (Louis M.			
Martini) 12½% alcohol	3 fl. oz.	63	TR.
MEXICALI DOGS, frozen			
(Hormel)	5-oz. serving	400	41.0
MEXICAN DINNER, frozen:			
(Banquet):			
Regular	12-oz. dinner	483	62.0
Combination	12-oz. dinner	518	72.0
Extra Helping	21¼-oz. dinner	777	105.0
(Morton)	10-oz. dinner	294	43.0
(Patio):			
Regular	13¼-oz. meal	533	63.0
Combination	13-oz. meal	468	58.0
Fiesta	12¼-oz. meal	461	55.0
(Swanson):			
4-course	16-oz. dinner	580	67.0
Hungry Man	22-oz. dinner	920	99.0
(Van de Kamp's)	11½-oz. dinner	420	45.0
MILK BREAK BARS			
(Pillsbury):			
Chocolate	1 bar	230	22.0
Chocolate mint	1 bar	230	21.0
Natural	1 bar	230	21.0
Peanut butter	1 bar	220	21.0
MILK, CONDENSED,			
sweetened, canned:			
(USDA)	1 T. (.7 oz.)	61	10.4
(Carnation)	1 fl. oz.	123	20.8
Eagle Brand (Borden)	1 T. (.7 oz.)	60	10.4

(USDA): United States Department of Agriculture
(HEW/FAO): Health, Education and Welfare/Food and Agriculture
    Organization
* Prepared as Package Directs

Food and Description	Measure or Quantity	Calories	Carbo-hydrates (grams)
(Milnot) *Dairy Sweet*	1 fl. oz. (1.3 oz.)	119	19.3
MILK, DRY:			
Whole (USDA) packed cup	1 cup (5.1 oz.)	728	55.4
*Nonfat, instant:			
(USDA)	8 fl. oz.	82	10.8
(Alba):			
Regular	8 fl. oz.	81	11.6
Chocolate flavor	8 fl. oz.	80	12.9
(Carnation)	8 fl. oz.	80	12.0
(Pet)	1 cup	80	12.0
(Sanalac)	1 cup	80	11.0
MILK, EVAPORATED:			
Regular:			
(Carnation)	½ cup (4 fl. oz.)	170	12.2
(Pet)	½ cup (4 fl. oz.)	170	12.0
Filled, *Dairymate*	½ cup	150	12.0
Low fat (Carnation)	½ cup	110	12.0
Skimmed:			
(Carnation)	½ cup	100	14.0
Pet 99	½ cup	100	14.0
MILK, FRESH:			
Buttermilk (Friendship) low fat	1 cup	120	12.0
Chocolate:			
(Borden) *Dutch Blend,*			
lowfat	1 cup	180	25.0
(Hershey's)	1 cup	190	29.0
(Johanna):			
Regular	1 cup	200	26.0
Lowfat	1 cup	150	26.0
(Nestlé) *Quik*	1 cup	220	30.0
Lowfat:			
(Borden):			
1% milkfat	1 cup	100	11.0
2% milkfat, *Hi-Protein*			
Brand	1 cup	140	13.0
(Johanna):			
Regular:			
1% lowfat, protein			
fortified	1 cup	110	13.0
2% lowfat, *Mighty Milk*	1 cup	140	13.0
Buttermilk	1 cup	120	11.0

Food and Description	Measure or Quantity	Calories	Carbo-hydrates (grams)
Nonfat (Johanna)	1 cup	80	11.0
Skim (USDA)	1 cup	88	12.5
Whole (USDA)	1 cup	159	12.0
MILK, GOAT (USDA) whole	1 cup	163	11.2
MILK, HUMAN (USDA)	1 oz. (by wt.)	22	2.7
MILNOT	½ cup	151	12.2
MINERAL WATER (See also **VICHY WATER**) (Schwepps)	6 fl. oz.	0	0.
MINI-WHEATS, cereal (Kellogg's)	1 biscuit	28	6.0
MINT, LEAVES, raw, trimmed (HEW/FAO)	½ oz.	4	.8
MIRACLE WHIP (See **SALAD DRESSING**)			
MOLASSES:			
Barbados (USDA)	1 T. (.7 oz.)	51	13.3
Blackstrap (USDA)	1 T. (.7 oz.)	40	10.4
Dark (Brer Rabbit)	1 T. (.7 oz.)	33	10.6
Light (USDA)	1 T. (.7 oz.)	48	12.4
Medium (USDA)	1 T.	44	11.4
Unsulphured (Grandma's)	1 T.	60	15.0
MORTADELLA, sausage (USDA)	1 oz.	89	.2
MOST, cereal (Kellogg's)	½ cup (1 oz.)	100	22.0
MOSTACCIOLI, frozen (Banquet) *Buffet Supper,* & sauce	2-lb. pkg.	1004	36.0

(USDA): United States Department of Agriculture
(HEW/FAO): Health, Education and Welfare/Food and Agriculture Organization
* Prepared as Package Directs

Food and Description	Measure or Quantity	Calories	Carbo-hydrates (grams)
MOUSSE, canned, dietetic (Featherweight) chocolate	½ cup (4 oz.)	100	22.0
MÜESLIX, cereal (Kellogg's):			
Bran	½ cup (1.4 oz.)	130	31.0
Five grain	½ cup (1.4 oz.)	150	31.0
MUFFIN:			
Apple (Pepperidge Farm)	1 muffin	170	23.0
Blueberry:			
Home recipe (USDA)	1.4-oz. muffin	112	16.8
(Hostess)	1¾-oz. muffin	127	21.9
(Morton):			
Regular	1.6-oz. muffin	120	23.0
Rounds	1.5-oz. muffin	110	21.0
(Pepperidge Farm)	1.9-oz. muffin	180	27.0
Bran:			
Home recipe (USDA)	1.4-oz. muffin	104	17.2
(Pepperidge Farm)	1 muffin	180	28.0
Carrot walnut (Pepperidge Farm)	1 muffin	170	27.0
Chocolate chip (Pepperidge Farm)	1 muffin	200	28.0
Cinnamon swirl (Pepperidge Farm)	1 muffin	190	30.0
Corn:			
Home recipe (USDA) prepared with whole-ground cornmeal	1.4-oz. muffin	115	17.0
(Morton)	1.7-oz. muffin	130	17.0
(Pepperidge Farm)	1.9-oz. muffin	180	27.0
English:			
Millbrook (Interstate Brands):			
Regular	2-oz. muffin	130	23.0
Cinnamon raisin	2-oz. muffin	130	24.0
Sourdough	2-oz. muffin	120	23.0
Whole wheat	2-oz. muffin	120	23.0
(Pepperidge Farm):			
Plain	2-oz. muffin	140	26.0
Cinnamon raisin	2-oz. muffin	150	28.0
(Pritikin)	2.3-oz. muffin	150	28.0
Roman Meal	2.3-oz. muffin	150	29.8
Sunmaid (Interstate Brands) raisin	2.3-oz. muffin	180	33.0

Food and Description	Measure or Quantity	Calories	Carbo-hydrates (grams)
(Thomas'):			
Regular or frozen	2-oz. muffin	133	25.7
Honey wheat	2-oz. muffin	135	27.0
Raisin	2.2-oz. muffin	153	30.4
Sourdough	2-oz. muffin	133	25.8
Plain (USDA) home recipe	1.4-oz. muffin	118	16.9
Raisin:			
(Arnold)	2½-oz. muffin	170	35.0
(Wonder)	2-oz. muffin	150	27.8
Sourdough (Wonder)	2-oz. muffin	131	25.6
MUFFIN MIX:			
*Apple cinnamon (Betty Crocker)	1 muffin	120	19.0
*Banana nut (Betty Crocker)	1/12 of pkg.	150	21.0
Blueberry:			
*(Betty Crocker) wild	1 muffin	120	18.0
(Duncan Hines)	1/12 of pkg.	99	17.0
Bran:			
(Duncan Hines)	1/12 of pkg.	97	16.3
(Elam's) natural	1 T. (.25 oz.)	23	5.3
*Carrot nut (Betty Crocker)	1/12 of pkg.	150	22.0
*Cherry (Betty Crocker)	1/12 of pkg.	120	18.0
*Chocolate chip (Betty Crocker)	1/12 of pkg.	150	22.0
*Cinnamon streusel (Betty Crocker)	1/10 of pkg.	200	27.0
Corn:			
*(Dromedary)	1 muffin	120	20.0
*(Flako)	1 muffin	140	23.0
*Oatmeal raisin (Betty Crocker)	1/12 of pkg.	140	22.0
MULLIGAN STEW, canned, *Dinty Moore, Short Orders,* (Hormel)	7½-oz. can	230	14.0
MUSCATEL WINE (Gallo) 14% alcohol	3 fl. oz.	86	7.9

(USDA): United States Department of Agriculture
(HEW/FAO): Health, Education and Welfare/Food and Agriculture Organization
* Prepared as Package Directs

Food and Description	Measure or Quantity	Calories	Carbo- hydrates (grams)
MUSHROOM:			
Raw (USDA):			
Whole	½ lb. (weighed untrimmed)	62	9.7
Trimmed, sliced	½ cup (1.2 oz.)	10	1.5
Canned (Green Giant) solids & liq., whole or sliced,	¼ cup	12	2.0
Frozen (Birds Eye)	⅓ of 8-oz. pkg.	19	4.0
MUSHROOM, CHINESE, dried (HEW/FAO):			
Dry	1 oz.	81	18.9
Soaked, drained	1 oz.	12	2.4
MUSKELLUNGE, raw (USDA):			
Whole	1 lb. (weighed whole)	242	0.
Meat only	4 oz.	234	0.
MUSKMELON (See CANTALOUPE, CASABA or HONEYDEW)			
MUSKRAT, roasted (USDA)	4 oz.	174	0.
MUSSEL (USDA):			
Atlantic & Pacific, raw:			
In Shell	1 lb. (weighed in shell)	153	7.2
Meat only	4 oz.	108	3.7
Pacific, canned, drained	4 oz.	129	1.7
MUSTARD:			
Powder (French's)	1 tsp. (1.5 grams)	9	.3
Prepared:			
Brown (French's; Gulden's)	1 tsp.	5	.3
Chinese (Chun King)	1 tsp.	5	.3
Cream salad (French's)	1 tsp.	3	.3
Dijon, *Grey Poupon*	1 tsp. (.2 oz.)	6	Tr.
Horseradish (French's)	1 tsp. (.2 oz.)	5	.3
Medford (French's)	1 tsp.	5	.3
Onion (French's)	1 tsp.	8	1.6
Unsalted (Featherweight)	1 tsp.	5	.3
Yellow (Gulden's)	1 tsp.	5	.4

Food and Description	Measure or Quantity	Calories	Carbo-hydrates (grams)
MUSTARD GREENS:			
Raw (USDA) whole	1 lb. (weighed untrimmed)	98	17.8
Boiled (USDA) drained	1 cup (7.8 oz.)	51	8.8
Canned (Allen's) chopped, solids & liq.	½ cup (4.1 oz.)	20	2.0
Frozen, chopped:			
(Birds Eye)	⅓ of 10-oz. pkg.	25	3.2
(Frosty Acres)	3.3-oz. serving	20	3.0
(McKenzie)	⅓ of 10-oz. pkg.	25	3.0
(Southland)	⅕ of 16-oz. pkg.	20	3.0
MUSTARD SPINACH (USDA):			
Raw	1 lb.	100	17.7
Boiled, drained, no added salt	4-oz. serving	18	3.2

Food and Description	Measure or Quantity	Calories	Carbo-hydrates (grams)

N

NATHAN'S:
French fries	1 reg. order	550	60.0
Hamburger	4½-oz. sandwich	360	18.0
Hot dog	3.4-oz. serving	290	19.0

NATURAL CEREAL:
Familia:
Regular	½ cup (1.8 oz.)	187	34.8
With bran	½ cup (1.7 oz.)	166	29.0
With granola	½ cup (2.0 oz.)	257	37.2
No added salt	½ cup (1.8 oz.)	181	32.1

Heartland:
Plain, coconut or raisin	¼ cup (1 oz.)	130	18.0
Trail mix	¼ cup (1 oz.)	120	19.0

(Quaker):
Hot, whole wheat	⅓ cup (1 oz.)	106	21.8
100% natural	¼ cup (1 oz.)	138	17.4
100% natural, with apple & cinnamon	¼ cup (1 oz.)	135	18.0
100% natural with raisins & dates	¼ cup (1 oz.)	134	18.0

NATURE SNACKS (Sun-Maid):
Carob Crunch	1 oz.	143	16.8
Carob Peanut	1¼ oz.	190	18.0
Carob Raisin or Yogurt Raisin	1¼ oz.	160	25.0
Nuts Galore	1 oz.	170	5.0
Raisin Crunch or Rocky Road	1 oz.	126	19.1
Sesame Nut Crunch	1 oz.	154	14.6
Tahitian Treat or Yogurt Crunch	1 oz.	123	19.4
Yogurt Peanut	1¼ oz.	200	18.0

Food and Description	Measure or Quantity	Calories	Carbo- hydrates (grams)
NECTARINE, fresh (USDA):			
Whole	1 lb. (weighed with pits)	267	71.4
Flesh only	4 oz.	73	19.4
NOODLE (See also **SPAGHETTI**). Plain noodle products are essentially the same in caloric value and carbohydrate content on the same weight basis. The longer they are cooked, the more water is absorbed and this affects the nutritive values. Also, the longer they are cooked, the amount of calories decreases somewhat. (USDA):			
Dry	1 oz.	110	20.4
Dry, 1½" strips	1 cup (2.6 oz.)	283	52.6
Cooked	1 oz.	35	6.6
NOODLES & BEEF:			
Canned (Hormel) *Short Orders*	7½-oz. can	230	16.0
Frozen (Banquet) *Buffet Supper*	2-lb. pkg.	754	83.6
NOODLES & CHICKEN:			
Canned (Hormel) *Dinty Moore, Short Orders*	7½-oz. can	210	15.0
Frozen (Swanson)	10½-oz. dinner	270	37.0
NOODLES, CHOW MEIN:			
(Chun King)	1 oz.	139	16.5
(La Choy)	½ cup (1 oz.)	150	16.0
NOODLE MIX:			
*(Betty Crocker):			
Fettucini Alfredo	¼ of pkg.	220	23.0

(USDA): United States Department of Agriculture
(HEW/FAO):   Health, Education and Welfare/Food and Agriculture
                         Organization
* Prepared as Package Directs

Food and Description	Measure or Quantity	Calories	Carbo-hydrates (grams)
Parisienne	¼ of pkg.	160	26.0
Romanoff	¼ of pkg.	230	23.0
Stroganoff	¼ of pkg.	240	26.0
*(Lipton) & Sauce:			
Alfredo:			
Regular	¼ of pkg.	146	22.1
Carbonara	¼ of pkg.	140	20.2
Beef	¼ of pkg.	125	22.6
Butter	¼ of pkg.	152	23.1
Butter & herb	¼ of pkg.	140	22.8
Cheese	¼ of pkg.	141	24.8
Chicken	¼ of pkg.	131	22.8
Chicken broccoli	¼ of pkg.	129	22.4
Parmesan	¼ of pkg.	143	21.1
Sour cream & chive	¼ of pkg.	147	23.5
Stroganoff	¼ of pkg.	110	19.1
Noodle Roni, parmesano	⅕ of 6-oz. pkg.	130	21.0
NOODLES, RICE (La Choy)	1 oz.	130	21.0
NOODLE ROMANOFF, frozen (Stouffer's)	⅓ of 12-oz. pkg.	170	15.0
NUT, MIXED:			
Dry roasted:			
(Flavor House) salted	1 oz.	172	5.4
(Planters)	1 oz.	160	7.0
Oil roasted (Planters) with or without peanuts	1 oz.	180	6.0
NUT & HONEY CRUNCH, cereal (Kellogg's)	⅔ cup (1 oz.)	110	24.0
NUTMEG (French's)	1 tsp. (1.9 grams)	11	.9
NUTRIFIC, cereal (Kellogg's)	1 cup (1.3 oz.)	120	28.0
NUTRI-GRAIN, cereal (Kellogg's):			
Corn	½ cup (1 oz.)	100	24.0

Food and Description	Measure or Quantity	Calories	Carbo-hydrates (grams)
Nuggets	¼ cup (1 oz.)	90	23.0
Wheat	⅔ cup (1 oz.)	100	24.0
Wheat & Raisin	⅔ cup (1.4 oz.)	130	32.0
NUTRIMATO (Mott's)	6 fl. oz.	70	17.0

Food and Description	Measure or Quantity	Calories	Carbohydrates (grams)

OAT FLAKES, cereal (Post) | ⅔ cup (1 oz.) | 107 | 20.6

OATMEAL:
  Dry:
    Regular:
      (USDA) | ½ cup (1.2 oz.) | 140 | 44.5
      (Elam's):
        Scotch style or stone
          ground | 1 oz. | 108 | 18.2
        Steel cut, whole grain | ¼ cup (1.6 oz.) | 174 | 30.4
      (H-O) old fashioned | 1 T. (.14 oz.) | 15 | 2.6
      (Quaker) old fashioned | ⅓ cup (1 oz.) | 109 | 18.5
      (3-Minute Brand) | ⅓ cup (1 oz.) | 110 | 18.1
    Instant:
      (Harvest Brand):
        Regular | 1 oz. | 108 | 17.3
        Apple & cinnamon | 1¼ oz. | 136 | 25.7
        Cinnamon & spice | 1⅝ oz. | 183 | 35.5
        Maple & brown sugar | 1.5 oz. | 171 | 25.6
        Peaches & cream | ⅓ cup (1¼ oz.) | 140 | 25.6
      (H-O):
        Regular, boxed | 1 T. | 15 | 2.6
        Regular, packets | 1-oz. packet | 105 | 17.9
        With bran & spice | 1½-oz. packet | 157 | 29.0
        Country apple & brown
          sugar | 1.1-oz. packet | 121 | 22.7
        With maple & brown
          sugar flavor | 1½-oz. packet | 160 | 31.8
        Sweet & mellow | 1.4-oz. packet | 149 | 28.7
      (Quaker):
        Regular | 1-oz. packet | 105 | 18.1
        Apple & cinnamon | 1¼-oz. packet | 134 | 26.0
        Bran & raisin | 1.5-oz. packet | 153 | 29.2
        Cinnamon & spice | 1⅝-oz. packet | 176 | 34.8
        Honey & graham | 1¼-oz. packet | 136 | 26.6
        Maple & brown sugar | 1.5-oz. packet | 163 | 31.9

Food and Description	Measure or Quantity	Calories	Carbo-hydrates (grams)
Raisins & spice	1½-oz. packet	159	31.4
(3-Minute Brand)	1½-oz. packet	162	25.9
Quick:			
(Harvest Brand)	⅓ cup (1 oz.)	110	18.1
(H-O)	½ cup (1.2 oz.)	129	22.2
(Quaker)	⅓ cup (1 oz.)	109	18.5
(Ralston Purina)	⅓ cup (1 oz.)	110	18.0
(3-Minute Brand)	⅓ cup	110	18.1
Cooked, regular (USDA)	1 cup (8.5 oz.)	132	23.3
OCTOPUS, raw (USDA) meat only	4 oz.	83	0.
OIL, SALAD OR COOKING:			
(USDA) all kinds, including olive	1 T. (.5 oz.)	124	0.
(USDA) all kinds, including olive	½ cup (3.9 oz.)	972	0.
(Bertoli) olive	1 T.	120	0.
(Calavo) avocado	1 T.	120	0.
Crisco, Fleischmann's; Mazola	1 T. (.5 oz.)	120	0.
(Golden Thistle; *Goya*)	1 T. (.5 oz.)	130	0.
Mrs. Tucker's, corn or soybean	1 T.	130	0.
(Planters) peanut or popcorn	1 T.	130	0.
Sunlite; Wesson	1 T.	120	0.
OKRA:			
Raw (USDA) whole	1 lb. (weighed untrimmed)	140	29.6
Boiled (USDA) drained:			
Whole	½ cup (3.1 oz.)	26	5.3
Pods	8 pods (3 oz.)	25	5.1
Slices	½ cup (2.8 oz.)	23	4.8
Frozen:			
(Birds Eye)			
Whole, baby	⅓ of 10-oz. pkg.	36	6.7
Cut	⅓ of 10-oz. pkg.	30	5.7
(Frosty Acres):			
Cut	3.3-oz. serving	25	6.0
Whole	3.3-oz. serving	30	7.0

(USDA): United States Department of Agriculture
(HEW/FAO): Health, Education and Welfare/Food and Agriculture Organization
* Prepared as Package Directs

Food and Description	Measure or Quantity	Calories	Carbo- hydrates (grams)
(McKenzie):			
Cut	3.3 oz.	30	6.0
Whole	3.3 oz.	35	7.0
(Southland):			
Cut	⅓ of 16-oz. pkg.	25	6.0
Whole	⅓ of 16-oz. pkg.	30	7.0
OLD-FASHIONED COCKTAIL			
(Hiram Walker) 62 proof	3 fl. oz.	165	3.0
OLIVE:			
Greek style (USDA):			
With pits, drained	1 oz.	77	2.0
Pitted, drained	1 oz.	96	2.5
Green (USDA)	1 oz.	33	.4
Ripe, by variety (USDA):			
Ascalano, any size, pitted & drained	1 oz.	37	.7
Manzanilla, any size	1 oz.	37	.7
Mission	3 small or 2 large	18	.3
Mission, slices	½ cup (2.2 oz.)	26	6.1
Ripe, by size (Lindsay):			
Colossal	1 olive	9	.6
Extra large	1 olive	6	.3
Jumbo	1 olive	7	.5
Large	1 olive	6	.4
Medium	1 olive	3	.2
Super colossal	1 olive	11	.8
ONION (See also **ONION, GREEN** and **ONION, WELCH**):			
Raw (USDA):			
Whole	1 lb. (weighed untrimmed)	157	35.9
Whole	3.9-oz. onion (2½" dia.)	38	8.7
Chopped	½ cup (3 oz.)	33	7.5
Chopped	1 T. (.4 oz.)	4	1.0
Grated	1 T. (.5 oz.)	5	1.2
Slices	½ cup (2 oz.)	21	4.9
Boiled, drained (USDA):			
Whole	½ cup (3.7 oz.)	30	6.8
Whole, pearl onions	½ cup (3.2 oz.)	27	6.0

Food and Description	Measure or Quantity	Calories	Carbo-hydrates (grams)
Halves or pieces	½ cup (3.2 oz.)	26	5.8
Canned, *O & C* (Durkee):			
Boiled	1-oz. serving	8	2.0
In cream sauce	1-oz. serving	143	17.0
Dehydrated:			
Flakes:			
(USDA)	1 tsp. (1.3 grams)	5	1.1
(Gilroy)	1 tsp.	5	1.2
Powder (Gilroy)	1 tsp.	9	2.0
Frozen:			
(Birds Eye):			
Chopped	1 oz.	8	2.0
Small, whole	¼ of 16-oz. pkg.	44	9.6
Small, with cream sauce	⅓ of 9-oz. pkg.	118	11.2
(Frosty Acres) chopped	1 oz.	8	2.0
(McKenzie) chopped	1 oz.	8	2.0
(Mrs. Paul's) rings, breaded & fried	½ of 5-oz. pkg.	167	22.2
(Southland) chopped	⅕ of 10-oz. pkg.	15	4.0
ONION BOUILLON:			
(Herb-Ox):			
Cube	1 cube	10	1.3
Packet	1 packet	14	2.1
MBT	1 packet	16	2.0
ONION, COCKTAIL (Vlasic) lightly spiced	1 oz.	4	1.0
ONION, GREEN, raw (USDA):			
Whole	1 lb. (weighed untrimmed)	157	35.7
Bulb & entire top	1 oz.	10	2.3
Bulb without green top	3 small onions (.9 oz.)	11	2.6
Slices, bulb & white portion of top	½ cup (1.8 oz.)	22	5.2
Tops only	1 oz.	8	1.6

(USDA): United States Department of Agriculture
(HEW/FAO): Health, Education and Welfare/Food and Agriculture Organization
* Prepared as Package Directs

Food and Description	Measure or Quantity	Calories	Carbo-hydrates (grams)
ONION SALAD SEASONING (French's) instant	1 T.	15	3.0
ONION SALT (French's)	1 tsp.	6	1.0
ONION SOUP (See **SOUP,** Onion)			
ONION, WELCH, raw (USDA):			
Whole	1 lb. (weighed untrimmed)	100	19.2
Trimmed	4 oz.	39	7.4
OPOSSUM (USDA) roasted, meat only	4 oz.	251	0.
ORANGE, fresh (USDA):			
California Navel:			
Whole	1 lb. (weighed with rind & seeds)	157	39.3
Whole	6.3-oz. orange (2⅖″ dia.)	62	15.5
Sections	1 cup (8.5 oz.)	123	30.6
California Valencia:			
Whole	1 lb. (weighed with rind & seeds)	174	42.2
Fruit, including peel	6.3-oz. orange (2⅝″ dia.)	72	27.9
Sections	1 cup (8.6 oz.)	123	29.9
Florida, all varieties:			
Whole	1 lb. (weighed with rind & seeds)	158	40.3
Whole	7.4-oz. orange (3″ dia.)	73	18.6
Sections	1 cup (8.5 oz.)	113	28.9
ORANGE DRINK:			
Canned:			
(Ardmore Farms)	6 fl. oz.	86	20.9
(Borden) *Bama*	8.45-fl.-oz. container	120	29.0

Food and Description	Measure or Quantity	Calories	Carbo-hydrates (grams)
(Hi-C)	6 fl. oz.	95	23.3
(Johanna Farms) *Ssips*	8.45-fl.-oz. container	130	32.0
(Lincoln)	6 fl. oz.	90	23.0
*Mix:			
Dietetic:			
Crystal Light	6 fl. oz.	4	.4
(Sunkist)	8 fl. oz.	8	2.0
ORANGE EXTRACT (Virginia Dare) 79% alcohol	1 tsp.	22	0.
ORANGE-GRAPEFRUIT JUICE:			
Canned:			
(Del Monte):			
Sweetened	6 fl. oz.	91	21.1
Unsweetened	6 fl. oz.	79	18.3
(Libby's) unsweetened	6 fl. oz.	80	19.0
*Frozen (Minute Maid) unsweetened	6 fl. oz.	76	19.1
ORANGE JUICE:			
Fresh (USDA):			
California Navel	½ cup (4.4 oz.)	60	14.0
California Valencia	½ cup (4.4 oz.)	58	13.0
Florida, early or midseason	½ cup (4.4 oz.)	50	11.4
Florida Temple	½ cup (4.4 oz.)	67	16.0
Florida Valencia	½ cup (4.4 oz.)	56	13.0
Canned, unsweetened:			
(USDA)	½ cup (4.4 oz.)	60	13.9
(Ardmore Farms)	6 fl. oz.	84	20.1
(Borden) *Sippin' Pak*	8.45-fl.-oz. container	110	26.0
(Del Monte)	6 fl. oz. (6.5 oz.)	80	19.0
(Johanna Farms)	6 fl. oz.	84	19.5
Canned, sweetened:			
(USDA)	6 fl. oz.	66	15.4
(Del Monte)	6 fl. oz.	76	17.4

(USDA): United States Department of Agriculture
(HEW/FAO):   Health, Education and Welfare/Food and Agriculture
              Organization
* Prepared as Package Directs

Food and Description	Measure or Quantity	Calories	Carbo-hydrates (grams)
Chilled:			
(Citrus Hill):			
Regular	6 fl. oz.	90	20.0
Lite	6 fl. oz.	60	14.0
(Minute Maid):			
Regular	6 fl. oz.	91	21.9
Calcium Fortified	6 fl. oz.	93	21.9
Reduced Acid	6 fl. oz.	89	21.9
(Sunkist)	6 fl. oz.	76	17.7
*Dehydrated crystals (USDA)	½ cup (4.4 oz.)	57	13.4
*Frozen:			
(USDA)	½ cup (4.4 oz.)	56	13.3
(Birds Eye) *Orange Plus*	6 fl. oz.	99	24.0
(Citrus Hill):			
Regular	6 fl. oz.	90	20.0
Lite	6 fl. oz.	60	14.0
(Minute Maid) regular	6 fl. oz.	91	21.9
(Sunkist)	6 fl. oz.	84	20.1
ORANGE JUICE BAR, frozen			
(Sunkist)	3-fl.-oz. bar	72	17.6
ORANGE, MANDARIN (See TANGERINE)			
ORANGE PEEL, CANDIED			
(USDA)	1 oz.	90	22.9
ORANGE-PINEAPPLE DRINK, canned (Lincoln)	6 fl. oz.	90	23.0
ORANGE-PINEAPPLE JUICE, canned (Texsun)	8 fl. oz.	89	21.0
ORCHARD BLEND JUICE, canned (Welch's):			
Apple grape	6 fl. oz.	100	24.0
Harvest or North Country	6 fl. oz.	90	22.0
Vineyard	6 fl. oz.	120	30.0
OREGANO (French's)	1 tsp.	6	1.0
OVALTINE:			
Chocolate	¾ oz.	78	17.9

Food and Description	Measure or Quantity	Calories	Carbo-hydrates (grams)
Malt	¾ oz.	88	17.6
OVEN FRY (General Foods):			
Crispy crumb for chicken	4.2-oz. envelope	460	82.4
Crispy crumb for pork	4.2-oz. envelope	484	78.0
Homestyle flour recipe	3.2-oz. envelope	304	64.8
OYSTER:			
Raw (USDA):			
Eastern, meat only	19–31 small or 13–19 med.	158	8.2
Pacific & Western, meat only	6–9 small or 4–6 med. (8.5 oz.)	218	15.4
Canned (Bumble Bee) shelled, whole, solids & liq.	1 cup (8.5 oz.)	218	15.4
Fried (USDA) dipped in milk, egg & breadcrumbs	4 oz.	271	21.1
OYSTER STEW (USDA):			
Home recipe:			
1 part oysters to 1 part milk by volume	1 cup (8.5 oz., 6–8 oysters)	245	14.2
1 part oysters to 2 parts milk by volume	1 cup (8.5 oz.)	233	10.8
1 part oysters to 3 parts milk by volume	1 cup (8.5 oz.)	206	11.3
Frozen:			
Prepared with equal volume milk	1 cup (8.5 oz.)	201	14.2
Prepared with equal volume water	1 cup (8.5 oz.)	122	8.2

(USDA): United States Department of Agriculture
(HEW/FAO):   Health, Education and Welfare/Food and Agriculture
                        Organization
* Prepared as Package Directs

Food and Description	Measure or Quantity	Calories	Carbo-hydrates (grams)

P

PAC-MAN CEREAL
(General Mills) | 1 cup (1 oz.) | 110 | 25.0

*PANCAKE BATTER			
FROZEN (Aunt Jemima):			
Plain	4" pancake	70	14.1
Blueberry or buttermilk	4" pancake	68	13.8
Buttermilk	4" pancake	68	14.2
PANCAKE DINNER OR			
ENTREE, frozen			
(Swanson):			
& blueberries, in sauce,	7-oz. entree	400	70.0
& sausage	6-oz. entree	460	52.0
& strawberries	7-oz. entree	430	82.0
*PANCAKE & WAFFLE MIX:			
Plain:			
(Aunt Jemima):			
Original	4" pancake	73	8.7
Complete	4" pancake	80	15.7
(Log Cabin):			
Regular	4" pancake	60	8.7
Complete	4" pancake	58	11.2
(Pillsbury) *Hungry Jack:*			
Complete:			
Bulk	4" pancake	63	13.0
Packets	4" pancake	70	10.0
Extra Lights	4" pancake	70	10.0
Golden Blend:			
Regular	4" pancake	67	8.7
Complete	4" pancake	80	14.3
Panshakes	4" pancake	83	14.3
Blueberry (Pillsbury)			
Hungry Jack	4" pancake	107	9.7

Food and Description	Measure or Quantity	Calories	Carbo-hydrates (grams)
Buckwheat (Aunt Jemima)	4″ pancake	67	8.3
Buttermilk:			
(Aunt Jemima):			
Regular	4″ pancake	100	13.3
Complete	4″ pancake	80	15.3
(Betty Crocker):			
Regular	4″ pancake	93	13.0
Complete	4″ pancake	70	13.7
(Pillsbury) *Hungry Jack:*			
Regular	4″ pancake	80	9.7
Complete	4″ pancake	63	13.0
Whole wheat (Aunt Jemima)	4″ pancake	83	10.7
Dietetic:			
(Estee)	3″ pancake	33	7.0
(Featherweight) low sodium	4″ pancake	43	8.0
PANCAKE & WAFFLE SYRUP (See **SYRUP**, Pancake & Waffle)			
PANCREAS, raw (USDA):			
Beef, lean only	4 oz.	160	0.
Calf	4 oz.	183	0.
Hog or hog sweetbread	4 oz.	274	0.
PAPAW, fresh (USDA):			
Whole	1 lb. (weighed with rind & seeds)	289	57.2
Flesh only	4 oz.	96	19.1
PAPAYA, fresh (USDA):			
Whole	1 lb. (weighed with skin & seeds)	119	30.4
Cubed	1 cup (6.4 oz.)	71	18.2
PAPAYA JUICE, canned (HEW/FAO)	4 oz.	77	19.6

(USDA): United States Department of Agriculture
(HEW/FAO):   Health, Education and Welfare/Food and Agriculture
             Organization
* Prepared as Package Directs

Food and Description	Measure or Quantity	Calories	Carbo-hydrates (grams)
PAPRIKA, domestic (French's)	1 tsp.	7	1.1
PARSLEY, fresh (USDA):			
Whole	½ lb.	100	19.3
Chopped	1 T. (4 grams)	2	.3
PARSLEY FLAKES, dehydrated (French's)	1 tsp. (1.1 grams)	4	.6
PARSNIP (USDA):			
Raw, whole	1 lb. (weighed unprepared)	293	67.5
Boiled, drained, cut in pieces	½ cup (3.7 oz.)	70	15.8
PASSION FRUIT, fresh (USDA):			
Whole	1 lb. (weighed with shell)	212	50.0
Pulp & seeds	4 oz.	102	24.0
PASSION FRUIT JUICE, fresh (HEW/FAO)	4 oz.	50	11.5
PASTA frozen (see also **NOODLE** and **SPAGHETTI**):			
(Birds Eye):			
Continental style	½ of 10-oz. pkg.	164	16.0
Mexicana	½ of 10-oz. pkg.	115	21.0
Primavera	5-oz. pkg.	204	21.7
(Stouffer's):			
Carbonara	9 ¾-oz. meal	620	34.0
Casino	9 ¼-oz. meal	300	44.0
Mexicali	10-oz. meal	490	36.0
Oriental	9⅞-oz. meal	300	35.0
Primavera	10 ⅝-oz. meal	270	13.0
*PASTA SALAD, mix (Betty Crocker) *Suddenly Salad:*			
Classic	⅙ of pkg.	150	19.0
Italian	⅙ of pkg.	160	20.0

Food and Description	Measure or Quantity	Calories	Carbo-hydrates (grams)
*PASTA & SAUCE, mix			
(Lipton):			
Cheddar broccoli with fusilli	¼ of pkg.	135	23.9
Cheese supreme	¼ of pkg.	139	23.8
Garlic, creamy	¼ of pkg.	144	25.3
Mushroom & chicken	¼ of pkg.	124	23.4
Mushroom, creamy	¼ of pkg.	143	24.8
Oriental with fusilli	¼ of pkg.	130	25.5
Tomato, herb	¼ of pkg.	130	26,0
PASTINA, DRY (USDA):			
Carrot	1 oz.	105	21.5
Egg	1 oz.	109	20.4
Spinach	1 oz.	104	21.2
PASTOSO (Petri) 12% alcohol	3 fl. oz.	71	1.2
PASTRAMI, packaged:			
(Carl Buddig) smoked, sliced	1 oz.	40	Tr.
(Eckrich) sliced	1-oz. slice	47	1.3
*Hebrew National,*1st cut	1 oz.	44	<1.0
PASTRY SHEET, PUFF, frozen			
(Pepperidge Farm)	1 sheet	1150	88.0
PASTRY SHELL, frozen			
(Pepperidge Farm)	1 shell (1.7 oz.)	210	17.0
PÂTÉ:			
De foie gras (USDA)	1 T. (.5 oz.)	69	.7
Liver:			
(Hormel)	1 T.	35	.3
(Sell's)	½ of 4.8-oz. can	223	2.7
PEA, GREEN:			
Raw (USDA):			
In pod	1 lb. (weighed in pod)	145	24.8
Shelled	1 lb.	381	65.3
Shelled	½ cup (2.4 oz.)	58	9.9

(USDA): United States Department of Agriculture
(HEW/FAO):   Health, Education and Welfare/Food and Agriculture
                    Organization
* Prepared as Package Directs

Food and Description	Measure or Quantity	Calories	Carbo-hydrates (grams)
Boiled (USDA) drained	½ cup (2.9 oz.)	58	9.9
Canned, regular pack:			
(USDA):			
Alaska, early or June:			
Solids & liq.	½ cup (4.4 oz.)	82	15.5
Solids only	½ cup (3 oz.)	76	14.4
Sweet:			
Solids & liq.	½ cup (4.4 oz.)	71	12.9
Solids only	½ cup (3 oz.)	69	12.9
Drained liquid	4 oz.	25	4.9
(Del Monte) seasoned or sweet, regular size solids & liq.	½ cup	60	11.0
(Larsen) *Freshlike*	½ cup (4.4 oz.)	50	10.0
(Libby's) sweet, solids & liq.	½ cup (4.2 oz.)	66	11.6
Canned, dietetic pack:			
(USDA):			
Alaska, early or June:			
Solids & liq.	4 oz.	62	11.1
Solids only	4 oz.	88	16.2
Sweet:			
Solids & liq.	4 oz.	53	9.5
Solids only	4 oz.	82	14.7
(Del Monte) No Salt Added, sweet, solids & liq.	½ cup (4.3 oz.)	60	11.0
(Diet Delight) solids & liq.	½ cup (4.3 oz.)	50	8.0
(Featherweight) sweet, solids & liq.	½ cup (4 oz.)	70	12.0
(Larsen) *Fresh-Lite,* no salt added	½ cup (4.4 oz.)	50	10.0
(S&W) *Nutradiet,* green label, solids & liq.	½ cup	40	8.0
Frozen:			
(Birds Eye):			
Regular	⅓ of 10-oz. pkg.	78	13.3
In butter sauce	⅓ of 10-oz. pkg.	85	12.6
In cream sauce	⅓ of 8-oz. pkg.	84	14.3
Tiny, tender, deluxe	⅓ of 10-oz. pkg.	64	10.7
(Frosty Acres):			
Regular	3.3-oz. serving	80	13.0
Tiny	3.3-oz. serving	60	11.0
(McKenzie):			
Regular	3.3 oz.	80	13.0

Food and Description	Measure or Quantity	Calories	Carbohydrates (grams)
Tiny	3.3 oz.	60	10.0
PEA & CARROT:			
Canned, regular pack, solids & liq.:			
(Del Monte)	½ cup (4 oz.)	50	10.0
(Larsen) *Freshlike*	½ cup (4.6 oz.)	50	12.0
(Libby's)	½ cup (4.2 oz.)	56	10.3
(Veg-All)	½ cup	50	12.0
Canned, dietetic pack, solids & liq.:			
(Diet Delight)	½ cup (4.3 oz.)	40	6.0
(Larsen) *Fresh-Like,* no salt added	½ cup (4.6 oz.)	50	12.0
(S&W) *Nutradiet,* green label	½ cup	35	7.0
Frozen:			
(Birds Eye)	⅓ of 10-oz. pkg.	61	11.2
(Frosty Acres)	3.3-oz. serving	60	11.0
(McKenzie)	3.3-oz. serving	60	11.0
PEA, CROWDER, frozen:			
(Birds Eye)	⅕ of 16-oz. pkg.	130	22.6
(McKenzie)	3-oz. serving	130	23.0
(Southland)	⅕ of 16-oz. pkg.	130	23.0
PEA, MATURE SEED, dry (USDA):			
Whole	1 lb.	1542	272.5
Whole	1 cup	680	120.6
Split	1 lb.	1579	284.4
Split	1 cup (7.2 oz.)	706	127.3
Cooked, split, drained solids	½ cup (3.4 oz.)	112	20.2
PEA & ONION:			
Canned (Larsen)	½ cup	60	12.0
Frozen (Birds Eye)	⅓ of 10-oz. pkg.	67	11.7

(USDA): United States Department of Agriculture
(HEW/FAO):   Health, Education and Welfare/Food and Agriculture Organization
* Prepared as Package Directs

Food and Description	Measure or Quantity	Calories	Carbo-hydrates (grams)
PEA POD:			
Raw (USDA) edible podded or Chinese	1 lb. (weighed untrimmed)	228	51.7
Boiled (USDA) drained	4 oz.	49	10.8
Frozen (La Choy)	6-oz. pkg.	70	12.0
PEA PUREE, canned (Larsen) no salt added	½ cup	50	10.0
PEACH:			
Fresh (USDA):			
Whole, without skin	1 lb. (weighed unpeeled)	150	38.3
Whole	4-oz. peach (2″ dia.)	38	9.6
Diced	½ cup (4.7 oz.)	51	12.9
Sliced	½ cup (3 oz.)	31	8.2
Canned, regular pack, solids & liq.:			
(USDA):			
Extra heavy syrup	4 oz.	110	28.5
Heavy syrup	2 med. halves & 2 T. syrup (4.1 oz.)	91	23.5
Juice pack	4 oz.	51	13.2
Light syrup	4 oz.	66	17.1
(Del Monte):			
Cling:			
Halves or slices	½ cup (4 oz.)	80	22.0
Spices	3½ oz.	80	20.0
Freestone	½ cup (4 oz.)	90	23.0
(Hunt's) *Snack Pack,* diced	5-oz. container	110	29.0
(Libby's) heavy syrup:			
Halves	½ cup (4.5 oz.)	105	25.4
Slices	½ cup (4.5 oz.)	102	24.7
Canned, dietetic pack, solids & liq.:			
(Del Monte) Lite:			
Cling	½ cup (4 oz.)	50	13.0
Freestone	½ cup (4 oz.)	60	13.0
(Diet Delight) Cling:			
Juice pack	½ cup (4.4 oz.)	50	14.0
Water pack	½ cup (4.3 oz.)	30	2.0

Food and Description	Measure or Quantity	Calories	Carbo- hydrates (grams)
(Featherweight):			
Cling or Freestone,			
juice pack	½ cup	50	12.0
Cling, water pack	½ cup	30	8.0
(S&W) *Nutradiet*, Cling:			
Juice pack	½ cup	60	14.0
Water pack	½ cup	30	8.0
Dehydrated (USDA):			
Uncooked	1 oz.	96	24.9
Cooked, with added sugar,			
solids & liq.	½ cup (5.4 oz.)	184	47.6
Dried (USDA):			
Uncooked	½ cup	231	60.1
Cooked:			
Unsweetened	½ cup	111	28.9
Sweetened	½ cup (5.4 oz.)	181	46.8
Frozen (Birds Eye) quick thaw	5-oz. serving	141	34.1
PEACH BUTTER (Smucker's)	1 T. (.7 oz.)	45	12.0
PEACH LIQUEUR (DeKupyer)	1 fl. oz.	82	8.3
PEACH NECTAR, canned			
(Ardmore Farms)	6 fl. oz.	90	23.4
PEACH PRESERVE OR JAM:			
Sweetened (Smucker's)	1 T. (.7 oz.)	53	13.5
Dietetic (Dia-Mel)	1 T.	6	0.
PEACH, STRAINED, canned			
(Larsen) no salt added	½ cup	65	17.0
PEANUT:			
Raw (USDA):			
In shell	1 lb. (weighed in shell)	1868	61.6
With skins	1 oz.	160	5.3
Without skins	1 oz.	161	5.0

(USDA): United States Department of Agriculture
(HEW/FAO): Health, Education and Welfare/Food and Agriculture
          Organization
* Prepared as Package Directs

Food and Description	Measure or Quantity	Calories	Carbo-hydrates (grams)
Roasted:			
(USDA):			
Whole	1 lb. (weighed in shell)	1769	62.6
Chopped	½ cup	404	13.0
Halves	½ cup	421	13.5
(Adams):			
Regular	1 oz.	170	5.0
Butter toffee	1 oz.	140	20.0
(Beer Nuts)	1 oz.	180	7.0
(Eagle) Honey Roast	1 oz.	170	7.0
(Fisher):			
In shell, salted	1 oz.	105	3.7
Shelled:			
Dry roasted, salted or unsalted	1 oz.	160	6.0
Oil roasted, salted	1 oz.	166	5.3
(Planters):			
Dry roasted	1 oz. (jar)	160	6.0
Oil roasted	¾-oz. bag	170	5.0
(Tom's):			
In shell	1 oz.	120	3.4
Shelled:			
Dry roasted	1 oz.	160	5.0
Hot flavored	1 oz.	170	4.0
Redskin or toasted	1 oz.	170	5.0
Spanish roasted:			
(Adams)	1 oz.	170	5.0
(Frito-Lay's)	1 oz.	168	6.6
(Planter's):			
Dry roasted	1 oz. (jar)	175	3.4
Oil roasted	1 oz. (can)	182	3.4
PEANUT BUTTER:			
Regular:			
(Adams) creamy or crunchy	1 T. (.6 oz.)	95	2.5
(Algood) *Cap'n Kid*	1 T.	85	3.0
(Bama)	1 T.	100	3.0
(Elam's) natural, with defatted wheatgerm	1 T. (.6 oz.)	109	2.1
(Estee) low sodium	1 T.	100	3.0
(Home Brands)	1 T.	105	2.5
(Peter Pan):			
Crunchy	1 T. (.6 oz.)	95	2.9
Smooth	1 T. (.6 oz.)	95	2.5

Food and Description	Measure or Quantity	Calories	Carbo- hydrates (grams)
(Skippy):			
Creamy or super chunk	1 T.	95	2.1
Dietetic:			
(Adams) low sodium	1 T. (.6 oz.)	95	2.5
(Featherweight) low sodium	1 T. (.5 oz.)	90	2.0
(Peter Pan) low sodium	1 T.	95	2.6
(Smucker's) no salt added	1 T.	100	3.0
PEANUT BUTTER BOPPERS:			
(General Mills):			
Cookie crunch or fudge chip	1 bar	170	15.0
Fudge graham	1 bar	160	15,0
Honey crisp	1 bar	160	14.0
Peanut crunch	1 bar	170	13.0
PEANUT BUTTER MORSELS:			
(Nestlé)	1 oz.	160	12.0
(Reese's)	1 oz.	153	21.3
PEAR:			
Fresh (USDA):			
Whole	1 lb. (weighed with stems & core)	252	63.2
Whole	6.4-oz. pear (3″ × 2½″ dia.)	101	25.4
Quartered	1 cup (6.8 oz.)	117	29.4
Slices	½ cup (6.8 oz.)	50	12.5
Canned, regular pack, solids & liq.:			
(USDA):			
Extra heavy syrup	4 oz.	104	26.8
Heavy syrup	½ cup	87	22.3
Juice pack	4 oz.	52	13.4
Light syrup	4 oz.	69	17.7
(Del Monte) Bartlett, halves or slices	½ cup (4. oz.)	80	22.0
(Libby's) halves, heavy syrup	½ cup (4.5 oz.)	102	25.1

(USDA): United States Department of Agriculture
(HEW/FAO):   Health, Education and Welfare/Food and Agriculture
          Organization
* Prepared as Package Directs

Food and Description	Measure or Quantity	Calories	Carbo-hydrates (grams)
Canned, dietetic pack, solids & liq.:			
(Del Monte) Lite, Bartlett halves or slices	½ cup (4 oz.)	50	14.0
(Diet Delight):			
Juice pack	½ cup	60	16.0
Water pack	½ cup	35	9.0
(Featherweight) Bartlett, halves:			
Juice pack	½ cup	60	15.0
Water pack	½ cup	40	10.0
(Libby's) water pack	½ cup	60	15.0
(S&W) *Nutradiet,* halves, quarters or slices, white or blue label	½ cup	35	10.0
Dried (Sun-Maid)	½ cup (3.5 oz.)	260	70.0
PEAR-APPLE JUICE (Tree Top) canned or frozen	6 fl. oz.	90	23.0
PEAR, CANDIED (USDA)	1 oz.	86	21.5
PEAR-GRAPE JUICE (Tree Top) canned or frozen	6 fl. oz.	100	26.0
PEAR NECTAR, canned:			
(Del Monte)	6 fl. oz. (6.6 oz.)	122	11.5
(Libby's)	6 fl. oz.	100	25.0
PEAR-PASSION FRUIT NECTAR, canned (Libby's)	6 fl. oz.	60	14.0
PEAR, STRAINED, canned (Larsen) no salt added	½ cup	65	17.0
PEBBLES, cereal (Post):			
Cocoa	⅞ cup (1 oz.)	117	24.4
Fruity	⅞ cup (1 oz.)	116	24.5
PECAN:			
In shell (USDA)	1 lb. (weighed in shell)	1652	35.1
Shelled (USDA):			
Whole	1 lb.	3116	66.2

Food and Description	Measure or Quantity	Calories	Carbo-hydrates (grams)
Chopped	½ cup (1.8 oz.)	357	7.6
Chopped	1 T. (7 grams)	48	1.0
Halves	12–14 halves (.5 oz.)	96	2.0
Halves	½ cup (1.9 oz.)	371	7.9
Oil dipped (Fisher) salted	¼ cup	410	8.9
Roasted, dry:			
(Fisher) salted	1 oz.	170	3.0
(Flavor House)	1 oz.	195	4.1
(Planters)	1 oz.	206	3.5
PECTIN, FRUIT:			
Certo	6-oz. pkg.	19	4.8
Sure-Jell:			
Regular	1¾-oz. pkg.	170	42.6
Light	1¾-oz. pkg.	160	40.0
PEPPER, BANANA (Vlasic)			
hot rings	1 oz.	4	1.0
PEPPER, BLACK (French's):			
Regular	1 tsp. (2.3 grams)	9	1.5
Seasoned	1 tsp.	8	1.0
PEPPER, CHERRY (Vlasic)			
mild	1 oz.	8	2.0
PEPPER, CHILI:			
Raw, green (USDA) without seeds	4 oz.	42	10.3
Canned:			
(Del Monte):			
Green, whole	½ cup (4 oz.)	20	5.0
Jalapeno or chili, whole	½ cup (4 oz.)	30	6.0
(La Victoria):			
Marinated	1 T.	4	1.0
Nacho	1 T.	2	1.0
Old El Paso, green, chopped or whole	1 oz.	7	1.4
(Ortega):			
Green, diced, strips or whole	1 oz.	10	2.6

(USDA): United States Department of Agriculture
(HEW/FAO):   Health, Education and Welfare/Food and Agriculture
            Organization
* Prepared as Package Directs

Food and Description	Measure or Quantity	Calories	Carbo-hydrates (grams)
Jalapeno, diced or whole	1 oz.	9	1.7
(Vlasic) Jalapeno	1 oz.	8	2.0
PEPPERMINT EXTRACT			
(Durkee) imitation	1 tsp.	15	DNA
PEPPERONCINI (Vlasic)			
Greek, mild	1 oz.	4	1.0
PEPPERONI:			
(Eckrich)	1-oz. serving	135	1.0
(Hormel):			
Regular, chub, Rosa or Rosa Grande	1 oz.	140	0.
Canned bits	1 T.	35	0.
Leoni Brand	1 oz.	130	0.
Packaged, sliced	1 slice	40	0.
PEPPER & ONION, frozen			
(Southland)	2-oz. serving	15	2.0
PEPPER STEAK, frozen:			
(Armour) *Classic Lite* beef	10½-oz. meal	260	28.0
(Blue Star) *Dining Lite,* with rice	9¼-oz. meal	267	32.5
(La Choy) Fresh & Lite, with rice & vegetables	10-oz. meal	280	33.1
(Le Menu)	11½-oz. meal	360	32.0
(Stouffer's)	10½-oz. pkg.	330	36.0
*PEPPER STEAK MIX (Chun King) stir fry	6-oz. serving	249	8.6
PEPPER, STUFFED:			
Home recipe (USDA) with beef & crumbs	2¾″ × 2½″ pepper with 1⅛ cups stuffing	314	31.1
Frozen:			
(Armour) *Dinner Classics,* green	12-oz. meal	390	41.0
(Celentano) red, with beef, in sauce	12½-oz. pkg.	290	21.0

Food and Description	Measure or Quantity	Calories	Carbo- hydrates (grams)
(Stouffer's) green with beef in tomato sauce	7¾-oz. serving	200	19.0
(Weight Watchers) with veal stuffing	11¾-oz. meal	270	29.0
PEPPER, SWEET:			
Raw (USDA):			
Green:			
Whole	1 lb. (weighed untrimmed)	82	17.9
Without stem & seeds	1 med. pepper (2.6 oz.)	13	2.9
Chopped	½ cup (2.6 oz.)	16	3.6
Slices	½ cup (1.4 oz.)	9	2.0
Red:			
Whole	1 lb. (weighed untrimmed)	112	25.8
Without stem & seeds	1 med. pepper (2.2 oz.)	19	2.4
Boiled, green, without salt, drained	1 med. pepper (2.6 oz.)	13	2.8
Frozen:			
(Frosty Acres):			
Green	1-oz. serving	6	1.0
Red & green	2-oz. serving	15	2.0
(McKenzie)	1-oz. serving	6	1.0
(Southland):			
Green, diced	2-oz. serving	10	2.0
Red & green, cut	2-oz. serving	15	2.0
PERCH, OCEAN:			
Raw Atlantic, (USDA):			
Whole	1 lb. (weighed whole)	124	0.
Meat only	4 oz.	108	0.
Pacific, raw, whole	1 lb. (weighed whole)	116	0.
Frozen:			
(Banquet)	8¾-oz. dinner	434	49.8

(USDA): United States Department of Agriculture
(HEW/FAO): Health, Education and Welfare/Food and Agriculture
            Organization
* Prepared as Package Directs

Food and Description	Measure or Quantity	Calories	Carbo-hydrates (grams)
(Frionor) *Norway Gourmet*	4-oz. piece	120	0.
(Gorton's) *Fishmarket Fresh*	4 oz.	100	1.0
(Mrs. Paul's) fillet, breaded & fried	2-oz. piece	145	10.5
(Van de Kamp's):			
Regular batter, dipped, french fried	2-oz. piece	135	10.0
Light & crispy	2-oz. piece	170	10.0
Today's Catch	4 oz.	110	0.
PERNOD (Julius Wile)	1 fl. oz.	79	1.1
PERSIMMON (USDA):			
Japanese or Kaki, fresh:			
With seeds	4.4-oz. piece	79	20.1
Seedless	4.4-oz. piece	81	20.7
Native, fresh, flesh only	4-oz. serving	144	38.0
PETIT SIRAH WINE (Louis M. Martini):			
Regular, 12½% alcohol	3 fl. oz.	62	Tr.
White, 12.3% alcohol	3 fl. oz.	54	Tr.
PHEASANT, raw (USDA) meat only	4-oz. serving	184	0.
PICKLE:			
Cucumber, fresh or bread & butter			
(USDA)	3 slices (.7 oz.)	15	3.8
(Fannings)	1.2-oz. serving	17	3.9
(Featherweight) low sodium	1-oz. pickle	12	3.0
(Nalley's) chip	1-oz. serving	27	6.5
(Vlasic):			
Chips	1-oz. serving	30	7.0
Chunks	1-oz. serving	25	6.0
Stix	1-oz. serving	18	5.0
Dill:			
(USDA)	4.8-oz. pickle	15	3.0
(Claussen) halves	2 oz.	7	1.3
(Featherweight) low sodium, whole kosher	1-oz. serving	4	1.0

Food and Description	Measure or Quantity	Calories	Carbo-hydrates (grams)
(Smucker's):			
Candied sticks	4" piece (.8 oz.)	45	11.0
Hamburger, sliced	1 slice (.13 oz.)	Tr.	0.
Polish, whole	3½" pickle		
	(1.8 oz.)	8	1.0
Spears	3½" spear		
	(1.4 oz.)	6	1.0
(Vlasic):			
No garlic	1-oz. serving	4	1.0
Original	1-oz. serving	2	1.0
Hamburger (Vlasic) chips	1-oz. serving	2	1.0
Hot & spicy (Vlasic) garden mix	1-oz. serving	4	1.0
Kosher dill:			
(Claussen) halves or whole	2-oz. serving	7	1.3
(Featherweight) low sodium	1-oz. serving	4	1.0
(Smucker's):			
Baby	2¾"-long pickle	4	.5
Slices	1 slice (.1 oz.)	Tr.	0.
Whole	3½"-long pickle (.5 oz.)	8	1.0
(Vlasic):			
Deli	1-oz. serving	4	1.0
Spear, regular or half-the-salt	1-oz. serving	4	1.0
Sour (USDA) cucumber	1 oz.	3	.6
Sweet:			
(Nalley's) Nubbins	1-oz. serving	28	7.9
(Smucker's):			
Candied mix	1 piece (.3 oz.)	14	3.3
Gherkins	2" long pickle (9 grams)	15	3.5
Slices	1 slice (.2 oz.)	11	2.3
Whole	2½" long pickle	18	4.0
(Vlasic) butter chips, half-the-salt	1-oz. serving	30	7.0
Sweet & sour (Claussen) slices	1 slice	3	.8

(USDA): United States Department of Agriculture
(HEW/FAO): Health, Education and Welfare/Food and Agriculture
Organization
* Prepared as Package Directs

Food and Description	Measure or Quantity	Calories	Carbo-hydrates (grams)
PIE:			
Regular, non-frozen:			
Apple:			
Home recipe (USDA), two crust	1/6 of 9" pie	404	60.2
(Dolly Madison)	4½-oz. pie	490	59.0
(Hostess)	4½-oz. pie	409	51.1
Banana, home recipe (USDA), cream or custard	1/6 of 9" pie	336	46.7
Berry (Hostess)	4½-oz. pie	404	51.1
Blackberry, home recipe (USDA) two crust	1/6 of 9" pie	384	54.4
Blueberry:			
Home recipe (USDA), two-crust	1/6 of 9" pie	382	55.1
(Dolly Madison)	4½-oz. pie	430	56.0
(Hostess)	4½-oz. pie	394	49.9
Boston cream (USDA), home recipe	1/12 of 8" pie	208	34.4
Butterscotch (USDA), home recipe, 1-crust	1/6 of 9" pie	406	58.2
Cherry:			
Home recipe (USDA), 2-crust	1/6 of 9" pie	412	60.7
(Dolly Madison):			
Regular	4½-oz. pie	470	53.0
N' cream	4½-oz. pie	440	63.0
(Hostess)	4½-oz. pie	429	56.2
Chocolate (Dolly Madison):			
Regular	4½-oz. pie	560	74.0
Pudding	4½-oz. pie	500	53.0
Chocolate chiffon (USDA) home recipe, made with vegetable shortening	1/6 of 9" pie	459	61.2
Chocolate meringue (USDA), home recipe, made with vegetable shortening	1/6 of 9" pie	353	46.9
Coconut custard (USDA), home recipe	1/6 of 9" pie	357	37.8
Lemon (Dolly Madison)	4½-oz. pie	460	60.0
Lemon Meringue (USDA) one-crust	1/6 of 9" pie	357	52.8
Mince, home recipe, (USDA) 2-crust	1/6 of 9" pie	428	65.1

Food and Description	Measure or Quantity	Calories	Carbo-hydrates (grams)
Peach (Dolly Madison)	4½-oz. pie	460	54.0
Pecan:			
Home recipe (USDA) 1-crust, made with lard or vegetable shortening	⅙ of 9″ pie	577	70.8
Pineapple, custard, home recipe (USDA) made with lard or vegetable shortening	⅙ of 9″ pie (5.4 oz.)	400	60.2
Pineapple, home recipe (USDA) 1 crust, made with lard or vegetable shortening	⅙ of 9″ pie	344	48.8
Pumpkin, home recipe (USDA) 2-crust, made with lard or vegetable shortening	⅙ of 9″ pie (5.4 oz.)	321	37.2
Raisin, home recipe (USDA) 2-crust, made with lard or vegetable shortening	⅙ of 9″ pie (5.6 oz.)	427	67.9
Rhubarb, home recipe (USDA) 2-crust, made with lard or vegetable shortening	⅙ of 9″ pie (5.6 oz.)	400	60.4
Strawberry, home recipe (USDA) made with lard or vegetable shortening	⅙ of 9″ pie (5.6 oz.)	313	48.8
Vanilla (Dolly Madison) pudding	4½-oz. pie	500	52.0
Frozen:			
Apple:			
(Banquet) Family size	⅙ of 20-oz. pie	253	37.0
(Morton):			
Regular	⅙ of 24-oz. pie	290	41.0
Great Little Desserts:			
Regular	8-oz. pie	590	88.0

(USDA): United States Department of Agriculture
(HEW/FAO):   Health, Education and Welfare/Food and Agriculture
                  Organization
* Prepared as Package Directs

Food and Description	Measure or Quantity	Calories	Carbo-hydrates (grams)
Dutch	7¾-oz. pie	600	94.0
(Sara Lee):			
Regular	⅙ of 31-oz. pie	376	43.2
Dutch	⅙ of 30-oz. pie	354	50.6
(Weight Watchers)	3-oz. serving	180	33.0
Banana cream:			
(Banquet)	⅙ of 14-oz. pie	177	21.0
(Morton):			
Regular	⅙ of 14-oz. pie	160	19.0
Great Little Desserts	3½-oz. pie	250	27.0
Blackberry (Banquet)	⅙ of 20-oz. pie	268	40.0
Blueberry:			
(Banquet)	⅙ of 20-oz. pie	266	40.0
(Morton):			
Great Little Desserts	8-oz. pie	580	86.0
Regular	⅙ of 24-oz. pie	280	39.0
(Sara Lee)	⅙ of 31-oz. pie	449	44.8
Cherry:			
(Banquet) Family size	⅙ of 24-oz. pie	252	36.0
(Morton):			
Regular	⅙ of 24-oz. pie	300	423.0
Great Little Desserts	8-oz. pie	590	87.0
(Sara Lee)	⅙ of 31-oz. pie	397	48.0
(Weight Watchers)	3-oz. serving	200	38.0
Chocolate (Morton)	⅙ of 14-oz. pie	180	20.0
Chocolate cream:			
(Banquet)	⅙ of 14-oz. pie	185	24.0
(Morton) *Great Little Desserts*	3½-oz. pie	270	29.0
Coconut cream:			
(Banquet)	⅙ of 14-oz. pie	187	22.0
(Morton) *Great Little Desserts*	3½-oz. pie	270	25.0
Coconut custard (Morton) *Great Little Desserts*	6½-oz. pie	370	53.0
Lemon (Morton)	⅙ of 14-oz. pie	160	18.0
Lemon cream:			
(Banquet)	⅙ of 14-oz. pie	173	23.0
(Morton) *Great Little Desserts*	3½-oz. pie	250	27.0
Mince:			
(Banquet)	⅙ of 20-oz. pie	258	38.0
(Morton)	⅙ of 24-oz. pie	310	46.0
Peach:			
(Banquet) Family size	⅙ of 20-oz. pie	244	35.0

Food and Description	Measure or Quantity	Calories	Carbo-hydrates (grams)
(Morton):			
Regular	⅙ of 24-oz. pie	280	39.0
Great Little Desserts	8-oz. pie	590	91.0
(Sara Lee)	⅙ of 31-oz. pie	458	56.2
Pumpkin:			
(Banquet)	⅙ of 20-oz. pie	197	29.0
(Morton) regular	⅙ of 24-oz. pie	230	36.0
(Sara Lee)	⅛ of 45-oz. pie	354	49.4
Strawberry cream (Banquet)	⅙ of 14-oz. pie	168	22.0
PIECRUST:			
Home recipe (USDA), 9″ pie, baked, made with vegetable shortening	1 crust	900	78.8
(Empire Kosher)	7 oz.	1001	105.0
Refrigerated (Pillsbury)	2 crusts	1920	184
***PIECRUST MIX:**			
(Betty Crocker):			
Regular	1/16 of pkg.	120	10.0
Stick	⅛ of stick	120	10.0
(Flako)	⅙ of 9″ pie shell	245	25.2
(Pillsbury) mix or stick	⅙ of 2-crust pie	270	25.0
PIE FILLING (See also PUDDING OR PIE FILLING):			
Apple:			
(Comstock)	⅙ of 21-oz. can	110	24.0
(Thank You Brand)	3½ oz.	91	23.0
(White House)	½ cup (4.8 oz.)	163	39.0
Apple rings or slices (See **APPLE,** canned)			
Apricot (Comstock)	⅙ of 21-oz. can	110	24.0
Banana cream (Comstock)	⅙ of 21-oz. can	110	22.0
Blueberry (Comstock)	⅙ of 21-oz. can	120	26.0
Cherry:			
(Comstock)	⅙ of 21-oz. can	120	26.0
(Thank You Brand):			
Regular	3½ oz.	99	24.8

(USDA): United States Department of Agriculture
(HEW/FAO): Health, Education and Welfare/Food and Agriculture Organization
* Prepared as Package Directs

Food and Description	Measure or Quantity	Calories	Carbo-hydrates (grams)
Sweet	3½ oz.	115	29.0
(White House)	½ cup (4.8 oz.)	190	45.0
Chocolate (Comstock)	⅙ of 21-oz. can	140	27.0
Coconut cream (Comstock)	⅙ of 21-oz. can	120	24.0
Coconut custard (USDA) home recipe, made with egg yolk & milk	5 oz. (inc. crust)	288	41.3
Lemon (Comstock)	⅙ of 21-oz. can	160	33.0
Mincemeat (Comstock)	⅙ of 21-oz. can	170	36.0
Peach (Comstock)	⅙ of 21-oz. can	130	27.0
Pineapple (Comstock)	⅙ of 21-oz. can	110	25.0
Pumpkin (See also PUMPKIN, canned):			
(Libby's)	1 cup	210	58.0
(Comstock)	⅙ of 27-oz. can	170	38.0
Raisin (Comstock)	⅙ of 21-oz. can	140	30.0
Strawberry (Comstock)	⅙ of 21-oz. can	130	28.0
Dietetic (Thank You Brand):			
Apple	3¼ oz.	60	.3
Cherry	3⅓ oz.	83	20.8
*PIE MIX:			
Boston cream (Betty Crocker)	⅛ of pie	270	50.0
Chocolate (Royal) No Bake	⅛ of pie	260	25.0
PIEROGIES, frozen (Empire Kosher):			
Cheese	1½-oz. serving	110	13.0
Onion	1½-oz. serving	90	13.0
PIGEON, (See SQUAB)			
PIGEON PEA (USDA):			
Raw, immature seeds in pods	1 lb.	207	37.7
Dry seeds	1 lb.	1551	288.9
PIGNOLI (See PINE NUT)			
PIGS FEET, pickled (USDA):			
Blue:			
Whole	1 lb. (weighed whole)	180	0.
Meat only	4 oz.	102	0.
Northern:			
Whole	1 lb. (weighed whole)	104	0.
Meat only	4 oz.	100	0.

Food and Description	Measure or Quantity	Calories	Carbo-hydrates (grams)
Walleye:			
Whole	1 lb. (weighed whole)	140	0.
Meat only	4 oz.	105	0.
PIMIENTO, canned:			
(Dromedary) drained	1-oz. serving	10	2.0
(Ortega) drained	¼ cup	6	1.3
(Sunshine) diced or sliced,			
solids & liq.	1 T.	4	.9
***PIÑA COLADA COCKTAIL:**			
Canned (Mr. Boston)			
12½% alcohol	3 fl. oz.	249	34.2
*Mix (Bar-Tender's)	5 fl. oz.	254	24.0
PINEAPPLE:			
Fresh (USDA):			
Whole	1 lb. (weighed untrimmed)	123	32.3
Diced	½ cup (2.8 oz.)	41	10.7
Sliced	¾″ × 3½″ slice (3 oz.)	44	11.5
Canned, regular pack, solids & liq.:			
(USDA):			
Heavy syrup:			
Crushed	½ cup (5.6 oz.)	97	25.4
Slices	1 large slice & 2 T. syrup (4.3 oz.)	90	23.7
Tidbits	½ cup (4.6 oz.)	95	25.0
Juice pack	4 oz.	66	17.1
Light syrup	5 oz.	76	17.5
(Del Monte):			
Juice pack:			
Chunks, slice or tidbits	½ cup (4 oz.)	70	18.0
Spears	2 spears (3.1 oz.)	50	14.0
Syrup pack	½ cup (4 oz.)	90	23.0

(USDA): United States Department of Agriculture
(HEW/FAO): Health, Education and Welfare/Food and Agriculture
Organization
* Prepared as Package Directs

Food and Description	Measure or Quantity	Calories	Carbohydrates (grams)
(Dole)			
Juice pack, chunk, crushed or sliced	½ cup (4 oz.)	70	17.5
Heavy syrup, chunk, crushed or sliced	½ cup	95	24.8
Canned, unsweetened or dietetic, solids & liq.:			
(Diet Delight) juice pack	½ cup (4.4 oz.)	70	18.0
(Featherweight):			
Juice pack	½ cup	70	18.0
Water pack	½ cup	60	15.0
(Libby's) Lite	½ cup (4.4 oz.)	60	16.0
(S&W) *Nutradiet,* blue label	1 slice	30	7.5
PINEAPPLE, CANDIED			
(USDA)	1-oz. serving	90	22.7
PINEAPPLE FLAVORING			
(Durkee) imitation	1 tsp.	6	DNA
PINEAPPLE & GRAPEFRUIT JUICE DRINK, canned:			
(Del Monte) regular or pink	6 fl. oz.	90	24.0
(Dole) pink	6 fl. oz.	101	25.4
(Texsun)	6 fl. oz.	91	22.0
PINEAPPLE JUICE:			
Canned:			
(Ardmore Farms)	6 fl. oz.	102	25.2
(Del Monte) unsweetened	6 fl. oz.		
	(6.6 oz.)	100	25.0
(Dole) unsweetened	6 fl. oz.	103	25.4
*Frozen (Minute Maid)	6 fl. oz.	92	22.7
PINEAPPLE-ORANGE DRINK, canned (Hi-C)	6 fl. oz.	94	23.0
PINEAPPLE-ORANGE JUICE:			
Canned (Del Monte)	6 fl. oz.		
	(6.6 oz.)	90	24.0
*Frozen (Minute Maid)	6 fl. oz.	94	23.0
PINEAPPLE PRESERVE OR JAM, sweetened (Smucker's)	1 T. (.7 oz.)	53	13.5

Food and Description	Measure or Quantity	Calories	Carbo-hydrates (grams)
PINE NUT (USDA):			
Pignoli, shelled	4 oz.	626	13.2
Pinon, whole	4 oz. (weighed in shell)	418	13.5
Pinon, shelled	4 oz.	720	23.2
PINOT CHARDONNAY WINE			
(Paul Masson) 12% alcohol	3 fl. oz.	71	2.4
PISTACHIO NUT:			
Raw (USDA):			
In shell	4 oz. (weighed in shell)	337	10.8
Shelled	½ cup (2.2 oz.)	368	11.8
Shelled	1 T. (8 grams)	46	1.5
Roasted:			
(Fisher) Salted:			
In shell	1 oz.	84	2.7
Shelled	1 oz.	174	5.4
(Flavor House) dry roasted	1 oz.	168	5.4
(Frito-Lay's)	1 oz.	175	4.8
(Planters) dry roasted	1 oz.	170	6.0
PITANGA, Fresh (USDA)			
Whole	1 lb. (weighed whole)	187	45.9
Flesh only	4 oz.	58	14.2
PIZZA PIE (See also **SHAKEY'S**):			
Regular, non-frozen:			
Home recipe (USDA) with cheese topping	⅛ of 14″ pie	177	21.2
(*Domino's*:)			
Beef, ground:			
Plain:			
Small	⅛ of 12″ pizza	180	24.3
Large	1/12 of 16″ pizza	263	28.5
With pepperoni:			
Small	⅛ of 12″ pizza	216	24.3
Large	1/12 of 16″ pizza	303	24.5

(USDA): United States Department of Agriculture
(HEW/FAO): Health, Education and Welfare/Food and Agriculture Organization
* Prepared as Package Directs

Food and Description	Measure or Quantity	Calories	Carbo-hydrates (grams)
Cheese:			
Plain:			
Small	⅛ of 12″ pizza	157	24.3
Large	1/12 of 16″ pizza	239	28.4
Double:			
Small	⅛ of 12″ pizza	240	24.7
Large	1/12 of 16″ pizza	350	29.1
Double, with pepperoni:			
Small	⅛ of 12″ pizza	227	24.8
Large	1/12 of 16″ pizza	389	29.1
Mushroom & sausage:			
Small	⅛ of 12″ pizza	183	24.6
Large	1/12 of 16″ pizza	266	28.9
Pepperoni:			
Plain:			
Small	⅛ of 12″ pizza	192	24.3
Large	1/12 of 16″ pizza	278	28.5
With mushroom:			
Small	⅛ of 12″ pizza	194	24.5
Large	1/12 of 16″ pizza	280	28.8
With sausage:			
Small	⅛ of 12″ pizza	215	48.9
Large	1/12 of 16″ pizza	303	57.3
Sausage:			
Small	⅛ of 12″ pizza	180	24.4
Large	1/12 of 16″ pizza	264	28.6
(Godfather's):			
Cheese:			
Original:			
Mini	¼ of pizza (2.8 oz.)	190	31.0
Small	⅙ of pizza (3.6 oz.)	240	32.0
Medium	⅛ of pizza (4 oz.)	270	36.0
Large:			
Regular	1/10 of pizza (4.4 oz.)	297	39.0
Hot slice	⅛ of pizza (5½ oz.)	370	48.0
Stuffed:			
Small	⅙ of pizza (4.4 oz.)	310	38.0
Medium	⅛ of pizza (4.8 oz.)	350	42.0

Food and Description	Measure or Quantity	Calories	Carbo-hydrates (grams)
Large	1/10 of pizza (5.2 oz.)	381	44.0
Thin crust:			
Small	1/6 of pizza (2.6 oz.)	180	21.0
Medium	1/8 of pizza (3 oz.)	310	26.0
Large	1/10 of pizza (3.4 oz.)	228	28.0
Combo:			
Original:			
Mini	1/4 of pizza (3.8 oz.)	240	32.0
Small	1/6 of pizza (5.6 oz.)	360	35.0
Medium	1/8 of pizza (6.2 oz.)	400	39.0
Large:			
Regular	1/10 of pizza (6.8 oz.)	437	42.0
Hot Slice	1/8 of pizza (8.5 oz.)	550	52.0
Stuffed:			
Small	1/6 of pizza (6.3 oz.)	430	41.0
Medium	1/8 of pizza (7 oz.)	480	45.0
Large	1/10 of pizza (7.6 oz.)	521	47.0
Thin crust:			
Small	1/6 of pizza (4.3 oz.)	270	23.0
Medium	1/8 of pizza (4.9 oz.)	310	29.0
Large	1/10 of pizza (5.4 oz.)	336	31.0
Frozen:			
Bagel (Empire Kosher)	2-oz. serving	140	17.0

(USDA): United States Department of Agriculture
(HEW/FAO): Health, Education and Welfare/Food and Agriculture
Organization
* Prepared as Package Directs

Food and Description	Measure or Quantity	Calories	Carbohydrates (grams)
Canadian style bacon:			
(Celeste):			
Small	8-oz. pie	483	50.5
Large	¼ of 19-oz. pie	288	30.0
(Stouffer's) French Bread	½ of 11⅝-oz. pkg.	360	41.0
Cheese:			
(Celentano):			
Nine-slice	2.7-oz. piece	157	20.0
Thick crust	⅓ of 13-oz. pizza	238	31.0
(Empire Kosher):			
Regular	⅓ of 10-oz. pie	195	27.0
Family size	⅕ of 15-oz. pie	215	30.0
3-pack	⅑ of 27-oz. pie	215	30.0
(Stouffer's) French Bread:			
Regular:			
Plain	½ of 10⅜-oz. pkg.	340	41.0
Double cheese	½ of 11¾-oz. pkg.	410	43.0
Lean Cuisine:			
Plain	5⅛-oz. serving	310	40.0
Extra Cheese	5½-oz. serving	350	39.0
(Weight Watchers)	6-oz. pie	350	37.0
Combination:			
(Celeste) Chicago style	¼ of 24-oz. pie	360	36.2
(La Pizzeria)	½ of 13½-oz. pie	420	43.0
(Weight Watchers) deluxe	7¼-oz. pie	340	38.0
Deluxe:			
(Celeste):			
Small	½ of 9-oz. pie	281	31.3
Large	¼ of 23½-oz. pie	368	37.4
(Stouffer's) French Bread:			
Regular	6.2-oz. serving	430	41.0
Lean Cuisine	6 ⅛-oz. serving	350	40.0
English muffin (Empire Kosher)	2-oz. serving	140	17.0
Hamburger (Stouffer's) French Bread	½ of 12¼-oz. pkg.	410	40.0
Pepperoni:			
(Celeste):			
Regular:			

Food and Description	Measure or Quantity	Calories	Carbohydrates (grams)
Small	7¼-oz. pie	568	54.1
Large	¼ of 20-oz. pie	347	34.8
Chicago style	¼ of 24-oz. pie	374	36.7
(Stouffer's) French Bread:			
Regular	½ of 11¼-oz pkg.	410	41.0
Lean Cuisine	5½-oz. serving	340	40.0
(Weight Watchers)	6¼-oz. serving	370	38.0
Sausage:			
(Celeste):			
Regular:			
Small	½ of 8-oz. pie	262	29.8
Large	¼ of 22-oz. pie	359	34.7
Chicago style	¼ of 24-oz. pie	382	36.6
(Stouffer's) French Bread	½ of 12-oz. pkg.	420	41.0
(Weight Watchers) veal	6¾-oz. pie	350	35.1
Sausage & mushroom:			
(Celeste):			
Small	9-oz. pie	555	56.8
Large	¼ of 24-oz. pie	365	34.1
(Stouffer's) French Bread	½ of 12½-oz. pkg.	410	42.0
Sausage & pepperoni (Stouffer's) French Bread	½ of 12½-oz. pkg.	450	40.0
Vegetable (Stouffer's) French Bread	½ of 12¾-oz. pkg.	420	41.0
*Mix (Ragu) *Pizza Quick*	¼ of pie	300	37.0
PIZZA PIE CRUST, refrigerated (Pillsbury)	⅛ of crust	90	16.0
PIZZA SAUCE:			
(Contadina):			
Regular or with cheese	½ cup (4.2 oz.)	80	10.0
With pepperoni	½ cup (4.2 oz.)	90	10.0
With tomato chunks	½ cup (4.2 oz.)	50	10.0

(USDA): United States Department of Agriculture
(HEW/FAO): Health, Education and Welfare/Food and Agriculture Organization
* Prepared as Package Directs

Food and Description	Measure or Quantity	Calories	Carbo-hydrates (grams)
(Ragu):			
Regular	15½-oz. jar	250	30.0
Pizza Quick:			
Chunky	14-oz. jar	332	44.2
Mushroom, sausage or			
traditional	14-oz. jar	329	32.9
Pepperoni	14-oz. jar	412	32.9
PIZZA SEASONING SPICE			
(French's)	1 tsp. (.1 oz.)	5	1.0
PLANTAIN, raw (USDA):			
Whole	1 lb. (weighed with skin)	389	101.9
Flesh only	4 oz.	135	35.4
PLUM:			
Fresh (USDA):			
Damson:			
Whole	1 lb. (weighed with pits)	272	73.5
Flesh only	4 oz.	75	20.2
Japanese & hybrid:			
Whole	1 lb. (weighed with pits)	205	52.5
	2.1-oz. plum (2" dia.)	27	6.9
Diced	½ cup (2.9 oz.)	39	10.1
Halves	½ cup (3.1 oz.)	42	10.8
Slices	½ cup (3 oz.)	40	10.3
Prune type:			
Whole	1 lb. (weighed with pits)	320	84.0
Halves	½ cup (2.8 oz.)	60	52.8
Canned, purple, regular pack solids & liq.:			
(USDA):			
Extra heavy syrup	4 oz.	116	30.3
Heavy syrup, with pits	½ cup (4.5 oz.)	106	27.6
Heavy syrup, without pits	½ cup (4.2 oz.)	100	25.9
Light syrup	4 oz.	71	18.8

Food and Description	Measure or Quantity	Calories	Carbo-hydrates (grams)
(Stokely-Van Camp)	½ cup	120	30.0
(Thank You Brand):			
Heavy syrup	½ cup (4.8 oz.)	109	27.2
Light syrup	½ cup (4.7 oz.)	80	20.0
Canned, unsweetened or low calorie, solids & liq.:			
(Diet Delight) purple:			
Juice pack	½ cup (4.4 oz.)	70	19.0
Water pack	½ cup (4.4 oz.)	50	13.0
(Featherweight) purple:			
Juice pack	½ cup	80	18.0
Water pack	½ cup	40	9.0
(S&W) *Nutradiet,* purple,			
juice pack	½ cup	80	20.0
(Thank You Brand)	½ cup (4.8 oz.)	49	12.2
PLUM JELLY:			
Sweetened (Bama)	1 T. (.7 oz.)	45	12.0
Dietetic or low calorie			
(Featherweight)	1 T.	16	4.0
PLUM PRESERVE or JAM,			
Sweetened (Smucker's)	1 T. (.7 oz.)	53	13.5
PLUM PUDDING (Richardson & Robbins)	2″ wedge (3.6 oz.)	270	61.0
POLISH-STYLE SAUSAGE (See **SAUSAGE**)			
POLYNESIAN-STYLE DINNER, frozen (Swanson)			
4-compartment	12-oz. dinner	360	52.0

(USDA): United States Department of Agriculture
(HEW/FAO):   Health, Education and Welfare/Food and Agriculture
                Organization
* Prepared as Package Directs

Food and Description	Measure or Quantity	Calories	Carbo-hydrates (grams)
POMEGRANATE, raw (USDA):			
Whole	1 lb. (weighed whole)	160	41.7
Pulp only	4 oz.	71	18.6
PONDEROSA RESTAURANT:			
A-1 Sauce	1 tsp.	4	1.0
Beef, chopped patty only (See also Bun):			
Regular	3½ oz.	209	0.
Big	4.8 oz.	295	0.
Double Deluxe	5.9 oz.	362	0.
Junior (*Square Shooter*)	1.6 oz.	98	0.
Steakhouse Deluxe	2.96 oz.	181	0.
Beverages:			
Coca-Cola	8 fl. oz.	96	24.0
Coffee	6 fl. oz.	2	.5
Dr Pepper	8 fl. oz.	96	24.8
Lemon	8 fl. oz.	110	28.5
Milk:			
Regular	8 fl. oz.	159	12.0
Chocolate	8 fl. oz.	208	25.9
Orange drink	8 fl. oz.	110	30.0
Root beer	8 fl. oz.	104	25.6
Sprite	8 fl. oz.	95	24.0
Tab	8 fl. oz.	1	.1
Bun:			
Regular	2.4-oz. bun	190	35.0
Hot dog	1 bun	108	18.9
Junior	1.4-oz. bun	118	21.0
Steakhouse deluxe	2.4-oz. bun	190	35.0
Chicken strips:			
Adult portion	2¾ oz.	282	15.8
Children's portion	1.4 oz.	141	7.9
Cocktail sauce	1½ oz.	57	.2
Filet Mignon	3.8 oz. (edible portion)	152	.2
Filet of sole, fish only (See also Bun)	3-oz. piece	125	4.4
Fish, baked	4.9-oz. serving	268	11.6
Gelatin dessert	½ cup	97	23.5

Food and Description	Measure or Quantity	Calories	Carbo-hydrates (grams)
Gravy, au jus	1 oz.	3	Tr.
Ham & cheese:			
Bun (See Bun)			
Cheese, Swiss	2 slices (.8 oz.)	76	.5
Ham	2½ oz.	184	1.4
Hot dog, child's, meat only			
(See also Bun)	1.6-oz. hot dog	140	2.0
Margarine:			
Pat	1 pat	36	Tr.
On potato, as served	½ oz.	100	.1
Mustard sauce, sweet & sour	1 oz.	50	9.5
New York strip steak	6.1 oz. (edible portion)	362	0.
Onion, chopped	1 T. (.4 oz.)	4	.9
Pickle, dill	3 slices (.7 oz.)	2	.2
Potato:			
Baked	7.2-oz. potato	145	32.8
French fries	3-oz. serving	230	30.2
Prime ribs:			
Regular	4.2 oz. (edible portion)	286	0.
Imperial	8.4 oz. (edible portion)	572	0.
King	6 oz. (edible portion)	409	0.
Pudding:			
Butterscotch	4½ oz.	200	27.4
Chocolate	4½ oz.	213	27.1
Vanilla	4½ oz.	195	27.5
Ribeye	3.2 oz. (edible portion)	197	0.
Ribeye & Shrimp:			
Ribeye	3.2 oz.	197	0.
Shrimp	2.2 oz.	139	0.
Roll, kaiser	2.2-oz. roll	184	33.0
Salad bar:			
Bean sprouts	1 oz.	13	1.5
Beets	1 oz.	5	.9

(USDA): United States Department of Agriculture
(HEW/FAO):   Health, Education and Welfare/Food and Agriculture
                        Organization
* Prepared as Package Directs

Food and Description	Measure or Quantity	Calories	Carbo-hydrates (grams)
Broccoli	1 oz.	9	1.7
Cabbage, red	1 oz.	9	2.0
Carrots	1 oz.	12	2.8
Cauliflower	1 oz.	8	1.5
Celery	1 oz.	4	1.1
Chickpeas (Garbanzos)	1 oz.	102	17.3
Cucumber	1 oz.	4	.7
Mushrooms	1 oz.	8	1.2
Onion, white	1 oz.	11	2.6
Pepper, green	1 oz.	6	1.4
Radish	1 oz.	5	1.0
Tomato	1 oz.	6	1.3
Salad dressing:			
Blue cheese	1 oz.	129	2.1
Italian, creamy	1 oz.	138	2.8
Low calorie	1 oz.	14	.8
Oil & vinegar	1 oz.	124	.9
Sweet'n Tart	1 oz.	129	9.2
Thousand Island	1 oz.	117	6.7
Shrimp dinner	7 pieces (3½ oz.)	220	9.8
Sirloin:			
Regular	3.3 oz. (edible portion)	197	0.
Super	6½ oz. (edible portion)	383	0.
Tips	4 oz. (edible portion)	192	0.
Steak sauce	1 oz.	23	4.0
Tartar sauce	1.5 oz.	285	4.5
T-Bone	4.3 oz. (edible portion)	240	0.
Tomato (See also Salad Bar):			
Slices	2 slices (.9 oz.)	5	1.2
Whole, small	3.5 oz.	22	4.7
Topping, whipped	¼ oz.	19	1.2
Worcestershire sauce	1 tsp.	4	.9

POPCORN:

*Plain, popped fresh:			
(Jiffy Pop)	½ of 5-oz. pkg.	244	29.8
(Jolly Time):			
Regular, no added butter or salt:			
White	1 cup	19	4.0

Food and Description	Measure or Quantity	Calories	Carbo-hydrates (grams)
Yellow	1 cup	22	4.7
Microwave:			
Natural	1 cup	53	5.0
Butter flavor	1 cup	53	5.3
Cheese flavor	1 cup	60	5.7
(Orville Redenbacher's)			
Original:			
Plain	1 cup (.2 oz.)	22	4.5
With oil & salt	1 cup (.3 oz.)	40	5.3
Caramel crunch	1 cup	140	19.0
Hot air corn	1 cup	25	4.5
Microwave:			
Regular, butter flavored	1 cup	27	2.5
Regular, natural	1 cup	27	2.7
Flavored:			
Caramel	1 cup	96	11.6
Cheese	1 cup	50	4.0
Sour cream & onions	1 cup	50	4.3
(Pillsbury) Microwave			
Popcorn:			
Regular	1 cup	70	6.5
Butter flavor, regular or			
frozen	1 cup	70	6.7
Salt free, frozen	1 cup	57	7.7
Butter flavor	1 cup	65	6.0
Pop-Secret (General Mills)	1 cup	140	16.0
(Super Pop):			
Dry popped	1 oz.	100	20.0
Oil popped	1 oz.	220	20.0
Packaged:			
Plain: (Bachman)	1 oz.	160	13.0
Caramel-coated:			
(Bachman)	1-oz. serving	110	25.0
(Old Dutch)	1 oz.	109	DNA
(Old London) without			
peanuts	1¾-oz. serving	195	43.6
Cheese flavored (Bachman)	1-oz. serving	180	14.0
Cracker Jack	1-oz. serving	120	22.0
(Snyder's) cheese flavored	1 oz.	150	13.0
(Wise) butter flavored	1 oz.	140	16.0

(USDA): United States Department of Agriculture
(HEW/FAO): Health, Education and Welfare/Food and Agriculture
Organization
* Prepared as Package Directs

Food and Description	Measure or Quantity	Calories	Carbo-hydrates (grams)
POPCORN POPPING OIL			
(Orville Redenbacher's)			
Gourmet, buttery flavor	1 T.	120	0.
POPOVER:			
Home recipe (USDA)	1 average popover (2 oz.)	128	14.7
*Mix (Flako)	1 popover	170	25.0
POPPY SEED (French's)	1 tsp.	13	.8
POPSICLE, twin	3-fl.-oz. pop	70	17.0
PORGY, raw (USDA):			
Whole	1 lb. (weighed whole)	208	0.
Meat only	4 oz.	127	0.
PORK, medium-fat:			
Fresh (USDA):			
Boston butt:			
Raw:	1 lb. (weighed with bone & skin)	1220	0.
Roasted, lean & fat	4 oz.	400	0.
Roasted, lean only	4 oz.	277	0.
Chop:			
Broiled, lean & fat	1 chop (4 oz., weighed with bone)	295	0.
Broiled, lean & fat	1 chop (4 oz., weighed with bone)	332	0.
Broiled, lean & fat	1 chop (3 oz., weighed without bone)	230	0.
Fat, separable cooked	1 oz.	219	0.
Ham (see also **HAM**):			
Raw	1 lb. (weighed with bone & skin)	1188	0.
Roasted, lean & fat	4 oz.	424	0.

Food and Description	Measure or Quantity	Calories	Carbo-hydrates (grams)
Roasted, lean only	4 oz.	246	0.
Loin:			
Raw	1 lb. (weighed with bone)	1065	0.
Roasted, lean & fat	4 oz.	411	0.
Roasted, lean only	4 oz.	288	0.
Picnic:			
Raw	1 lb. (weighed with bone & skin)	1083	0.
Simmered, lean & fat	4 oz.	424	0.
Simmered, lean only	4 oz.	240	0.
Spareribs:			
Raw, with bone	1 lb. (weighed with bone)	976	0.
Braised, lean & fat	4 oz.	499	0.
Cured, light commercial cure:			
Bacon (see **BACON**)			
Bacon butt (USDA):			
Raw	1 lb. (weighed with bone & skin)	1227	0.
Roasted, lean & fat	4 oz.	374	0.
Roasted, lean only	4 oz.	276	0.

PORK & BEANS (See BEAN, BAKED)

PORK, CANNED, chopped luncheon meat (USDA):			
Regular	1 oz.	83	.4
Chopped	1 cup (4.8 oz.)	400	1.8
Diced	1 cup	415	1.8
PORK DINNER, frozen (Swanson) loin of	11¼-oz. dinner	290	26.0
PORK, PACKAGED (Eckrich)	1-oz. serving	45	1.0
PORK RINDS (Old Dutch)	1-oz. serving	154	1.0

(USDA): United States Department of Agriculture
(HEW/FAO): Health, Education and Welfare/Food and Agriculture Organization
* Prepared as Package Directs

Food and Description	Measure or Quantity	Calories	Carbo-hydrates (grams)
PORK STEAK, BREADED, FROZEN (Hormel)	3-oz. serving	220	11.0
PORK, SWEET & SOUR, frozen (Chun King)	13-oz. meal	324	56.0
PORT WINE:			
(Gallo) 16% alcohol	3 fl. oz.	94	7.8
(Louis M. Martini) 19½% alcohol	3 fl. oz.	165	2.0
POSTUM, instant, regular or coffee flavored	6 fl. oz.	11	2.6
POTATO:			
Cooked (USDA)			
Au gratin, with cheese	½ cup (4.3 oz.)	177	16.6
Baked, peeled	2½" dia. potato (3.5 oz.)	92	20.9
Boiled, peeled before boiling, no salt	4.3-oz. potato	79	17.7
French-fried in deep fat, no salt	10 pieces (2 oz.)	156	20.5
Hash-browned, home recipe, after holding overnight	½ cup (3.4 oz.)	223	28.4
Mashed, milk & butter added	½ cup (3.5 oz.)	92	12.1
Canned, solids & liq.:			
(Allen's) Butterfield	½ cup	45	10.0
(Del Monte) sliced or whole	½ cup (4 oz.)	45	10.0
(Larsen) *Freshlike*	½ cup	60	13.0
(Sunshine) whole	½ cup (4.4 oz.)	51	10.5
Frozen:			
(Birds Eye):			
Cottage fries	2.8-oz. serving	119	17.3
Crinkle cuts:			
Regular	3-oz. serving	115	18.4
Deep Gold	3-oz. serving	138	25.5
French fries:			
Regular	3-oz. serving	113	16.8
Deep Gold	3-oz. serving	161	24.4
Hash browns:			
Regular	4-oz. serving	74	16.5
Shredded	¼ of 12-oz. pkg.	61	13.1
Steak fries	3-oz. serving	109	17.9

Food and Description	Measure or Quantity	Calories	Carbo-hydrates (grams)
Tasti Fries	2½-oz. serving	136	16.5
Tasti Puffs	¼ of 10-oz. pkg.	192	19.4
Tiny Taters	⅕ of 16.oz. pkg.	204	22.0
Whole, peeled	3.2-oz. serving	59	12.8
(Empire Kosher) french fries	3-oz. serving	110	18.0
(Larsen) diced	4-oz. serving	80	19.0
(McKenzie) whole, white, boiled	3-oz. serving	70	15.0
(Stouffer's):			
Au gratin	⅓ of 11½-oz. pkg.	110	10.0
Scalloped	⅓ of 11½-oz. pkg.	90	11.0
POTATO & BACON, canned (Hormel) *Short Orders,* au gratin	7½ oz. can	240	20.0
POTATO & BEEF, canned, *Dinty Moore* (Hormel) *Short Orders*	7½-oz. can	250	25.0
POTATO CHIPS:			
(Bachman):			
Regular	1 oz.	160	14.0
BBQ or sour cream & onion	1 oz.	150	14.0
(Cottage Fries) unsalted	1 oz.	160	14.0
Delta Gold	1 oz.	160	14.0
(Laura Scudder's):			
Barbecue	1 oz.	150	15.0
Sour cream & onion	1 oz.	150	14.0
Lays:			
All flavors except sour cream & onion	1 oz.	150	15.0
Sour cream & onion	1 oz.	160	15.0
Ruffles:			
Regular:			
All flavors	1 oz.	150	15.0
Light	1 oz.	130	19.0

(USDA): United States Department of Agriculture
(HEW/FAO):   Health, Education and Welfare/Food and Agriculture Organization
* Prepared as Package Directs

Food and Description	Measure or Quantity	Calories	Carbo-hydrates (grams)
Cottage fries:			
BBQ	1 oz.	150	14.0
Sour cream & chive or			
unsalted	1 oz.	160	14.0
(New York Deli)	1 oz.	160	14.0
(Old Dutch) *O'Grady's:*	1 oz.	150	16.0
All flavors except BBQ	1 oz.	150	16.0
BBQ	1 oz.	140	16.0
(Snyder's)	1 oz.	150	15.0
(Tom's):			
Regular, BBQ, rippled or			
sour cream & onion	1 oz.	160	14.0
Hot or vinegar and salt	1 oz.	160	15.0
(Wise):			
Regular:			
Barbecue, garlic & onion	1 oz.	150	14.0
Lightly salted, natural or			
salt & vinegar	1 oz.	160	14.0
Cottage Fries:			
BBQ	1 oz.	150	14.0
No salt added or sour			
cream & chives	1 oz.	160	14.0
Ridgies	1 oz.	160	14.0
POTATO & HAM, canned (Hormel) *Short Orders,* scalloped	7½-oz. can	250	19.0
*POTATO MIX:			
Au gratin:			
(Betty Crocker)	½ cup	150	21.0
(French's) tangy	½ cup	130	20.0
(Libby's) *Potato Classics*	¾ cup	130	22.0
(Lipton) & sauce	¼ of pkg.	108	22.4
Beef & mushroom (Lipton)	½ cup	95	20.4
Casserole (French's) cheddar cheese & bacon	½ cup	130	18.0
Cheddar bacon (Lipton) & sauce	½ cup	106	20.5
Cheddar broccoli (Lipton)	½ cup	104	20.5
Chicken flavored mushroom (Lipton) & sauce	½ cup	90	19.2
Chicken & herb (Betty Crocker)	½ cup	120	19.0
Creamed (Betty Crocker)	½ cup	180	22.0

Food and Description	Measure or Quantity	Calories	Carbo-hydrates (grams)
Hash browns (Betty Crocker)			
with onion	½ cup	160	24.0
Italian (Lipton)	½ cup	107	20.8
Julienne (Betty Crocker)	½ cup	140	19.0
Mashed:			
(Betty Crocker) *Buds*	½ cup	130	17.0
(French's):			
Big Tate	½ cup	140	16.0
Idaho	½ cup	120	16.0
(Pillsbury) *Hungry Jack,*			
flakes	½ cup	140	17.0
Nacho (Lipton) & sauce	½ cup	103	20.9
Scalloped:			
(Betty Crocker)	½ cup	140	19.0
(French's):			
Creamy Italian	½ cup	120	19.0
Crispy top or real cheese	½ cup	140	19.0
(Lipton) & sauce	½ cup	102	19.5
Sour cream & chive:			
(Betty Crocker)	½ cup	160	21.0
(French's)	½ cup	150	19.0
(Lipton)	¼ pkg.	113	21.0
*POTATO PANCAKE MIX			
(French's)	3″ pancake	30	5.3
POTATO SALAD:			
Home recipe (USDA):			
With cooked salad dressing			
seasonings	4 oz.	112	18.5
With mayonnaise & French dressing, hard-cooked			
eggs, seasonings	4 oz.	164	15.2
Canned (Nally's):			
Regular	4-oz. serving	139	17.0
German style	4-oz. serving	143	18.2
*Mix (Betty Crocker)			
Suddenly Salads, creamy	⅙ of pkg.	250	21.0

(USDA): United States Department of Agriculture
(HEW/FAO):   Health, Education and Welfare/Food and Agriculture
              Organization
* Prepared as Package Directs

Food and Description	Measure or Quantity	Calories	Carbo-hydrates (grams)
POTATO STARCH (Manischewitz)	½ cup	315	DNA
POTATO STICKS (Durkee) *O & C*	1½-oz. serving	231	22.0
POTATO, STUFFED, BAKED, frozen (Green Giant):			
With cheese flavored topping	½ of 10-oz. pkg.	200	33.0
With sour cream & chives	½ of 10-oz. pkg.	230	31.0
POTATO TOPPERS (Libby's)	1 T.	30	4.0
POT ROAST, frozen (Stouffer's) *Right Course*	9 ¼-oz. meal	220	22.0
POUND CAKE (See **CAKE,** Pound)			
PRESERVE OR JAM (See individual flavors)			
PRETZELS:			
(Eagle) *A & Eagle*	1 oz.	110	22.0
(Estee) unsalted	1 piece (1.3 grams)	5	1.0
(Nabisco) *Mister Salty:*			
Regular:			
Dutch	1 piece	55	11.0
Logs	1 piece	12	2.3
Mini	1 piece	7	1.3
Mini mix or nuggets	1 piece	5	1.0
Rings	1 piece	5	.9
Rods	1 piece	55	10.5
Sticks	1 piece	1	.2
Twists	1 piece	22	4.2
Juniors	1 piece	4	.7
(Old Dutch)	1-oz. serving	120	23.0
(Pepperidge Farm):			
Nuggets	1¼-oz. serving	148	26.3
Sticks, thin	1¼-oz. serving	145	26.3
Twists, tiny	1-oz. serving	116	21.6
(Rokeach) Dutch style:			
Regular	1 oz.	110	24.0
Unsalted	1 oz.	110	20.0

Food and Description	Measure or Quantity	Calories	Carbo-hydrates (grams)
Rold Gold	1 oz.	110	22.0
(Seyfert's) rods, butter	1 oz.	110	21.0
(Snyder's)			
Hard	1 oz.	102	22.7
Sticks or thins	1 oz.	110	22.0
(Tom's) twists	1 oz.	100	22.0
(Wise) nuggets	1 oz.	110	21.0
PRICKLY PEAR, fresh			
(USDA):			
Whole	1 lb. (weighed with rind & seeds)	84	21.8
Flesh only	4 oz.	48	12.4
PRODUCT 19, cereal (Kellogg's)	1 cup (1 oz.)	100	24.0
PRO GRAIN, cereal			
(Kellogg's)	¾ cup (1 oz.)	100	24.0
PROSCIUTTO (Hormel)			
boneless	1 oz.	90	0.
PRUNE:			
Canned:			
(Featherweight) stewed,			
water pack	½ cup	130	35.0
(Sunsweet) stewed	½ cup (4.6 oz.)	120	32.0
Dried:			
(Del Monte):			
Moist Pak	2 oz.	120	30.0
Uncooked:			
With pits	2 oz.	120	31.0
Pitted	2 oz.	140	35.0
(Sunsweet):			
Whole	2 oz.	120	31.0
Pitted	2 oz.	140	36.0
PRUNE JUICE:			
(Algood) *Lady Betty*	6 fl. oz.	130	30.0

(USDA): United States Department of Agriculture
(HEW/FAO): Health, Education and Welfare/Food and Agriculture Organization
* Prepared as Package Directs

Food and Description	Measure or Quantity	Calories	Carbo-hydrates (grams)
(Ardmore Farms)	6 fl. oz.	148	36.6
(Del Monte)	6 fl. oz.		
	(6.7 oz.)	120	33.0
(Mott's) regular	6 fl. oz.	140	34.0
(Sunsweet):			
Regular	6 fl. oz.	140	33.0
Home style with pulp	6 fl. oz.	130	32.0
PRUNE NECTAR, canned			
(Mott's)	6 fl. oz.	100	25.0
PRUNE WHIP (USDA) home			
recipe	1 cup (4.8 oz.)	211	49.8
PUDDING OR PIE FILLING			
(See also **CUSTARD**):			
Home recipe (USDA):			
Bread (See **BREAD PUDDING**)			
Rice, made with raisins	½ cup (4.7 oz.)	1983	35.2
Tapioca:			
Apple	½ cup (4.4 oz.)	146	36.8
Cream	½ cup (2.9 oz.)	110	14.0
Canned, regular pack:			
Banana:			
(Del Monte) *Pudding Cup*	5-oz. container	181	30.1
(Hunt's) *Snack Pack*	4¼-oz. container	180	22.0
(Thank You Brand)	½ cup	150	33.8
Butterscotch:			
(Del Monte) *Pudding Cup*	5-oz. container	184	30.8
(Hunt's) *Snack Pack*	4¼-oz. container	180	26.0
(Swiss Miss)	4-oz. container	160	23.0
(Thank You Brand)	½ cup	149	33.8
Chocolate:			
(Del Monte) *Pudding Cup*:			
Regular	5-oz. container	201	32.9
Fudge	5-oz. container	193	30.9
(Hunt's) *Snack Pack*:			
Regular	4¼-oz. container	160	28.0
Fudge	4¼-oz. container	170	24.0
German	4¼-oz. container	190	30.0
Marshmallow	4¼-oz. container	170	26.0
(Thank You Brand)	½ cup	191	36.4
Lemon (Thank You Brand)	½ cup	174	37.7

Food and Description	Measure or Quantity	Calories	Carbo-hydrates (grams)
Rice:			
(Betty Crocker)	4¼-oz. container	150	25.0
(Comstock; Menner's)	½ of 7½-oz. can	120	23.0
(Hunt's) *Snack Pack*	4¼-oz. container	190	23.0
Tapioca:			
(Del Monte) *Pudding Cup*	5-oz. container	172	30.1
(Hunt's) *Snack Pack*	4¼-oz. container	160	28.0
(Swiss Miss)	4-oz. container	150	26.0
(Thank You Brand)	½ cup	144	24.7
Vanilla:			
(Del Monte)	5-oz. container	188	32.1
(Hunt's) *Snack Pack*	4¼-oz. container	170	28.0
(Swiss Miss)	4-oz. container	160	26.0
(Thank You Brand)	½ cup	150	26.0
Canned, dietetic pack (Estee)	½ cup	70	13.0
Chilled, *Swiss Miss:*			
Butterscotch, chocolate malt or vanilla	4-oz. container	150	24.0
Chocolate or double rich	4-oz. container	160	24.0
Chocolate malt	4-oz. container	150	22.0
Chocolate sundae	4-oz. container	170	26.0
Rice	4-oz. container	150	24.0
Tapioca	4-oz. container	130	22.0
Vanilla sundae	4-oz. container	170	25.0
Frozen (Rich's):			
Butterscotch	4½-oz. container	198	27.2
Chocolate	4½-oz. container	212	27.4
Vanilla	4½-oz. container	194	27.4
*Mix, sweetened, regular & instant:			
Banana:			
(Jell-O) cream:			
Regular	½ cup	161	26.7
Instant	½ cup	174	30.0
(Royal) regular	½ cup	160	27.0
Butter pecan (Jell-O) instant	½ cup	175	29.1
Butterscotch:			
(Jell-O):			
Regular	½ cup	172	29.7
Instant	½ cup	175	30.0

(USDA): United States Department of Agriculture
(HEW/FAO): Health, Education and Welfare/Food and Agriculture
        Organization
* Prepared as Package Directs

Food and Description	Measure or Quantity	Calories	Carbo-hydrates (grams)
(My-T-Fine) regular	½ cup	143	28.0
(Royal) regular	½ cup	160	27.0
Chocolate:			
(Jell-O):			
Plain:			
Regular	½ cup	174	28.8
Instant	½ cup	181	30.6
Fudge:			
Regular	½ cup	169	27.8
Instant	½ cup	182	30.9
Milk:			
Regular	½ cup	171	28.2
Instant	½ cup	184	34.0
(My-T-Fine) regular	½ cup	169	27.0
(Royal)	½ cup	190	35.0
Coconut:			
(Jell-O) cream:			
Regular	½ cup	176	24.4
Instant	½ cup	182	26.1
(Royal) instant	½ cup	170	30.0
Flan (Royal) regular	½ cup	150	22.0
Lemon:			
(Jell-O):			
Regular	½ cup	181	38.8
Instant	½ cup	179	31.1
(My-T-Fine) regular	½ cup	164	30.0
Lime (Royal) Key Lime, regular	½ cup	160	30.0
Pineapple (Jell-O) cream, instant	½ cup	176	30.4
Pistachio (Jell-O) instant	½ cup	174	28.4
Raspberry (Salada) *Danish Dessert*	½ cup	130	32.0
Rice, *Jell-O Americana*	½ cup	176	29.9
Strawberry (Salada) *Danish Dessert*	½ cup	130	32.0
Tapioca:			
Jell-O Americana:			
Chocolate	½ cup	173	27.8
Vanilla	½ cup	162	27.4
(My-T-Fine) vanilla	½ cup	130	28.0
Vanilla:			
(Jell-O):			
Plain, instant	½ cup	179	31.0
French, regular	½ cup	172	29.7

Food and Description	Measure or Quantity	Calories	Carbo-hydrates (grams)
(Royal)	½ cup	180	29.0
*Mix, dietetic:			
Butterscotch:			
(Estee)	½ cup	50	9.0
(D-Zerta)	½ cup	68	12.0
(Estee)	½ cup	70	13.0
(Royal)	½ cup	100	16.0
Chocolate:			
(Estee)	½ cup	50	9.0
(D-Zerta)	½ cup (4.6 oz.)	68	11.5
(Estee)	½ cup	70	11.5
(Featherweight)	½ cup	60	9.0
(Louis Sherry)	½ cup (4.2 oz.)	50	9.0
Lemon (Estee)	½ cup	50	9.0
Vanilla:			
(Estee)	½ cup (4.2 oz.)	50	9.0
(D-Zerta)	½ cup	70	13.0
(Estee) instant	½ cup	70	13.0
(Royal)	½ cup	100	16.0

PUDDING POPS (See *JELL-O PUDDING POPS*)

PUDDING ROLL-UPS, *Fruit Corners* (General Mills):

Butterscotch	.5-oz. piece	60	11.0
Chocolate fudge or milk chocolate	.5-oz. piece	60	10.0

PUDDING SUNDAE
(Swiss Miss):

Caramel or mint	4-oz. container	170	25.0
Chocolate	4-oz. container	190	29.0
Peanut butter	4-oz. container	200	23.0
Vanilla	4-oz. container	180	28.0

PUFF PASTRY (See **PASTRY SHEET, PUFF**)

(USDA): United States Department of Agriculture
(HEW/FAO): Health, Education and Welfare/Food and Agriculture Organization
* Prepared as Package Directs

Food and Description	Measure or Quantity	Calories	Carbo-hydrates (grams)
PUFFED RICE:			
(Malt-O-Meal)	1 cup (.5 oz.)	50	12.0
(Quaker)	1 cup	55	12.7
PUFFED WHEAT:			
(Malt-O-Meal)	1 cup (.5 oz.)	50	11.0
(Quaker)	1 cup (.5 oz.)	54	10.8
PUMPKIN:			
Fresh (USDA):			
Whole	1 lb. (weighed with rind & seeds	83	20.6
Flesh only	4 oz.	29	7.4
Canned:			
(Del Monte)	½ cup (4.3 oz.)	35	9.0
(Festal)	½ cup	45	9.5
(Libby's) solid pack	½ of 16-oz. can	40	10.0
(Stokely-Van Camp)	½ cup (4.3 oz.)	45	9.5
PUMPKIN SEED, dry (USDA):			
Whole	4 oz. (weighed in hull)	464	12.6
Hulled	4 oz.	627	17.0

Food and Description	Measure or Quantity	Calories	Carbo-hydrates (grams)

Q

QUAIL, raw (USDA) meat & skin	4 oz.	195	0.
QUIK (Nestlé):			
Chocolate	1 tsp. (.4 oz.)	45	9.5
Strawberry	1 tsp. (.4 oz.)	45	11.0
QUISP, cereal	1⅙ cup (1 oz.)	121	23.1

(USDA): United States Department of Agriculture
(HEW/FAO):   Health, Education and Welfare/Food and Agriculture
                        Organization
* Prepared as Package Directs

Food and Description	Measure or Quantity	Calories	Carbo-hydrates (grams)

R

RABBIT (USDA)
  Domesticated:

Food and Description	Measure or Quantity	Calories	Carbo-hydrates (grams)
Raw, ready-to-cook	1 lb. (weighed with bones)	581	0.
Stewed, flesh only	4 oz.	245	0.
Wild, ready-to-cook	1 lb. (weighed with bones)	490	0.
RACCOON, roasted, meat only	4 oz.	289	0.

RADISH (USDA):
  Common, raw:

Food and Description	Measure or Quantity	Calories	Carbo-hydrates (grams)
Without tops	½ lb. (weighed untrimmed)	34	7.4
Trimmed, whole	4 small radishes (1.4 oz.)	7	1.4
Trimmed sliced	½ cup (2 oz.)	10	2.1
Oriental, raw, without tops	½ lb. (weighed unpared)	34	7.4
Oriental, raw, trimmed & pared	4 oz.	22	4.8

RAISIN:
  Dried:
   (USDA):

Food and Description	Measure or Quantity	Calories	Carbo-hydrates (grams)
Whole, pressed down	½ cup (2.9 oz.)	237	63.5
Chopped	½ cup (2.9 oz.)	234	62.7
Ground	½ cup (4.7 oz.)	387	103.7
(Del Monte):			
Golden	3 oz.	260	68.0
Thompson	3 oz.	250	68.0
(Sun-Maid) seedless, natural			
Thompson	1 oz.	96	23.0
Cooked, (USDA) added sugar solids & liq.	½ cup (4.3 oz.)	260	68.8

Food and Description	Measure or Quantity	Calories	Carbo-hydrates (grams)
RAISIN BRAN (See BRAN BREAKFAST CEREAL)			
RAISIN SQUARES, cereal (Kellogg's)	½ cup (1 oz.)	90	22.0
RALSTON, cereal, (Ralston Purina) regular or instant	¼ cup (1 oz.)	90	20.0
RASPBERRY:			
Black (USDA):			
Fresh:			
Whole	1 lb. (weighed with caps & stems)	160	34.6
Without caps & stems	½ cup (2.4 oz.)	49	10.5
Canned, water pack unsweetened, solids & liq.	4 oz.	58	12.1
Red:			
Fresh (USDA):			
Whole	1 lb. (weighed with caps & stems)	126	29.9
Without caps & stems	½ cup (2.5 oz.)	41	9.8
Canned, water pack, unsweetened or low calorie, solids & liq. (USDA)	4 oz.	40	10.0
Frozen (Birds Eye) quick thaw:			
Regular	5-oz. serving	155	37.0
In lite syrup	5-oz. serving	110	25.7
RASPBERRY PRESERVE OR JAM:			
Sweetened (Smucker's)	1 T. (.7 oz.)	53	13.5
Dietetic:			
(Estee; Louis Sherry)	1 T. (.6 oz.)	6	0.
(Featherweight) red	1 T.	16	4.0
(S&W) *Nutradiet*, red label	1 T.	12	3.0

(USDA): United States Department of Agriculture
(HEW/FAO): Health, Education and Welfare/Food and Agriculture
                      Organization
* Prepared as Package Directs

Food and Description	Measure or Quantity	Calories	Carbo-hydrates (grams)
RATATOUILLE, frozen (Stouffer's)	5-oz. serving	60	9.0
RAVIOLI:			
Canned, regular pack (Franco-American):			
Beef			
In meat sauce	7½-oz. can	230	36.0
RavioliOs	7½-oz. serving	210	34.0
Canned, dietetic:			
(Estee) beef	7½-oz. can	230	25.0
(Featherweight) beef	8-oz. serving	260	35.0
Frozen:			
(Buitoni):			
Regular, square:			
Cheese	4.8-oz. serving	331	45.2
Meat	4.8-oz. serving	318	44.9
Ravioletti:			
Cheese	2.6-oz. serving	221	36.9
Meat	2.6-oz. serving	233	37.1
(Celentano) cheese:			
Regular	½ of 13-oz. box	410	51.0
Mini	½ of 8-oz. box	250	37.0
(Weight Watchers) baked	8¹⁄₁₆-oz. meal	290	32.0
RED & GRAY SNAPPER, raw (USDA):			
Whole	1 lb. (weighed whole)	219	0.
Meat only	4 oz.	105	0.
RED LOBSTER RESTAURANT ("Lunch Portion" refers to a cooked serving weighing 5 oz. raw, unless otherwise noted):			
Calamari, breaded & fried	Lunch portion	360	30.0
Catfish	Lunch portion	170	0.
Chicken breast	4-oz. serving	120	0.
Clam, cherrystone	Lunch portion	130	11.0
Cod, Atlantic	Lunch portion	100	0.
Crab legs:			
King	16-oz. serving	170	6.0
Snow	16-oz. serving	150	1.0
Flounder	Lunch portion	100	1.0

Food and Description	Measure or Quantity	Calories	Carbo-hydrates (grams)
Grouper	Lunch portion	110	0.
Haddock	Lunch portion	100	2.0
Halibut	Lunch portion	110	1.0
Hamburger, without bun	5.3 oz.	320	0.
Lobster:			
Maine	1 lobster (edible portion)	240	5.0
Rock	1 tail	230	2.0
Mackerel	Lunch portion	190	1.0
Monkfish	Lunch portion	110	0.
Mussels	3-oz. serving	70	3.0
Oysters	6 raw oysters	110	11.0
Perch, Atlantic Ocean	Lunch portion	130	1.0
Pollock	Lunch portion	120	1.0
Rockfish, red	Lunch portion	90	0.
Salmon:			
Norwegian	Lunch portion	230	3.0
Sockeye	Lunch portion	160	3.0
Scallop:			
Calico	Lunch portion	180	8.0
Deep sea	Lunch portion	130	2.0
Shark:			
Blacktip	Lunch portion	150	0.
Mako	Lunch portion	140	0.
Shrimp	8-12 pieces	120	0.
Snapper, red	Lunch portion	110	0.
Sole, lemon	Lunch portion	120	1.0
Steak:			
Porterhouse	18-oz. serving	1420	0.
Sirloin	7-oz. serving	570	0.
Strip	7-oz. serving	690	0.
Swordfish	Lunch portion	100	0.
Tilefish	Lunch portion	100	0.
Trout, rainbow	Lunch portion	170	0.
Tuna, yellowfin	Lunch portion	180	0.
RELISH:			
Dill (Vlasic)	1 oz.	2	1.0
Hamburger:			
(Heinz)	1 T.	30	8.0

(USDA): United States Department of Agriculture
(HEW/FAO):   Health, Education and Welfare/Food and Agriculture
              Organization
* Prepared as Package Directs

Food and Description	Measure or Quantity	Calories	Carbo-hydrates (grams)
(Vlasic)	1 oz.	40	9.0
Hot dog:			
(Heinz)	1 oz.	35	8.0
(Vlasic)	1 oz.	40	8.0
India (Heinz)	1 oz.	35	9.0
Sour (USDA)	1 T. (.5 oz.)	3	.4
Sweet:			
(Heinz)	1 oz.	25	6.6
(Smucker's)	1 T. (.6 oz.)	23	4.8
(Vlasic)	1 oz.	30	8.0
RENNET MIX (Junket):			
*Powder, any flavor:			
Made with skim milk	½ cup	90	15.0
Made with whole milk	½ cup	120	15.0
Tablet	1 tablet	1	0.
RHINE WINE:			
(Great Western) 12% alcohol	3 fl. oz.	73	2.9
(Taylor) 12½% alcohol	3 fl. oz.	75	.3
RHUBARB (USDA)			
Cooked, sweetened, solids & liq.	½ cup (4.2 oz.)	169	43.2
Fresh:			
Partly trimmed	1 lb. (weighed with part leaves, ends & trimmings)	54	12.6
Trimmed	4 oz.	18	4.2
Diced	½ cup (2.2 oz.)	10	2.3
*RICE:			
Brown (Uncle Ben's) parboiled, with added butter & salt	⅔ cup	152	26.4
White:			
(USDA) instant or pre-cooked	⅔ cup (3.3 oz.)	101	22.5
(Minute Rice) instant, no added butter	⅔ cup (4.3 oz.)	120	27.4
(River)	½ cup	100	22.0
(Success) long grain	½ cup	110	23.0
*(Uncle Ben's):			
Cooked without butter or salt	⅔ cup	129	28.9
Cooked with butter and salt	⅔ cup	148	28.9
White & wild (Carolina)	½ cup	90	20.0

Food and Description	Measure or Quantity	Calories	Carbo-hydrates (grams)
RICE BRAN (USDA)	1 oz.	78	14.4
RICE CAKE, dietetic (Pritikin)	1 cake	35	6.0
RICE, FRIED (See also **RICE MIX**):			
*Canned (La Choy)	⅓ of 11-oz. can	190	40.0
Frozen:			
(Birds Eye)	3.7-oz. serving	104	22.8
(Chun King):			
Chicken	8 oz.	254	40.0
Pork	8 oz.	263	43.0
(La Choy) & meat	8-oz. serving	280	52.0
RICE, FRIED, SEASONING MIX:			
*(Durkee)	1 cup	213	46.5
(Kikkoman)	1-oz. pkg.	91	15.6
RICE KRINKLES, cereal			
(Post) frosted	⅞ cup (1 oz.)	109	25.9
RICE KRISPIES, cereal			
(Kellogg's):			
Regular	1 cup (1 oz.)	110	25.0
Cocoa	¾ cup (1 oz.)	110	25.0
Frosted	¾ cup (1 oz.)	110	25.0
Marshmallow	1¼ cups	140	33.0
Strawberry	¾ cup (1 oz.)	110	25.0
RICE MIX:			
Beef:			
(Lipton) & sauce	¼ of pkg.	120	25.9
*(Minute Rice) rib roast	½ cup (4.1 oz.)	149	25.1
Rice-A-Roni	⅙ of 8-oz. pkg.	130	26.0
*Cajun (Lipton) & sauce	¼ of pkg.	123	26.0
Chicken:			
*(Lipton) & sauce	½ cup	125	25.4
*(Minute Rice) drumstick	½ cup (3.8 oz.)	153	25.4

(USDA): United States Department of Agriculture
(HEW/FAO):   Health, Education and Welfare/Food and Agriculture
                    Organization
 * Prepared as Package Directs

Food and Description	Measure or Quantity	Calories	Carbo-hydrates (grams)
Rice-A-Roni	⅙ of 8-oz. pkg.	130	27.0
*Fried (Minute Rice)	½ cup (3.4 oz.)	156	25.2
*Herb & butter (Lipton) & sauce	½ cup	124	24.1
*Long grain & wild (Lipton) & sauce:			
Original	½ cup	121	26.1
Mushroom & herb	½ cup	125	26.4
(Minute Rice)	½ cup (4.1 oz.)	148	25.0
(Uncle Ben's):			
Without butter	½ cup	97	20.6
With butter	½ cup	112	20.6
*Medley (Lipton) & sauce	½ cup	150	26.0
*Mushroom (Lipton) & sauce	½ cup	123	26.1
*Pilaf (Lipton) & sauce	½ cup	117	24.7
Spanish (See also RICE, SPANISH):			
*(Carolina) Bake-It-Easy	¼ of pkg.	110	23.0
*(Lipton) & sauce	½ cup	120	25.7
*(Minute Rice)	½ cup (5.2 oz.)	150	25.6
Rice-A-Roni	⅐ of 7½-oz. pkg.	110	22.0

RICE PUDDING (See **PUDDING OR PIE FILLING**)

*RICE SEASONING, Spice Your Rice (French's):			
Beef flavor & onion, cheese & chives or chicken flavor & parmesan	½ cup	160	27.0
Buttery herb	½ cup	170	27.0
Chicken flavor & herb	½ cup	160	26.0

RICE, SPANISH:			
Home recipe (USDA)	4 oz.	99	18.8
Canned:			
Regular pack (Comstock; Menner's)	½ of 7½-oz. can	140	27.0
Dietetic (Featherweight) low sodium	7½-oz. serving	140	30.0
Frozen (Birds Eye)	3.7-oz. serving	122	26.1

RICE & VEGETABLE, frozen:			
(Birds Eye):			
For One:			
& broccoli, au gratin	5-oz. pkg.	229	25.0

Food and Description	Measure or Quantity	Calories	Carbo-hydrates (grams)
with green beans & almonds	5½-oz. pkg.	200	23.6
Mexican, with corn	5½-oz. pkg.	158	29.9
Pilaf	5½-oz. pkg.	215	27.6
Internationals:			
Country style	⅓ of 10-oz. pkg.	87	19.0
French style	⅓ of 10-oz. pkg.	106	23.0
Spanish style	⅓ of 10-oz. pkg.	111	24.0
(Green Giant):			
One Serving Vegetable:			
& broccoli in cheese sauce	4½-oz. pkg.	180	25.0
with peas & mushrooms with sauce	5½-oz. pkg.	130	27.0
Rice Originals:			
& broccoli in cheese sauce	*4 oz.*	*120*	*18.0*
Medley	*4 oz.*	*100*	*19.0*
& wild rice	*4 oz.*	*130*	*24.0*
RICE WINE (HEW/FAO):			
Chinese, 20.7% alcohol	1 fl. oz.	38	1.1
Japanese, 10.6% alcohol	1 fl. oz.	72	13.1
ROCK & RYE (Mr. Boston) 27% alcohol	1 fl. oz.	75	6.8
ROE (USDA):			
Raw:			
Carp, cod haddock, herring, pike or shad	4 oz.	147	1.7
Salmon, sturgeon or turbot	4 oz.	235	1.6
Baked or broiled, cod & shad	4 oz.	143	2.2
Canned, cod, haddock or herring, solids & liq.	4 oz.	134	.3
ROLL OR BUN:			
Commercial type, non-frozen:			
Apple (Dolly Madison)	2-oz. piece	180	33.0
Biscuit (Wonder)	1¼-oz. piece	99	17.0

(USDA): United States Department of Agriculture
(HEW/FAO): Health, Education and Welfare/Food and Agriculture Organization
* Prepared as Package Directs

Food and Description	Measure or Quantity	Calories	Carbo-hydrates (grams)
Brown & serve:			
(Interstate Brands) *Merita*	1-oz. roll	70	14.0
(Pepperidge Farm)	1 roll	100	20.0
(Roman Meal)	1-oz. piece	78	12.6
(Wonder):			
Buttermilk	1-oz. piece	84	13.1
French	1-oz. piece	87	13.6
Gem style	1-oz. piece	72	13.1
Half & Half	1-oz. piece	81	12.8
Home bake	1-oz. piece	73	12.8
Cherry (Dolly Madison)	2-oz. piece	180	33.0
Cinnamon (Dolly Madison)	1¾-oz. piece	180	28.0
Crescent (Pepperidge Farm) butter	1-oz. piece	110	13.0
Croissant (Pepperidge Farm):			
Almond or Walnut	2-oz. piece	210	21.0
Butter	2-oz. piece	200	19.0
Chocolate	2.4-oz. piece	260	25.0
Cinnamon	2-oz. piece	200	23.0
Honey sesame	2-oz. piece	200	22.0
Raisin	2-oz. piece	200	24.0
Danish (Dolly Madison)			
Danish Twirls:			
Apple	2-oz. piece	240	28.0
Cheese, cream	3½-oz. piece	380	43.0
Cherry	2-oz. piece	230	28.0
Cinnamon raisin	2-oz. piece	250	28.0
Dinner:			
Butternut	1-oz. roll	90	15.0
Eddy's	1-oz. roll	75	14.0
Holsum	1-oz. roll	90	15.0
Home Pride	1-oz. piece	85	14.2
(Wonder)	1¼-oz. piece	99	17.0
Dinner party rounds (Arnold)	.7-oz. piece	55	10.0
Egg, *Weber's*	1-oz. bun	70	12.0
Frankfurter:			
(Arnold) Hot Dog	1.3-oz. piece	110	20.0
(Pepperidge Farm)	1¾-oz. piece	110	18.0
(Wonder)	2-oz. piece	157	28.4
French (Arnold) *Francisco:*			
Regular	2-oz. roll	160	31.0
Sourdough	1.1-oz. piece	90	16.0
Golden Twist (Pepperidge Farm)	1-oz. piece	110	14.0

Food and Description	Measure or Quantity	Calories	Carbo-hydrates (grams)
Hamburger:			
(Arnold)	1.4-oz. piece	110	21.0
(Pepperidge Farm)	1.5-oz. piece	130	21.0
(Roman Meal)	1.8-oz. piece	193	36.1
(Wonder)	2-oz. piece	157	28.4
Hard (USDA)	1.8-oz. piece	156	29.8
Hoagie (Wonder)	6-oz. piece	465	81.8
Honey (Dolly Madison)	3½-oz. piece	420	47.0
Kaiser (Wonder)	6-oz. piece	465	81.8
Lemon (Dolly Madison)	2-oz. piece	180	31.0
Old fashioned (Pepperidge Farm)	.6-oz. piece	60	23.0
Pan (Wonder)	1¼-oz. piece	99	17.0
Parkerhouse (Pepperidge Farm)	.6-oz. piece	50	9.0
Party (Pepperidge Farm)	.4-oz. piece	30	5.0
Raspberry (Dolly Madison)	2-oz. piece	190	31.0
Sandwich:			
(Arnold):			
Francisco	2-oz. piece	160	30.0
Soft, plain or with poppy seed	1.3-oz. piece	110	18.0
Soft with sesame seeds	1.3-oz. piece	110	19.0
(Pepperidge Farm):			
Regular, with or without seeds	1.6-oz. piece	130	23.0
Onion with poppy seeds	1.9-oz. piece	150	26.0
Soft (Pepperidge Farm)	1¼-oz. piece	110	18.0
Sourdough french (Pepperidge Farm)	1.3-oz. piece	100	19.0
Steak, *Butternut*	1-oz. roll	80	14.0
Frozen:			
Apple crunch (Sara Lee)	1-oz. piece	102	13.5
Caramel pecan (Sara Lee)	1.3-oz. piece	161	17.4
Caramel sticky (Sara Lee)	1-oz. piece	116	15.2
Cinnamon (Sara Lee)	.9-oz. piece	100	13.9
Croissant (Sara Lee)	.9-oz. piece	109	11.2
Crumb (Sara Lee):			
Blueberry	1¾-oz. piece	169	26.8
French	1¾-oz. piece	188	29.9

(USDA): United States Department of Agriculture
(HEW/FAO):   Health, Education and Welfare/Food and Agriculture
            Organization
* Prepared as Package Directs

Food and Description	Measure or Quantity	Calories	Carbo-hydrates (grams)
Danish (Sara Lee):			
Apple	1.3-oz. piece	120	17.4
Apple country	1.8-oz. piece	156	22.9
Cheese	1.3-oz. piece	130	13.9
Cheese country	1.5-oz. piece	146	13.5
Cherry	1.3-oz. piece	125	16.4
Cinnamon raisin	1.3-oz. piece	147	17.3
Pecan	1.3-oz. piece	148	18.3
Honey (Morton):			
Regular	2.3-oz. piece	230	31.0
Mini	1.3-oz. piece	133	18.0
***ROLL OR BUN DOUGH:**			
Frozen (Rich's) home style	1 roll	75	14.0
Refrigerated (Pillsbury):			
Butterflake	1 piece	140	20.0
Caramel danish, with nuts	1 piece	160	19.0
Cinnamon:			
Regular	1 piece	210	29.0
With icing:			
Regular	1 piece	110	17.0
& raisin	1 piece	140	19.5
Crescent	1 piece	100	11.0
***ROLL MIX, HOT** (Pillsbury)	1 piece	100	17.0
***ROMAN MEAL CEREAL:**			
2- or 5-minute	⅓ cup (1 oz.)	103	20.0
5-minute with oats	⅓ cup (1 oz.)	105	15.5
ROSEMARY LEAVES			
(French's)	1 tsp	5	.8
ROSÉ WINE:			
Corbett Canyon (Glenmore)	3 fl. oz.	63	<1.0
(Great Western) 12% alcohol	3 fl. oz.	80	2.4
(Paul Masson):			
Regular, 11.8% alcohol	3 fl. oz.	76	4.2
Light, 7.1% alcohol	3 fl. oz.	49	3.9
ROY ROGERS:			
Bar Burger, R.R.	1 burger	611	28.0
Biscuit	1 biscuit	231	26.2

Food and Description	Measure or Quantity	Calories	Carbo-hydrates (grams)
Breakfast crescent sandwich:			
Regular	4.5-oz. sandwich	401	5.3
With bacon	4.7-oz. sandwich	431	25.5
With ham	5.8-oz. sandwich	557	25.3
With sausage	5.7-oz. sandwich	449	25.9
Brownie	1 piece	264	37.3
Cheeseburger:			
Regular	1 burger	563	27.4
With bacon	1 burger	581	25.0
Chicken:			
Breast	1 piece (5.1 oz.)	412	16.9
Breast & wing	6.9-oz. piece	604	25.4
Leg	1 piece (1.9 oz.)	140	5.5
Thigh	1 piece (3.5 oz.)	296	11.7
Thigh & leg	5.3-oz. piece	436	17.2
Wing	1 piece (1.8 oz.)	192	8.5
Cole slaw	3½-oz. serving	110	11.0
Danish:			
Apple	1 piece	249	31.6
Cheese	1 piece	254	31.4
Cherry	1 piece	271	31.7
Drinks:			
Coffee, black	6 fl. oz.	Tr.	Tr.
Coke:			
Regular	12 fl. oz.	145	37.0
Diet	12 fl. oz.	1	0.
Hot chocolate	6 fl. oz.	123	22.0
Milk	8 fl.oz.	150	11.4
Orange juice:			
Regular	7 fl. oz.	99	22.8
Large	10 fl. oz.	136	31.2
Shake:			
Chocolate	1 shake	358	61.3
Strawberry	1 shake	306	45.0
Vanilla	1 shake	315	49.4
Tea, iced, plain	8 fl.oz.	0	0.
Egg & biscuit platter:			
Regular	1 meal	394	21.9
With bacon	1 meal	435	22.1
With ham	1 meal	442	22.5

(USDA): United States Department of Agriculture
(HEW/FAO):   Health, Education and Welfare/Food and Agriculture
                        Organization
* Prepared as Package Directs

Food and Description	Measure or Quantity	Calories	Carbo-hydrates (grams)
With sausage	1 meal	550	21.9
Hamburger	1 burger	456	26.6
Pancake platter, with syrup & butter			
Plain	1 order	452	71.8
With bacon	1 order	493	72.0
With ham	1 order	506	72.4
With sausage	1 order	608	71.8
Potato:			
Baked, *Hot Topped:*			
Plain	1 potato	211	47.9
With bacon & cheese	1 potato	397	33.3
With broccoli & cheese	1 potato	376	39.6
With margarine	1 potato	274	47.9
With sour cream & chives	1 potato	408	47.6
With taco beef & cheese	1 potato	463	45.0
French fries:			
Regular	3 oz.	268	32.0
Large	4 oz.	357	42.7
Potato salad	3½-oz. order	107	10.9
Roast beef sandwich:			
Plain:			
Regular	1 sandwich	317	29.1
Large	1 sandwich	360	29.6
With cheese:			
Regular	1 sandwich	424	29.9
Large	1 sandwich	467	30.3
Salad bar:			
Bacon bits	1 T.	33	2.2
Beets, sliced	¼ cup	16	3.8
Broccoli	½ cup	20	3.5
Carrot, shredded	¼ cup	42	9.7
Cheese, cheddar	¼ cup	112	.8
Croutons	1 T.	35	7.0
Cucumber	1 slice	Tr.	.2
Egg, chopped	1 T.	27	.3
Lettuce	1 cup	10	4.0
Macaroni salad	1 T.	30	3.1
Mushrooms	¼ cup	5	.7
Noodle, Chinese	¼ cup	55	6.5
Pea, green	¼ cup	7	1.2
Pepper, green	1 T.	2	.5
Potato salad	1 T.	25	2.8
Sunflower seeds	1 T.	78	2.5
Tomato	1 slice	7	1.6

Food and Description	Measure or Quantity	Calories	Carbo- hydrates (grams)
Salad dressing:			
Regular:			
Bacon & tomato	1 T.	68	3.0
Bleu cheese	1 T.	75	1.0
Ranch	1 T.	77	2.0
1,000 Island	1 T.	80	2.0
Low calorie, Italian	1 T.	35	1.0
Strawberry shortcake	7.2-oz. serving	447	59.3
Sundae:			
Caramel	1 sundae	293	51.5
Hot fudge	1 sundae	337	53.3
Strawberry	1 sundae	216	33.1
RUM (See DISTILLED LIQUOR)			
RUTABAGA:			
Raw (USDA):			
Without tops	1 lb. (weighed with skin)	177	42.4
Diced	½ cup (2.5 oz.)	32	7.7
Boiled (USDA) drained, diced	½ cup (3 oz.)	30	7.1
Canned (Sunshine) solids & liq.	½ cup (4.2 oz.)	32	6.9
Frozen (Southland)	⅕ of 20-oz. pkg.	50	13.0
RYE, whole grain (USDA)	1 oz.	95	20.8
RYE FLOUR (See FLOUR)			
RYE WHISKEY (See DISTILLED LIQUOR)			

(USDA): United States Department of Agriculture
(HEW/FAO):   Health, Education and Welfare/Food and Agriculture
                    Organization
* Prepared as Package Directs

Food and Description	Measure or Quantity	Calories	Carbohydrates (grams)
SABLEFISH, raw (USDA):			
Whole	1 lb. (weighed whole)	362	0.
Meat only	4 oz.	215	0.
SAFFLOWER SEED (USDA) in hull	1 oz.	89	1.8
SAGE (French's)	1 tsp.	4	.6
SAKE WINE (HEW/FAO) 19.8% alcohol	1 fl. oz.	39	1.4
*SALAD BAR PASTA (Buitoni):			
Country buttermilk or homestyle	⅙ of pkg.	250	22.0
Italian:			
Creamy	⅙ of pkg.	290	20.0
Zesty	⅙ of pkg.	140	21.0
SALAD DRESSING:			
Regular:			
Bacon (Seven Seas) creamy	1 T.	60	1.0
Bacon & tomato (Henri's)	1 T.	70	4.0
Bleu or blue cheese:			
(USDA)	1 T. (.5 oz.)	76	1.1
(Bernstein's) Danish	1 T.	60	.6
(Henri's)	1 T.	60	3.0
Boiled (USDA) home recipe	1 T. (.6 oz.)	26	2.4
Caesar:			
(Pfeiffer)	1 T.	70	.5
(Wish-Bone)	1 T.	78	.9
Capri (Seven Seas)	1 T.	70	3.0
Dijon vinaigrette (Wish-Bone)	1 T.	60	1.1

Food and Description	Measure or Quantity	Calories	Carbo-hydrates (grams)
French:			
Home recipe (USDA)	1 T.	101	.6
(Bernstein's) creamy	1 T. (.5 oz.)	56	2.1
(Henri's):			
Hearty	1 T.	70	4.0
Original	1 T.	60	3.0
Sweet 'n saucy	1 T.	70	5.0
(Wish-Bone):			
Deluxe	1 T.	59	2.3
Garlic	1 T.	55	1.8
Garlic (Wish-Bone) creamy	1 T.	74	.5
Herb & spice (Seven Seas)	1 T.	60	1.0
Italian:			
(Henri's):			
Authentic	1 T.	80	1.0
Creamy garlic	1 T.	50	3.0
(Wish-Bone):			
Creamy	1 T.	56	1.7
Herbal	1 T.	70	1.2
Robusto	1 T.	70	1.3
Mayonnaise-type (Luzianne)			
Blue Plate	1 T.	70	3.0
Miracle Whip (Kraft)	1 T.	70	2.0
Ranchouse (Henri's) Chef's Recipe	1 T.	70	2.0
Red wine vinegar & oil (Wish-Bone)	1 T.	50	4.3
Roquefort:			
(USDA)	1 T. (.5 oz.)	76	1.1
(Bernstein's)	1 T.	65	.8
(Marie's)	1 T.	105	1.1
Russian:			
(USDA)	1 T.	74	1.6
(Henri's)	1 T.	60	4.0
(Wish-Bone)	1 T.	47	6.0
Spin Blend (Hellman's)	1 T. (.6 oz.)	57	2.6
Tas-Tee (Henri's)	1 T.	60	4.0
Thousand Island:			
(USDA)	1 T.	80	2.5
(Henri's)	1 T.	50	3.0

(USDA): United States Department of Agriculture
(HEW/FAO): Health, Education and Welfare/Food and Agriculture Organization
* Prepared as Package Directs

Food and Description	Measure or Quantity	Calories	Carbo-hydrates (grams)
(Pfeiffer)	1 T.	65	2.0
(Wish-Bone)	1 T.	61	32
Dietetic or low calorie:			
Bacon & tomato (Estee)	1 T.	8	1.0
Bleu or blue cheese:			
(Estee)	1 T. (.5 oz.)	8	1.0
(Henri's)	1 T.	35	5.0
Herb Magic (Luzianne Blue			
Plate) creamy	1 T.	8	2.0
(Walden Farms) chunky	1 T.	27	1.7
(Wish-Bone) chunky	1 T.	40	1.0
Buttermilk (Estee)	1 T.	6	1.0
Catalina (Kraft)	1 T.	16	3.0
Chef's Recipe			
Ranchhouse (Henri's)	1 T.	40	6.0
Cucumber:			
(Kraft) creamy	1 T.	30	1.0
(Wish-Bone) creamy	1 T.	40	1.0
Cucumber & onion			
(Henri's) creamy	1 T.	35	6.0
Dijon (Estee)	1 T.	8	<1.0
French:			
(Estee)	1 T. (.5 oz.)	4	1.0
(Henri's):			
Hearty	1 T.	30	5.0
Original	1 T.	40	6.0
(Pritikin)	1 T.	10	2.0
(Walden Farms)	1 T.	33	2.6
(Wish-Bone)	1 T.	31	2.1
Garlic (Estee)	1 T. (.5 oz.)	2	0.
Herb basket, *Herb Magic*			
(Luzianne Blue Plate)	1 T.	6	2.0
Italian:			
(Estee) regular or creamy	1 T. (.5 oz.)	4	0.
(Estee) spicy	1 T.	4	1.0
(Henri's) authentic	1 T.	20	2.0
Herb Magic (Luzianne			
Blue Plate)	1 T.	4	1.0
(Kraft) zesty	1 T.	6	1.0
(Pritikin):			
Regular	1 T.	6	2.0
Creamy	1 T.	16	3.0
(Walden Farm):			
Regular or low sodium	1 T.	9	1.5
No sugar added	1 T.	6	Tr.

Food and Description	Measure or Quantity	Calories	Carbo-hydrates (grams)
(Wish-Bone)	1 T	7	1.0
Miracle Whip	1 T.	45	2.0
Olive oil vinaigrette			
(Wish-Bone) lite	1 T.	16	2.0
Onion & chive (Wish-Bone)	1 T.	37	1.6
Ranch:			
Herb Magic (Luzianne			
Blue Plate)	1 T.	6	1.0
(Pritikin)	1 T.	18	4.0
(Wish-Bone)	1 T.	42	2.5
Red wine/vinegar			
(Estee)	1 T.	2	0.
Russian:			
(Pritikin)	1 T.	12	3.0
(Wish-Bone)	1 T. (.5 oz.)	25	5.0
Tas-Tee (Henri's)	1 T.	30	4.0
Thousand Island:			
(Estee)	1 T.	8	2.0
(Henri's)	1 T.	30	4.0
Herb Magic (Luzianne			
Blue Plate)	1 T.	8	2.0
(Kraft)	1 T.	30	2.0
(Walden Farms)	1 T.	24	3.1
(Wish-Bone)	1 T.	40	2.6
Vinaigrette (Pritikin)	1 T.	10	2.0
SALAD DRESSING MIX:			
*Regular (Good Seasons):			
Blue cheese	1 T. (.6 oz.)	84	.3
Buttermilk, farm style	1 T. (.6 oz.)	58	1.2
Classic herb	1 T.	83	.3
Farm style	1 T.	53	.7
French, old fashioned	1 T.	83	.5
Garlic, cheese	1 T.	85	.5
Garlic & herb	1 T.	84	.7
Italian:			
Regular, cheese or zesty	1 T. (.6 oz.)	84	.6
Mild	1 T. (.6 oz.)	86	1.2
Tomato & herb	1 T. (.6 oz.)	85	1.0

(USDA): United States Department of Agriculture
(HEW/FAO):   Health, Education and Welfare/Food and Agriculture
               Organization
* Prepared as Package Directs

Food and Description	Measure or Quantity	Calories	Carbo- hydrates (grams)
Dietetic:			
*Blue cheese			
(Weight Watchers)	1 T.	10	1.0
*French (Weight Watchers)	1 T.	4	1.0
Garlic (Estee) creamy	½-oz. pkg.	21	1.0
*Italian:			
(Good Seasons):			
Regular	1 T.	8	1.8
Lite	1 T.	27	.8
(Weight Watchers):			
Regular	1 T.	2	0.
Creamy	1 T.	4	1.0
*Russian (Weight Watchers)	1 T.	4	1.0
*Thousand Island			
(Weight Watchers)	1 T.	12	1.0
SALAD LIFT SPICE (French's)	1 tsp. (4 grams)	6	1.0
SALAD SEASONING (Durkee):			
Regular	1 tsp.	4	.7
Cheese	1 tsp.	10	.4
SALAD SUPREME			
(McCormick)	1 tsp. (.1 oz.)	11	.5
SALAMI:			
(USDA):			
Dry	1 oz.	128	.3
Cooked	1 oz.	88	.4
(Eckrich):			
For beer or cooked	1 oz.	70	1.0
Cotto:			
Beef	.7-oz. slice	50	1.0
Meat	1-oz. slice	70	1.0
Hard	1 oz.	130	1.0
Hebrew National	1 oz.	80	<1.0
(Hormel):			
Beef	1 slice	25	0.
Cotto:			
Chub	1 oz.	100	0.
Sliced	1 slice	52	5.
Genoa:			
Whole:			
Regular or Gran Value	1 oz.	110	0.
Di Lusso	1 oz.	100	0.

Food and Description	Measure or Quantity	Calories	Carbo-hydrates (grams)
Hard:			
Packaged, sliced	1 slice	40	0.
Whole:			
Regular	1 oz.	110	0.
National Brand	1 oz.	120	0.
Party slice	1 oz.	90	0.
Piccolo, stick	1 oz.	120	0.
(Ohse) cooked	1 oz.	65	1.0
(Oscar Mayer):			
For beer:			
Regular	.8-oz. slice	50	.3
Beef	.8-oz. slice	64	.3
Cotto:			
Regular	.8-oz. slice	53	.5
Beef	.5-oz. slice	29	.2
Beef	.8-oz. slice	46	.4
Genoa	.3-oz. slice	34	.1
Hard	.3-oz. slice	37	.1
SALISBURY STEAK, frozen:			
(Armour):			
Classic Lite	10-oz. meal	270	22.0
Dinner Classics	11-oz. meal	460	37.0
(Banquet):			
Dinner:			
American Favorites	11-oz. dinner	395	24.0
Extra Helping	19-oz. dinner	1024	72.0
Family Entree	2-lb. pkg.	1260	48.0
(Blue Star) *Dining Lite,* with creole sauce	9½-oz. meal	223	11.4
(Morton)	10-oz. dinner	294	23.0
(Stouffer's):			
Regular, with onion gravy	9⅞-oz. pkg.	250	9.0
Lean Cuisine, with Italian style sauce & vegetables	9½-oz. pkg.	280	12.0
(Swanson):			
Regular:			
Dinner, 4-compartment	11-oz. dinner	460	44.0
Entree	5½-oz. entree	340	19.0

(USDA): United States Department of Agriculture
(HEW/FAO): Health, Education and Welfare/Food and Agriculture
            Organization
* Prepared as Package Directs

Food and Description	Measure or Quantity	Calories	Carbo-hydrates (grams)
Hungry Man:			
Dinner	16½-oz. dinner	690	42.0
Entree	11¾-oz. entree	610	29.0
Main course entree	8½-oz. entree	380	26.0
(Weight Watchers) beef, Romana	8¾-oz. meal	300	24.0
SALMON:			
Atlantic (USDA):			
Raw:			
Whole	1 lb. (weighed whole)	640	0.
Meat only	4 oz.	246	0.
Canned, solids & liq., including bones	4 oz.	230	.9
Chinook or King (USDA)			
Raw:			
Steak	1 lb. (weighed whole)	886	0.
Meat only	4 oz.	252	0.
Canned, solids & liq., in-cluding bones	4 oz.	238	0.
Chum, canned (USDA), solids & liq., including bones	4 oz.	158	0.
Coho, canned (USDA) solids & liq., including bones	4 oz.	174	0.
Keta, canned (Bumble Bee) solids & liq., including bones	½ cup (3.9 oz.)	153	0.
Pink or Humpback (USDA):			
Raw:			
Steak	1 lb. (weighed whole)	475	0.
Meat only	4 oz.	135	0.
Canned, solids & liq.:			
(USDA) including bones	4 oz.	135	0.
(Bumble Bee) including bones	½ cup (4 oz.)	155	0.
(Del Monte)	7¾-oz. can	277	0.
Sockeye or Red or Blueback, canned, solids & liq.:			
(USDA)	4 oz.	194	0.
(Bumble Bee) including bones	½ cup (4 oz.)	155	0.

Food and Description	Measure or Quantity	Calories	Carbo-hydrates (grams)
(Del Monte)	½ of 7¾-oz. can	165	0.
Unspecified kind of salmon			
(USDA) baked or broiled	4.2 oz. steak (approx. 4" × 3" × ½")	218	0.
SALMON, SMOKED (USDA)	4 oz.	200	0.
SALT:			
Regular:			
Butter-flavored (French's) imitation	1 tsp. (3.6 grams)	8	0.
Garlic (Lawry's)	1 tsp. (4 grams)	5	1.0
Hickory smoke (French's)	1 tsp. (4 grams)	2	Tr.
Onion (Lawry's)	1 tsp.	4	.9
Seasoned (Lawry's)	1 tsp.	3	.6
Table:			
(USDA)	1 tsp.	0	0.
(Morton) iodized	1 tsp. (7 grams)	0	0.
Lite Salt (Morton) iodized	1 tsp. (6 grams)	0	0.
Substitute:			
(Adolph's):			
Regular	1 tsp. (6 grams)	1	Tr.
Packet	8-gram packet	<1	Tr.
Seasoned	1 tsp.	6	1.1
(Estee) *Salt-It*	½ tsp.	0	0.
(Morton):			
Regular	1 tsp. (6 grams)	Tr.	Tr.
Seasoned	1 tsp. (6 grams)	3	.5
SALT PORK, raw (USDA):			
With skin	1 lb. (weighed with skin)	3410	0.
Without skin	1 oz.	222	0.
SALT 'N SPICE SEASONING (McCormick)	1 tsp. (.1 oz.)	3	.5
SANDWICH SPREAD:			
(USDA)	1 T. (.5 oz.)	57	2.4

(USDA): United States Department of Agriculture
(HEW/FAO):   Health, Education and Welfare/Food and Agriculture
              Organization
* Prepared as Package Directs

Food and Description	Measure or Quantity	Calories	Carbo-hydrates (grams)
(USDA)	½ cup (4.3 oz.)	466	19.5
(Hellmann's)	1 T. (.5 oz.)	55	2.4
(Oscar Mayer)	1-oz. serving	67	3.6
SANGRIA (Taylor) 11.6% alcohol	3 fl. oz.	99	10.8
SARDINE:			
Raw (HEW/FAO):			
Whole	1 lb. (weighed whole)	321	0.
Meat only	4 oz.	146	0.
Canned:			
Atlantic:			
(USDA) in oil: Solids & liq.	3¾-oz. can	330	.6
(Drained solids, with skin & bones	3¾-oz. can	187	DNA
(Del Monte) in tomato sauce, solids & liq.	7½-oz. can	330	4.0
Imported (Underwood):			
In mustard sauce	3¾-oz. can	220	2.0
In tomato sauce	3¾-oz. can	220	2.0
Norwegian:			
(Granadaisa Brand) in tomato sauce	3¾-oz. can	195	0.
(King David Brand) brisling, in olive oil	3¾-oz. can	293	0.
King Oscar Brand:			
In mustard sauce, solids & liq.	3¾-oz. can	240	2.0
In oil, drained	3-oz. can	260	1.0
In tomato sauce, solids & liq.	3¾-oz. can	240	2.0
(Queen Helga Brand) sild, in sild oil	3¾-oz. can	310	0.
(Underwood) drained	3-oz. serving	230	1.0
Pacific (USDA) in brine or mustard, solids & liq.	4 oz.	222	1.9
SAUCE:			
Regular:			
A-1	1 T. (.6 oz.)	12	3.1
Barbecue:			
(USDA)	1 cup (8.8 oz.)	228	20.0

Food and Description	Measure or Quantity	Calories	Carbo- hydrates (grams)
Chris & Pitt's	1 T.	15	4.0
(French's) regular hot or smoky	1 T. (.6 oz.)	14	3.0
(Gold's)	1 T.	16	3.9
(Heinz):			
Regular	½ cup	160	27.0
Hickory smoked & hot	½ cup	160	31.0
(Hunt's) all natural:			
Country style, onion, original or southern style	1 T.	20	5.0
Hickory or hot & zesty	1 T.	25	6.0
(Kraft):			
Plain or hot	½ cup	160	DNA
Onion bits	½ cup	200	DNA
(La Choy) oriental	1 T.	16	3.8
Open Pit (General Foods):			
Original	1 T.	24	5.1
Original with minced onion	1 T.	25	5.7
Hot & spicy	1 T.	24	5.4
Smoke flavor	1 T.	24	5.5
Burrito (Del Monte)	¼ cup (2 oz.)	20	4.0
Cheese (Snow's) Welsh Rarebit	½ cup	170	10.0
Chili (See **CHILI SAUCE**)			
Cocktail (See also Seafood):			
(Gold's)	1 oz.	31	7.5
(Pfeiffer)	1-oz. serving	50	6.0
Hot (Gebhardt)			
Louisiana-style	1 tsp.	0	0.
Italian (See also **SPAGHETTI SAUCE** or **TOMATO SAUCE**):			
(Contadina)	4-fl.-oz. serving (4.4 oz.)	71	10.5
(Ragu) red cooking	3½-oz. serving	45	6.0
Newberg (Snow's)	⅓ cup	120	10.0
Picante (Pace)	1 tsp.	2	.3
Plum (La Choy) tangy	1 oz.	44	10.8
Salsa Brava (La Victoria)	1 T.	6	1.0

(USDA): United States Department of Agriculture
(HEW/FAO): Health, Education and Welfare/Food and Agriculture Organization
* Prepared as Package Directs

Food and Description	Measure or Quantity	Calories	Carbo-hydrates (grams)
Salsa Casera (La Victoria)	1 T.	4	1.0
Salsa Mexicana (Contadina)	4 fl. oz.		
	(4.4 oz.)	38	6.8
Salsa Picante (Del Monte):			
Regular	¼ cup (2 oz.)	20	4.0
Hot & chunky	¼ cup	15	3.0
Salsa Ranchera (La Victoria)	1 T.	6	1.0
Salsa Roja (Del Monte)	¼ cup (2 oz.)	20	4.0
Seafood cocktail			
(Del Monte)	1 T. (.6 oz.)	21	4.9
Soy:			
(USDA)	1 oz.	19	2.7
(Chun King)	1 tsp.	5	.7
(Gold's)	1 T.	10	1.0
(Kikkoman):			
Regular	1 T. (.6 oz.)	10	.9
Light, low sodium	1 T.	11	1.3
(La Choy)	1 T. (.5 oz.)	8	.9
Spare rib (Gold's)	1 oz.	60	14.0
Stir-fry (Kikkoman)	1 tsp.	6	2.3
Sweet & sour:			
(Chun King)	1.8-oz. serving	57	14.4
(Contadina)	4 fl. oz.		
	(4.4 oz.)	150	29.6
(Kikkoman)	1 T.	18	4.0
(La Choy)	1-oz. serving	30	7.0
Szechuan (La Choy)	1 oz.	48	12.0
Tabasco	¼ tsp.	Tr.	Tr.
Taco:			
(El Molino) red, mild	1 T.	5	1.0
(La Victoria):			
Green	1 T.	4	1.0
Red	1 T.	6	1.0
Old El Paso, hot or mild	1 T.	5	1.2
(Ortega) hot or mild	1 oz.	13	3.1
Tartar:			
(USDA)	1 T. (.5 oz.)	74	.6
(Hellmann's)	1 T. (.5 oz.)	70	.1
(Nalley's)	1 T.	89	.3
Teriyaki (Kikkoman)	1 T. (.6 oz.)	15	2.7
White (USDA) home recipe:			
Thin	¼ cup (2.2 oz.)	74	4.5
Medium	¼ cup (2.5 oz.)	103	5.6
Thick	¼ cup (2.2 oz.)	122	6.8
Worcestershire:			

Food and Description	Measure or Quantity	Calories	Carbo-hydrates (grams)
(French's) regular or smoky	1 T. (.6 oz.)	10	2.0
(Gold's)	1 T.	42	3.3
(Lea & Perrins)	1 T. (.6 oz.)	12	3.0
Dietetic:			
Barbecue (Estee)	1 T. (.6 oz.)	18	3.0
Cocktail (Estee)	1 T. (.5 oz.)	10	2.0
Mexican (Pritikin)	1 oz.	12	2.0
Picante (Estee)	1 T.	4	1.0
Soy:			
(Kikkoman) lite	1 T.	9	.3
(La Choy)	1 T.	<1	.8
Steak (Estee)	½ oz.	15	3.0
Taco (Estee)	1 oz.	14	3.0
Tartar (USDA)	1 T. (.5 oz.)	31	.9

SAUCE MIX:

Food and Description	Measure or Quantity	Calories	Carbo-hydrates (grams)
Regular:			
A la King (Durkee)	1.1-oz. pkg.	133	14.0
*Cheese:			
(Durkee)	½ cup	168	9.5
(French's)	½ cup	160	14.0
Hollandaise:			
(Durkee)	1-oz. pkg.	173	11.0
*(French's)	1 T.	15	.7
*Sour cream:			
(Durkee)	⅔ cup	214	15.0
(French's)	2½ T.	60	5.0
*Stroganoff (French's)	⅓ cup	110	11.0
Sweet & sour:			
*(Durkee)	½ cup	115	22.5
*(French's)	½ cup	55	14.0
(Kikkoman)	1 T.	18	4.0
Teriyaki:			
*(French's)	1 T.	17	3.5
(Kikkoman)	1.5-oz. pkg.	125	22.3
*White (Durkee)	½ cup	119	20.5
*Dietetic (Weight Watchers) lemon butter	1 T.	8	1.0

(USDA): United States Department of Agriculture
(HEW/FAO):   Health, Education and Welfare/Food and Agriculture
                        Organization
* Prepared as Package Directs

Food and Description	Measure or Quantity	Calories	Carbo-hydrates (grams)
SAUERKRAUT, canned:			
(USDA):			
Solids & liq.	½ cup (4.1 oz.)	21	4.7
Drained solids	½ cup (2.5 oz.)	15	3.1
(Claussen) drained	½ cup (2.7 oz.)	16	2.9
(Comstock) solids & liq.:			
Regular	½ cup (4.1 oz.)	30	4.0
Bavarian	½ cup (4.2 oz.)	35	7.0
(Del Monte) solids & liq.	½ cup (4 oz.)	25	6.0
(Silver Floss) solids & liq.:			
Regular, can	½ cup (4 oz.)	30	5.0
Regular, jar	½ cup (4 oz.)	25	5.0
Bavarian Kraut	½ cup	35	8.0
Krispy Kraut	½ cup	25	5.0
Polybag	½ cup	20	4.0
(Vlasic)	1 oz.	4	1.0
SAUERKRAUT JUICE, canned			
(USDA) 2% salt	½ cup (4.3 oz.)	12	2.8
SAUSAGE:			
*Brown & serve:			
(USDA)	1 oz.	120	.8
(Hormel)	1 sausage	70	0.
Country style (USDA) smoked	1 oz.	98	0.
Italian style, hot or mild			
(Hillshire Farms)	3-oz. serving	263	<1.0
Knockwurst (*Hebrew National,* hot)	1 oz.	79	.6
Links (Ohse) hot	1 oz.	80	4.0
Patty (Hormel) hot or mild	1 patty	150	0.
Polish-style:			
(Eckrich) meat:			
Regular	1 oz.	95	1.0
Skinless	1-oz. link	90	1.0
Skinless	1-oz. link	180	2.0
(Hormel):			
Regular	1 sausage	85	0.
Kielbasa, skinless	½ a link	180	1.0
Kolbase	3 oz.	220	1.0
(Ohse):			
Regular	1 oz.	80	1.0
Hot	1 oz.	70	3.0
(Vienna) beef	3 oz.	240	1.3

Food and Description	Measure or Quantity	Calories	Carbo-hydrates (grams)
Pork:			
*(USDA)	1 oz.	135	Tr.
(Eckrich):			
Links	1-oz. link	110	.5
Patty	2-oz. patty	240	1.0
Roll, hot	2-oz. serving	240	1.0
*(Hormel):			
Little Sizzlers	1 link	51	0.
Midget links	1 link	71	0.
Smoked	1 oz.	96	.3
(Jimmy Dean)	2-oz. serving	227	Tr.
*(Oscar Mayer) Little Friers	1 link	79	.3
Roll (Eckrich) minced	1-oz. slice	80	1.0
Smoked:			
(Eckrich):			
Beef:			
Regular	2 oz.	190	1.0
Smok-Y-Links	.8-oz. link	70	1.0
Cheese	2 oz.	180	2.0
Ham, Smok-Y-Links	.8-oz. link	75	1.0
Maple flavored, Smok-Y-Links	.8-oz. link	75	1.0
Meat:			
Regular	2 oz.	190	1.0
Hot	2.7-oz. link	240	3.0
Skinless:			
Regular	2-oz. link	180	2.0
Smok-Y-Links	.8-oz. link	75	1.0
(Hormel) Smokies:			
Regular	1 link	80	.5
Cheese	1 link	84	.5
(Okse)	1 oz.	80	1.0
(Oscar Mayer):			
Beef	1½-oz. link	126	.7
Cheese	1½-oz. link	127	.8
Little Smokies	1 link	28	.1
Meat	1.5-oz. link	126	.7
Thuringer (See THURINGER)			
Turkey (Louis Rich) links or tube	1-oz. serving	45	Tr.

(USDA): United States Department of Agriculture
(HEW/FAO): Health, Education and Welfare/Food and Agriculture
                Organization
* Prepared as Package Directs

Food and Description	Measure or Quantity	Calories	Carbo-hydrates (grams)
Vienna, canned:			
(USDA)	1 link (5-oz. can)	38	Tr.
(Hormel) drained:			
Regular	1 link	50	.3
Chicken	1 link	45	.3
(Libby's):			
In barbecue sauce	2½-oz. serving	180	2.0
In beef broth	1 link	46	.3
SAUTERNE:			
(Great Western)	3 fl. oz.	79	4.5
(Taylor)	3 fl. oz.	81	4.8
SAVORY (French's)	1 tsp.	5	1.0
SCALLION (See **ONION, GREEN**)			
SCALLOP:			
Raw (USDA) muscle only	4-oz. serving	92	3.7
Steamed (USDA)	4-oz. serving	127	DNA
Frozen:			
(Mrs. Paul's):			
Breaded & fried	3½-oz. serving	210	23.0
Mediterranean	11-oz. entree	250	36.0
(Stouffer's) *Lean Cuisine*, oriental, & vegetable with rice	11-oz. pkg.	230	32.0
SCALLOPS & SHRIMP MARINER frozen (Stouffer's) with rice	10¼-oz. pkg.	400	40.0
SCHNAPPS:			
Apple (Mr. Boston) 27% alcohol	1 fl. oz.	78	8.0
Cinnamon (Mr. Boston) 27% alcohol	1 fl. oz.	76	8.0
Peppermint:			
(De Kuyper)	1 fl. oz.	79	7.5
(Mr. Boston) 50% alcohol	1 fl. oz.	115	8.0
Spearmint (Mr. Boston)	1 fl. oz.	78	7.8
Strawberry (Mr. Boston)	1 fl. oz.	68	6.2
SCOTCH WHISKY (See **DISTILLED LIQUOR**)			

Food and Description	Measure or Quantity	Calories	Carbo-hydrates (grams)
SCREWDRIVER COCKTAIL (Mr. Boston) 12½% alcohol	3 fl. oz.	111	12.0
SCROD, frozen (Gorton's) *Light Recipe,* stuffed, baked	1 pkg.	260	4.0
SEA BASS, raw (USDA) meat only	4 oz.	109	0.
SEASON-ALL SEASONING (McCormick)	1 tsp.	4	.6
SEAFOOD DINNER OR ENTREE, frozen (Armour):			
Classic Lite, natural herbs	10½-oz. meal	220	30.0
Dinner Classics	11½-oz. meal	300	28.0
SEAFOOD NEWBERG, frozen:			
(Armour) *Dinner Classics*	10½-oz. meal	280	36.0
(Mrs. Paul's)	8½-oz. meal	310	34.0
SEAFOOD PLATTER, frozen (Mrs. Paul's) breaded & fried, combination	9-oz. serving	510	49.0
SEAWEED, dried (HEW/FAO):			
Agar	1 oz.	88	23.7
Lavar	1 oz.	67	12.6
SEGO DIET FOOD, canned:			
Regular:			
Very chocolate, very chocolate malt or very dutch chocolate	10 fl. oz.	225	43.0
Very strawberry or very vanilla	10 fl. oz.	225	34.0
Lite:			
Chocolate, chocolate jamocha almond, chocolate malt or dutch chocolate	10-fl.-oz. can	150	20.0
Double chocolate	10-fl.-oz. can	150	21.0
French vanilla, strawberry or vanilla	10-fl.-oz. can	150	17.0

(USDA): United States Department of Agriculture
(HEW/FAO):   Health, Education and Welfare/Food and Agriculture
                    Organization
* Prepared as Package Directs

Food and Description	Measure or Quantity	Calories	Carbo-hydrates (grams)
SELTZER (See **MINERAL WATER**)			
SESAME NUT MIX, canned (Planters) roasted	1 oz.	160	8.0
SESAME SEEDS, dry (USDA):			
Whole	1 oz.	160	6.1
Hulled	1 oz.	165	5.0
7 GRAIN CEREAL (Loma Linda):			
Crunchy	1 oz.	110	21.0
No sugar	1 oz.	110	20.0
SHAD (USDA):			
Raw:			
Whole	1 lb. (weighed whole)	370	0.
Meat only	4 oz.	193	0.
Cooked, home recipe:			
Baked with butter or margarine & bacon slices	4 oz.	228	0.
Creole	4 oz.	172	1.8
Canned, solids & liq.	4 oz.	172	0.
SHAD, GIZZARD, raw (USDA):			
Whole	1 lb. (weighed whole)	229	0.
Meat only	4 oz.	227	0.
SHAKE 'N BAKE:			
Oven Fry:			
Chicken:			
Extra Crispy	¼ pouch	110	20.0
Homestyle	¼ pouch	80	15.0
Pork, extra crispy	¼ pouch	120	21.0
Seasoning Mix:			
Chicken:			
Regular	¼ pouch	80	14.0
Barbecue	¼ pouch	90	18.0
Country mild	¼ pouch	80	10.0
Fish, original recipe	¼ pouch	70	14.0
Italian herb	¼ pouch	80	15.0
Pork:			
Regular	¼ pouch	80	16.0
Barbecue	¼ pouch	80	14.0

Food and Description	Measure or Quantity	Calories	Carbo-hydrates (grams)
SHAKEY'S:			
Chicken, fried, & potatoes:			
3-piece	1 order	947	51.0
5-piece	1 order	1700	130.0
Ham & cheese sandwich	1 sandwich	550	56.0
Pizza:			
Cheese:			
Homestyle pan crust	⅒ of 12″ pizza	303	31.0
Thick crust	⅒ of 12″ pizza	170	21.6
Thin crust	⅒ of 12″ pizza	133	13.2
Onion, green pepper, black olives & mushrooms:			
Homestyle pan crust	⅒ of 12″ pizza	320	32.1
Thick crust	⅒ of 12″ pizza	162	22.2
Thin crust	⅒ of 12″ pizza	125	13.8
Pepperoni:			
Homestyle pan crust	⅒ of 12″ pizza	343	31.1
Thick crust	⅒ of 12″ pizza	185	21.8
Thin crust	⅒ of 12″ pizza	148	13.2
Sausage & mushroom:			
Homestyle pan crust	⅒ of 12″ pizza	343	31.4
Thick crust	⅒ of 12″ pizza	178	21.8
Thin crust	⅒ of 12″ pizza	141	13.3
Sausage & pepperoni:			
Homestyle pan crust	⅒ of 12″ pizza	374	31.2
Thick crust	⅒ of 12″ pizza	177	21.7
Thin crust	⅒ of 12″ pizza	166	13.2
Special:			
Homestyle pan crust	⅒ of 12″ pizza	384	31.6
Thick crust	⅒ of 12″ pizza	208	22.3
Thin crust	⅒ of 12″ pizza	171	13.5
Potatoes	15-piece order	950	120.0
Spaghetti with meat sauce & garlic bread	1 order	940	134.0
Super hot hero	1 sandwich	810	67.0
SHELLS, PASTA, STUFFED, frozen:			
(Buitoni) jumbo:			
Cheese stuffed	5½-oz. serving	288	25.1

(USDA): United States Department of Agriculture
(HEW/FAO): Health, Education and Welfare/Food and Agriculture Organization
* Prepared as Package Directs

Food and Description	Measure or Quantity	Calories	Carbohydrates (grams)
Florentine (Celentano):	5½-oz. serving	264	23.1
Broccoli & cheese	11½-oz. pkg.	400	46.0
Cheese:			
Plain	½ of 12½-oz. pkg.	350	33.0
With sauce	½ of 16-oz. box	320	30.0
SHERBET OR SORBET:			
Cassis (Häagen-Dazs)	4 fl. oz.	128	32.0
Daiquiri Ice (Baskin-Robbins)	4 fl. oz.	140	35.0
Lemon (Häagen-Dazs)	4 fl. oz.	140	32.0
Orange:			
(USDA)	½ cup	129	29.7
(Baskin-Robbins)	4 fl. oz.	158	33.4
(Borden)	½ cup	110	25.0
(Häagen-Dazs)	4 fl. oz.	140	34.0
Rainbow (Baskin-Robbins)	4 fl. oz.	160	34.0
Raspberry:			
(Baskin-Robbins)	4 fl. oz.	140	34.0
(Häagen-Dazs)	4 fl. oz.	96	24.4
(Sealtest)	½ cup	140	30.0
SHREDDED WHEAT:			
(Nabisco):			
Regular	¾-oz. biscuit	90	19.0
& bran	1 oz.	110	23.0
Spoon Size	⅔ cup (1 oz.)	110	23.0
(Quaker)	1 biscuit (.6 oz.)	52	11.0
(Sunshine):			
Regular	1 biscuit	90	19.0
Bite size	⅔ cup (1 oz.)	110	22.0
SHRIMP:			
Raw (USDA):			
Whole	1 lb. (weighed in shell)	285	4.7
Meat only	4 oz.	103	1.7
Canned (Bumble Bee) solids & liq.	4½-oz. can	90	.9
Frozen:			
(Mrs. Paul's) fried	3-oz. serving	190	15.0
(Sau-Sea) cooked	5-oz. pkg.	90	0.

Food and Description	Measure or Quantity	Calories	Carbo-hydrates (grams)
SHRIMP & CHICKEN CANTONESE, frozen (Stouffer's) with noodles	10⅛-oz. meal	270	25.0
SHRIMP COCKTAIL, canned or frozen (Sau-Sea)	4 oz.	113	19.0
SHRIMP DINNER OR ENTREE, frozen:			
(Armour) *Classic Lite,* baby, in sherried cream sauce	10½-oz. meal	260	36.0
(Blue Star) *Dining Lite,* creole, with rice	10-oz. meal	210	37.0
(Conagra) *Light & Elegant*	10-oz. meal	218	36.0
(Gorton's) *Light Recipe:*			
Oriental	1 pkg.	350	72.0
& pasta medley	1 pkg.	370	30.0
Scampi	1 pkg.	350	15.0
Stuffed, baked	1 pkg.	340	36.0
(La Choy) Fresh & Lite, with lobster sauce	10-oz. meal	240	36.0
(Mrs. Paul's):			
Oriental	11-oz. meal	230	42.0
Parmesan	11-oz. meal	310	42.0
(Stouffer's) *Right Course,* primavera	9⅝-oz. serving	240	32.0
SHRIMP PASTE, canned (USDA)	1 oz.	51	.4
SKATE, raw (USDA) meat only	4 oz.	111	0.
SLENDER (Carnation):			
Bar:			
Chocolate or chocolate chip	1 bar	135	13.0
Chocolate peanut butter or vanilla	1 bar	135	12.0
Dry	1 packet	110	21.0
Liquid	10-fl.-oz. can	220	34.0

(USDA): United States Department of Agriculture
(HEW/FAO):   Health, Education and Welfare/Food and Agriculture Organization
* Prepared as Package Directs

Food and Description	Measure or Quantity	Calories	Carbo-hydrates (grams)
SLOPPY JOE:			
Canned:			
(Hormel) *Short Orders*	7½-oz. can	340	15.0
(Libby's):			
Beef	⅓ cup (2.5 oz.)	110	7.0
Pork	⅓ cup	120	6.0
Frozen (Banquet) *Cookin' Bag*	5-oz. pkg.	210	12.0
SLOPPY JOE SAUCE, canned			
(Ragú) *Joe Sauce*	3½-oz.	50	11.0
SLOPPY JOE SEASONING MIX:			
*(Durkee)			
Regular	1¼ cup	128	32.0
Pizza flavor	1¼ cup	746	26.0
(French's)	1.5-oz. pkg.	128	32.0
*(Hunt's) *Manwich*	5.9-oz. serving	320	31.0
(McCormick)	1.3-oz. pkg.	103	23.4
SMELT, Atlantic, jack & bar			
(USDA):			
Raw:			
Whole	1 lb. (weighed whole)	244	0.
Meat only	4 oz.	111	0.
Canned, solids & liq.	4 oz.	227	0.
S'MORES CRUNCH, cereal			
(General Mills)	¾ cup (1 oz.)	120	24.0
SMURF BERRY CRUNCH,			
cereal (Post)	1 cup (1 oz.)	116	25.4
SMOKED SAUSAGE (See SAUSAGE)			
SNACKS (See CRACKERS, PUFFS & CHIPS; *NATURE SNACKS*; POPCORN; POTATO CHIPS, PRETZELS, etc.)			
SNACK BAR			
(Pepperidge Farm):			

Food and Description	Measure or Quantity	Calories	Carbo-hydrates (grams)
Apple nut	1.7-oz. piece	170	33.0
Apricot raspberry or blueberry	1.7-oz. piece	170	36.0
Brownie nut or date nut	1½-oz. piece	190	30.0
Chocolate chip or coconut macaroon	1½-oz. piece	210	28.0
Raisin spice	1½-oz. piece	180	31.0
SNAIL, raw (USDA):			
Unspecified kind	4 oz.	102	2.3
Giant African	4 oz.	83	5.0
SNAPPER (See RED SNAPPER)			
SNO BALL (Hostess)	1½-oz. piece	148	27.3
SOAVE WINE (Antinori) 12% alcohol	3 fl. oz.	84	6.3
SOFT DRINK			
Sweetened:			
Apple (Slice)	6 fl. oz.	98	24.0
Birch beer (Canada Dry)	6 fl. oz.	82	21.0
Bitter lemon:			
(Canada Dry)	6 fl. oz. (6.5 oz.)	75	19.5
(Schweppes)	6 fl. oz. (6.5 oz.)	82	20.0
Bubble Up	6 fl. oz.	73	18.5
Cactus Cooler (Canada Dry)	6 fl. oz. (6.5 oz.)	90	21.8
Cherry:			
(Canada Dry) wild	6 fl. oz. (6.5 oz.)	98	24.0
(Shasta) black	6 fl. oz.	81	22.0
Cherry-lime (Spree) all natural	6 fl. oz.	79	21.5
Chocolate (Yoo-Hoo)	6 fl. oz.	93	18.0
Citrus Mist (Shasta)	6 fl. oz.	85	23.0
Club	Any quantity	0	0.

(USDA): United States Department of Agriculture
(HEW/FAO):   Health, Education and Welfare/Food and Agriculture Organization
* Prepared as Package Directs

Food and Description	Measure or Quantity	Calories	Carbo-hydrates (grams)
Cola:			
Coca-Cola:			
Regular, caffeine-free or			
cherry coke	6 fl. oz.	77	20.0
Classic	6 fl. oz.	72	19.0
Pepsi-Cola, regular or			
Pepsi Free	6 fl. oz.	80	19.8
RC 100, caffeine free	6 fl. oz.	86	21.4
(Royal Crown)	6 fl. oz.	86	21.4
(Shasta):			
Regular	6 fl. oz.	73	20.0
Cherry	6 fl. oz.	70	19.1
Shasta Free	6 fl. oz.	75	20.5
(Slice) cherry	6 fl. oz.	82	21.6
(Spree) all natural	6 fl. oz.	73	20.0
Collins mix (Canada Dry)	6 fl. oz. (6.5 oz.)	60	15.0
Cream:			
(Canada Dry) vanilla	6 fl. oz. (6.6 oz.)	97	24.0
(Shasta)	6 fl. oz.	77	21.0
Dr. Diablo (Shasta)	6 fl. oz.	70	19.0
Dr. Nehi (Royal Crown)	6 fl. oz.	82	20.4
Dr Pepper	6 fl. oz. (6.5 oz.)	75	19.4
Fruit punch:			
(Nehi)	6 fl. oz.	107	26.7
(Shasta)	6 fl. oz.	87	23.5
Ginger ale:			
(Canada Dry):			
Regular	6 fl. oz.	68	15.8
Golden	6 fl. oz.	75	18.0
(Fanta)	6 fl. oz.	63	16.0
(Nehi)	6 fl. oz.	76	19.0
(Schweppes)	6 fl. oz.	65	16.0
(Shasta)	6 fl. oz.	60	16.5
(Spree) all natural	6 fl. oz.	60	16.5
Ginger beer (Schweppes)	6 fl. oz.	70	17.0
Grape:			
(Canada Dry) concord	6 fl. oz. (6.6 oz.)	97	24.0
(Fanta)	6 fl. oz.	86	22.0
(Hi-C)	6 fl. oz.	74	19.5
(Nehi)	6 fl. oz.	97	24.4
(Schweppes)	6 fl. oz.	95	23.0
(Shasta)	6 fl. oz.	88	24.0

Food and Description	Measure or Quantity	Calories	Carbo-hydrates (grams)
Grapefruit:			
(Schweppes)	6 fl. oz.	80	20.0
(Spree) all natural	6 fl. oz.	77	21.0
Half & half (Canada Dry)	6 fl. oz. (6.5 oz.)	82	19.5
Hi-Spot (Canada Dry)	6 fl. oz. (6.5 oz.)	75	18.7
Island Lime (Canada Dry)	6 fl. oz. (6.6 oz.)	97	24.8
Kick (Royal Crown)	6 fl. oz.	99	24.8
Lemon (Hi-C)	6 fl. oz.	71	17.1
Lemon-lime:			
(Minute Maid)	6 fl. oz.	71	18.0
(Shasta)	6 fl. oz.	73	19.5
(Spree) all natural	6 fl. oz.	77	21.0
Lemon sour (Schweppes)	6 fl. oz.	79	19.0
Lemon-tangerine (Spree) all natural	6 fl. oz.	82	22.0
Manderin-lime (Spree) all natural	6 fl. oz.	77	21.0
Mello Yello	6 fl. oz.	87	22.0
Mr. PiBB	6 fl. oz.	71	19.0
Mt. Dew	6 fl. oz.	89	22.2
Orange:			
(Canada Dry) *Sunripe*	6 fl. oz. (6.6 oz.)	97	24.7
(Fanta)	6 fl. oz.	88	23.0
(Hi-C)	6 fl. oz.	74	19.5
(Minute Maid)	6 fl. oz.	87	22.0
(Nehi)	6 fl. oz.	104	26.0
(Schweppes) sparkling	6 fl. oz.	88	22.0
(Shasta)	6 fl. oz.	88	24.0
(Slice)	6 fl. oz.	97	25.2
Peach (Nehi)	6 fl. oz.	102	25.6
Punch (Hi-C)	6 fl. oz.	74	19.4
Quinine or tonic water			
(Schweppes)	6 fl. oz.	64	16.0
(Shasta)	6 fl. oz.	60	16.5
Red berry (Shasta)	6 fl. oz.	79	22.5
Red pop (Shasta)	6 fl. oz.	79	22.5
Root beer:			
(Fanta)	6 fl. oz.	78	20.0
(Nehi)	6 fl. oz.	97	24.4
(Ramblin')	6 fl. oz.	88	23.0

(USDA): United States Department of Agriculture
(HEW/FAO):   Health, Education and Welfare/Food and Agriculture
                        Organization
* Prepared as Package Directs

Food and Description	Measure or Quantity	Calories	Carbo-hydrates (grams)
(Schweppes)	6 fl. oz.	76	19.0
(Shasta)	6 fl. oz.	77	21.0
(Spree) all natural	6 fl. oz.	77	21.0
Seltzer	Any quantity	0	0.
7UP	6 fl. oz.	72	18.1
Slice	6 fl. oz.	76	19.8
Sprite	6 fl. oz.	71	18.0
Strawberry:			
(Nehi)	6 fl. oz.	97	24.3
(Shasta)	6 fl. oz.	73	20.0
Tropical blend (Spree) all natural	6 fl. oz.	73	20.5
Upper 10 (Royal Crown)	6 fl. oz.	85	21.1
Dietetic:			
Apple (Slice)	6 fl. oz.	10	2.4
Birch Beer (Shasta)	6 fl. oz.	2	.5
Blackberry (Schweppes) mid-calorie royal	6 fl. oz.	35	8.0
Cherry:			
Diet Rite	6 fl. oz.	2	.4
(Shasta) black	6 fl. oz.	Tr.	Tr.
Chocolate (Shasta)	6 fl. oz. (6.2 oz.)	0	0.
Cola:			
Coca Cola, regular, caffeine free or cherry	6 fl. oz.	Tr.	.1
Diet Rite (Royal Crown)	6 fl. oz.	Tr.	.2
Pepsi, diet, light or caffeine free	6 fl. oz.	Tr.	Tr.
RC	6 fl. oz.	Tr.	.2
(Shasta)	6 fl. oz.	0	0.
(Slice) cherry	6 fl. oz.	10	2.4
Cream:			
Diet Rite, caramel	6 fl. oz.	<1	.2
(Shasta)	6 fl. oz.	0	0.
Fresca	6 fl. oz.	2	.1
Frolic (Shasta)	6 fl. oz.	0	0.
Ginger ale:			
(Schweppes)	6 fl. oz.	2	<1.0
(Shasta)	6 fl. oz.	0	0.
Grape (Shasta)	6 fl. oz.	0	0.
Grapefruit, Diet Rite	6 fl. oz.	2	.4
Kiwi-passionfruit (Schweppes) mid-calorie royal	6 fl. oz.	35	8.0

Food and Description	Measure or Quantity	Calories	Carbo- hydrates (grams)
Lemon-lime:			
Diet Rite	6 fl. oz.	2	.6
(Minute Maid)	6 fl.oz.	10	2.0
(Shasta)	6 fl. oz.	0	0.
Orange:			
(Fanta)	6 fl. oz.	<1	.1
(Minute Maid)	6 fl. oz.	4	.4
(No-Cal)	6 fl. oz.	1	0.
(Shasta)	6 fl. oz.	0	0.
(Slice)	6 fl. oz.	10	2.1
Peach, *Diet Rite,* golden	6 fl. oz.	1	.3
Peaches 'n Cream (Schweppes) mid-calorie royal	6 fl. oz.	35	8.0
Quinine or tonic (Canada Dry: No-Cal)	6 fl. oz.	3	Tr.
Raspberry, *Diet Rite*	6 fl. oz.	2	.5
Root beer:			
(No-Cal)	6 fl. oz.	1	0.
(Shasta)	6 fl. oz.	0	0.
7UP	6 fl. oz.	2	0.
Slice	6 fl. oz.	13	3.0
Sprite	6 fl. oz.	2	Tr.
Strawberry (Shasta)	6 fl. oz.	0	0.
Strawberry-banana (Schweppes) mid-calorie royal	6 fl. oz.	35	8.0
Tab, regular or caffeine free	6 fl. oz.	Tr.	.2
Tangerine, *Diet Rite*	6 fl. oz.	2	.3
Tropical citrus (Schweppes) mid-calorie royal	6 fl. oz.	35	8.0
Upper 10 (RC)	6 fl. oz.	2	.6
SOLE, frozen:			
Raw, meat only (USDA)	4 oz.	90	0.
Frozen:			
(Frionor) Norway	4-oz. fillet	60	0.
(Gorton's):			
Fishmarket Fresh	4 oz.	90	1.0
Light Recipe, fillet, with			

(USDA): United States Department of Agriculture
(HEW/FAO):   Health, Education and Welfare/Food and Agriculture
                     Organization
* Prepared as Package Directs

Food and Description	Measure or Quantity	Calories	Carbo-hydrates (grams)
lemon butter sauce	1 pkg.	250	8.0
(Mrs. Paul's) fillets, breaded & fried	6-oz. serving	280	19.0
(Van de Kamp's):			
Regular, batter dipped, french fried	2-oz. piece	140	12.5
Lightly breaded	5-oz. piece	300	15.0
Today's Catch	4 oz.	80	0.
(Weight Watchers) in lemon sauce	9⅛-oz. meal	200	17.0
SOUFFLE:			
Cheese:			
Home recipe (USDA)	1 cup (collapsed)	207	5.9
Frozen (Stouffer's)	6-oz. serving	355	14.0
Corn, frozen (Stouffer's):	4-oz. serving	160	18.0
Spinach, frozen (Stouffer's)	4-oz. serving	140	8.0
SOUP:			
Canned, regular pack:			
*Asparagus (Campbell), condensed:			
Cream of	8-oz. serving	90	11.0
Creamy Natural	8-oz. serving	200	13.0
Bean:			
(Campbell):			
Chunky, with ham, old fashioned:			
Small	11-oz. can	290	37.0
Large	19¼-oz. can	530	66.0
*Condensed, with bacon	8-oz. serving	150	21.0
Semi-condensed, *Soup For One*, with ham	11-oz. serving	220	30.0
(Grandma Brown's)	8-oz. serving	182	29.1
Bean, black:			
*(Campbell) condensed	8-oz. serving	110	17.0
(Crosse & Blackwell) with sherry	6½-oz. serving	80	18.0
Beef:			
(Campbell):			
Chunky:			
Regular:			

Food and Description	Measure or Quantity	Calories	Carbo-hydrates (grams)
Small	10¾-oz. can	190	23.0
Large	19-oz. can	340	40.0
Stroganoff style	10¾-oz. can	300	28.0
*Condensed:			
Regular	8-oz. serving	80	10.0
Broth:	8-oz. serving	15	1.0
Consommé	8-oz. serving	25	2.0
Mushroom	8-oz. serving	60	5.0
Noodle:			
Regular	8-oz. serving	70	7.0
Homestyle	8-oz. serving	90	8.0
(College Inn) broth	1 cup (8.3 oz.)	18	1.0
(Swanson)	7¼-oz. can	20	1.0
Borscht (See **BORSCHT**)			
*Broccoli (Campbell) condensed, *Creamy Natural*	8-oz. serving	140	13.0
*Cauliflower (Campbell) condensed, *Creamy Natural*	8-oz. serving	200	18.0
Celery:			
*(Campbell) condensed, cream of	8-oz. serving	100	8.0
*(Rokeach):			
Prepared with milk	10-oz. serving	190	19.0
Prepared with water	10-oz. serving	90	12.0
*Cheddar cheese (Campbell)	8-oz. serving	130	10.0
Chicken:			
(Campbell):			
Chunky:			
Noodle, with mushrooms	10¾-oz. can	200	20.0
Old fashioned:			
Small	10¾-oz. can	170	21.0
Large	19-oz. can	300	36.0
With rice	19-oz. can	280	30.0
Vegetable	19-oz. can	340	38.0
*Condensed:			
Alphabet	8-oz. serving	80	10.0
Broth:			
Plain	8-oz. serving	35	3.0

(USDA): United States Department of Agriculture
(HEW/FAO):   Health, Education and Welfare/Food and Agriculture
                      Organization
* Prepared as Package Directs

Food and Description	Measure or Quantity	Calories	Carbo-hydrates (grams)
Noodles	8-oz. serving	60	8.0
& rice	8-oz. serving	50	8.0
Cream of	8-oz. serving	110	9.0
& dumplings	8-oz. serving	80	9.0
Gumbo	8-oz. serving	60	8.0
Mushroom, creamy	8-oz. serving	120	9.0
Noodle	8-oz. serving	70	8.0
NoodleOs	8-oz. serving	70	9.0
& rice	8-oz. serving	60	7.0
& stars	8-oz. serving	60	7.0
Vegetable	8-oz. serving	70	8.0
*Semi-condensed, *Soup For One:*			
& noodles, golden	11-oz. serving	120	14.0
Vegetable, full flavored	11-oz. serving	120	13.0
(College Inn) broth	1 cup (8.3 oz.)	35	0.
(Swanson) broth	7¼-oz. can	30	2.0
Chili beef (Campbell):			
Chunky:			
Small	11-oz. can	290	37.0
Large	19½-oz. can	520	66.0
*Condensed	8-oz. serving	130	17.0
Chowder:			
Beef'n vegetable (Hormel)			
Short Orders	7½-oz. can	120	15.0
Clam:			
Manhattan style:			
(Campbell):			
Chunky:			
Small	10¾-oz. can	160	24.0
Large	19-oz. can	300	44.0
*Condensed	8-oz. serving	70	11.0
(Crosse & Blackwell)	6½-oz. serving	50	9.0
*(Snow's) condensed	7½-oz. serving	70	9.0
New England Style:			
*(Campbell):			
Chunky:			
Small	10¾-oz. can	290	25.0
Large	19-oz. can	500	44.0
Condensed:			
Made with milk	8-oz. serving	150	17.0
Made with water	8-oz. serving	80	11.0
Semi-condensed, *Soup For One:*			

Food and Description	Measure or Quantity	Calories	Carbo-hydrates (grams)
Made with milk	11-oz. serving	190	22.0
Made with water	11-oz. serving	130	19.0
(Crosse & Blackwell)	6½-oz. serving	90	14.0
*(Gorton's)	1 can	560	68.0
*(Snow's) condensed, made with milk	7½-oz. serving	140	13.0
*Corn (Snow's) New England, condensed, made with milk	7½-oz. serving	150	18.0
*Fish (Snow's) New England, condensed, made with milk	7½-oz. serving	130	11.0
Ham'n potato (Hormel) *Short Orders*	7½-oz. can	130	14.0
*Seafood (Snow's) New England, condensed, made with milk	7½-oz. serving	130	11.0
Consommé madrilene (Crosse & Blackwell)	6½-oz. serving	25	4.0
Crab (Crosse & Blackwell)	6½-oz. serving	50	8.0
Gazpacho:			
*(Campbell) condensed	8-oz. serving	40	10.0
(Crosse & Blackwell)	6½-oz. serving	30	1.0
Ham'n butter bean (Campbell) *Chunky*	10¾-oz. can	280	34.0
Lentil (Crosse & Blackwell) with ham	6½-oz. serving	80	13.0
*Meatball alphabet (Campbell) condensed	8-oz. serving	100	11.0
Minestrone:			
(Campbell):			
Chunky	19-oz. can	280	42.0
*Condensed	8-oz. serving	80	12.0
(Crosse & Blackwell)	6½-oz. serving	90	18.0
Mushroom:			
*(Campbell) condensed:			
Cream of	8-oz. serving	100	9.0
Golden	8-oz. serving	80	10.0
(Crosse & Blackwell) cream of, bisque,	6½-oz. serving	90	8.0

(USDA): United States Department of Agriculture
(HEW/FAO): Health, Education and Welfare/Food and Agriculture Organization
* Prepared as Package Directs

Food and Description	Measure or Quantity	Calories	Carbo-hydrates (grams)
*(Rokeach) cream of, prepared with water	10-oz. serving	150	3.0
*Noodle (Campbell):			
Curly, & chicken	8-oz. serving	70	9.0
& ground beef	8-oz. serving	90	10.0
*Onion (Campbell):			
Regular	8-oz. serving	60	9.0
Cream of:			
Made with water	8-oz. serving	100	12.0
Made with water & milk	8-oz. serving	140	15.0
*Oyster stew (Campbell):			
Made with milk	8-oz. serving	150	10.0
Made with water	8-oz. serving	80	5.0
*Pea, green (Campbell) condensed	8-oz. serving	160	25.0
Pea, split:			
(Campbell):			
Chunky, with ham:			
Small	10¾-oz. can	230	33.0
Large	19-oz. can	400	58.0
*Condensed, with ham & bacon	8-oz. serving	160	24.0
(Grandma Brown's)	8-oz. serving	184	28.2
*Pepper pot (Campbell)	8-oz. serving	90	9.0
*Potato (Campbell):			
cream of, made with water	8-oz. serving	70	11.0
cream of, made with water & milk	8-oz. serving	110	14.0
Creamy Natural	8-oz. serving	220	16.0
*Scotch broth (Campbell) condensed	8-oz. serving	80	9.0
Shav (Gold's)	8-oz. serving	11	2.1
Shrimp:			
*(Campbell) condensed, cream of:			
Made with milk	8-oz. serving	160	13.0
Made with water	8-oz. serving	90	8.0
(Crosse & Blackwell)	6½-oz. serving	90	7.0
Sirloin burger (Campbell)			
Chunky:			
Small	10¾-oz. can	220	23.0
Large	19-oz. can	400	40.0
*Spinach (Campbell) condensed, *Creamy Natural*	8-oz. serving	160	14.0

Food and Description	Measure or Quantity	Calories	Carbo-hydrates (grams)
Steak & potato (Campbell)			
Chunky:			
Small	10¾-oz. can	200	24.0
Large	19-oz. can	340	42.0
Tomato:			
(Campbell):			
Condensed:			
Regular:			
Made with milk	8-oz. serving	160	22.0
Made with water	8-oz. serving	90	17.0
Bisque	8-oz. serving	120	23.0
Creamy Natural	8-oz. serving	190	26.0
& rice, old fashioned	8-oz. serving	110	22.0
Semi-condensed,			
Soup for One, Royale	11-oz. serving	180	35.0
*(Rokeach):			
Plain, made with water	10-oz. serving	90	20.0
& rice	10-oz. serving	160	25.0
Turkey (Campbell):			
Chunky	18¾-oz. can	360	32.0
*Condensed:			
Noodle	8-oz. serving	60	8.0
Vegetable	8-oz. serving	70	8.0
Vegetable:			
(Campbell):			
Chunky:			
Regular:			
Small	10¾-oz. can	140	23.0
Large	19-oz. can	260	42.0
Beef, old fashioned:			
Small	10¾-oz. can	180	20.0
Large	19-oz. can	320	36.0
Mediterranean	19-oz. can	320	48.0
*Condensed:			
Regular	8-oz. serving	80	13.0
Beef	8-oz. serving	70	8.0
Old fashioned	8-oz. serving	60	9.0
Vegetarian	8-oz. serving	80	13.0
*Semi-condensed,			
Soup For One:			

Food and Description	Measure or Quantity	Calories	Carbo- hydrates (grams)
Barley, with beef & bacon	11-oz. serving	160	20.0
Old world	11-oz. serving	130	18.0
*(Rokeach) vegetarian	10-oz. serving	90	15.0
Vichyssoise (Crosse & Blackwell) cream of	6½-oz. serving	70	5.0
*Won ton (Campbell)	8-oz. serving	40	5.0
Canned, dietetic pack:			
Bean (Pritikin) navy	½ of 14¾-oz. can	130	22.0
Beef (Campbell) *Chunky*, & mushroom, low sodium	10¾-oz. can	210	23.0
Chicken:			
(Campbell) low sodium:			
Chunky, regular	7½-oz. can	150	14.0
Vegetable	10¾-oz. can	240	20.0
(Estee) & vegetable	7¼-oz. serving	130	10.0
(Pritikin):			
Broth, defatted	½ of 13¾-oz. can	14	0.
Gumbo	½ of 14¾-oz. can	60	8.0
& ribbon pasta	½ of 14½-oz. can	60	8.0
Vegetable	½ of 14½-oz. can	70	12.0
Chowder, clam (Pritikin):			
Manhattan	½ of 14¾-oz. can	70	14.0
New England	½ of 14¾-oz. can	118	20.0
Lentil (Pritikin)	½ of 14¾-oz. can	100	17.0
Minestrone:			
(Estee)	7½-oz. can	165	19.0
(Pritikin)	½ of 14¾-oz. can	110	19.0
Mushroom:			
(Campbell) cream of, low sodium	10½-oz. can	200	17.0
(Pritikin)	½ of 14¾-oz. can	60	11.0
Onion (Campbell) french, low sodium	10½-oz. can	80	8.0
Pea, split:			
(Campbell) low sodium	10¾-oz. can	240	38.0

Food and Description	Measure or Quantity	Calories	Carbo-hydrates (grams)
(Pritikin)	½ of 15-oz. can	130	23.0
Tomato (Campbell) low sodium, with tomato pieces	10½-oz. can	180	29.0
Turkey (Pritikin) vegetable, with ribbon pasta	½ of 14¾-oz. can	50	7.0
Vegetable:			
(Campbell) low sodium, *Chunky*	10¾-oz. can	170	19.0
(Estee) & beef	7½-oz. serving	140	9.0
(Pritikin)	½ of 14¾-oz. can	70	14.0
Frozen:			
Asparagus (Kettle Ready) cream of	6 fl. oz.	62	5.1
*Barley & mushroom:			
(Empire Kosher)	½ of 15-oz. polybag	69	12.0
(Tabatchnick)	8 oz.	92	16.0
Bean & barley (Tabatchnick)	8 oz.	63	22.0
Bean & ham (Kettle Ready):			
Black	6 fl. oz.	154	23.0
Savory	6 fl. oz.	113	20.2
Beef (Kettle Ready) vegetable	6 fl. oz.	85	10.7
Broccoli, cream of:			
(Kettle Ready):			
Regular	6 fl. oz.	95	6.4
Cheddar	6 fl. oz.	137	4.7
(Tabatchnick)	7½ oz.	90	10.0
Cauliflower (Kettle Ready) cream of	6 fl. oz.	93	5.5
Cheese (Kettle Ready) cheddar, cream of	6 fl. oz.	158	7.3
Chicken:			
(Empire Kosher):			
Corn	½ of 15-oz. polybag	71	7.0
Noodle	½ of 15-oz. polybag	267	13.0

(USDA): United States Department of Agriculture
(HEW/FAO):   Health, Education and Welfare/Food and Agriculture
                      Organization
* Prepared as Package Directs

Food and Description	Measure or Quantity	Calories	Carbohydrates (grams)
(Kettle Ready):			
Cream of	6 fl. oz.	98	5.0
Gumbo	6 fl. oz.	93	12.1
Noodle	6 fl. oz.	94	12.0
Chili (Kettle Ready):			
Jalapeno	6 fl. oz.	173	14.7
Traditional	6 fl. oz.	161	13.8
Chowder:			
Clam:			
Boston (Kettle Ready)	6 fl. oz.	131	12.8
Manhattan:			
(Kettle Ready)	6 fl. oz.	69	7.9
(Tabatchnick)	7½ oz.	94	15.0
New England:			
(Kettle Ready)	6 fl. oz.	116	11.4
(Stouffer's)	8 oz.	180	16.0
(Tabatchnick)	7½-oz.	97	16.0
Corn & broccoli (Kettle Ready)	6 fl. oz.	101	12.8
Lentil (Tabatchnick)	8 oz.	173	27.0
Minestrone:			
(Kettle Ready)	6 fl. oz.	104	15.2
(Tabatchnick)	8 oz.	147	24.0
Mushroom (Kettle Ready) cream of	6 fl. oz.	85	6.2
Northern bean (Tabatchnick)	8 oz.	80	29.0
Onion (Kettle Ready) french	6 fl. oz.	42	4.9
Pea:			
(Empire Kosher)	7½ oz.	56	6.0
(Kettle Ready) split	6 fl. oz.	155	25.3
(Tabatchnick)	8 oz.	186	31.0
Potato (Tabatchnick)	8 oz.	95	19.0
Spinach, cream of:			
(Stouffer's)	8 oz.	210	12.0
(Tabatchnick)	7½ oz.	90	12.0
Tomato (Empire Kosher) with rice	7½ oz.	227	50.0
Turkey chili (Empire Kosher)	7½ oz.	200	DNA
Vegetable:			
(Empire Kosher)	7½ oz.	111	22.0
(Kettle Ready)	6 fl. oz.	85	12.3
(Tabatchnick)	8 oz.	97	18.0
Won ton (La Choy)	7½ oz.	50	6.0

Food and Description	Measure or Quantity	Calories	Carbo-hydrates (grams)
Chowder, clam, New England style (Stouffer's)	8-oz. serving	200	19.0
Pea, split:			
*(Mother's Own)	8-oz. serving	130	20.0
(Stouffer's) with ham	8¼-oz. serving	190	27.0
Spinach (Stouffer's) cream of	8-oz. serving	230	17.0
*Vegetable (Mother's Own)	8-oz. serving	40	Tr.
*Won ton (La Choy)	½ of 15-oz. pkg.	50	6.0
Mix, regular:			
Beef:			
*Carmel Kosher	6 fl. oz.	12	1.8
*(Lipton) Cup-A-Soup:			
Regular:			
Noodle	6 fl. oz.	45	8.0
Vegetable	6 fl. oz.	50	8.0
Lots-A-Noodles	7 fl. oz.	120	21.0
*Chicken:			
Carmel Kosher	6 fl. oz.	12	1.8
(Lipton):			
Regular, noodle	8 fl. oz.	70	9.0
Cup-A-Broth	6 fl. oz.	25	4.0
Cup-A-Soup:			
Regular:			
Cream of	6 fl. oz.	80	9.0
& noodles with meat	6 fl. oz.	45	6.0
& rice	6 fl. oz.	45	7.0
& vegetable	6 fl. oz.	40	7.0
Country style:			
Hearty	6 fl. oz.	70	10.0
Supreme	6 fl. oz.	100	11.0
Lots-A-Noodles:			
Regular	7 fl. oz.	120	23.0
Cream of	7 fl. oz.	150	22.0
*Minestrone (Manischewitz)	6 fl. oz.	50	9.0
*Mushroom:			
Carmel Kosher	6 fl. oz.	12	2.4
(Lipton):			
Regular:			
Beef	8 fl. oz.	40	7.0
Onion	8 fl. oz.	40	6.0

(USDA): United States Department of Agriculture
(HEW/FAO): Health, Education and Welfare/Food and Agriculture Organization
* Prepared as Package Directs

Food and Description	Measure or Quantity	Calories	Carbo-hydrates (grams)
Cup-A-Soup, cream of	6 fl. oz.	80	10.0
*Noodle (Lipton):			
With chicken broth	8 fl. oz.	70	10.0
Giggle Noodle	8 fl. oz.	80	12.0
Ring-O-Noodle	8 fl. oz.	60	9.0
*Onion:			
Carmel Kosher	6 fl. oz.	12	2.4
(Lipton):			
Regular:			
Plain	8 fl. oz.	35	6.0
Beefy	8 fl. oz.	30	4.0
Cup-A-Soup	6 fl. oz.	30	5.0
*Pea, green (Lipton)			
Cup-A-Soup:			
Regular, green	6 fl. oz.	120	16.0
Country style, Virginia	6 fl. oz.	140	18.0
*Pea, split (Manischewitz)	6 fl. oz.	45	8.0
*Tomato (Lipton):			
Cup-A-Soup:			
Regular	6 fl. oz.	80	17.0
Lots-A-Noodles, vegetable	7 fl. oz.	110	21.0
Hearty, vegetable noodle	8 fl. oz.	80	15.0
*Vegetable:			
(Lipton):			
Regular:			
Beef stock	8 fl. oz.	50	9.0
Country	8 fl. oz.	80	14.0
For dip	8 fl. oz.	45	8.0
Cup-A-Soup:			
Regular:			
Beef	6 fl. oz.	50	8.0
Spring	6 fl. oz.	40	7.0
Country Style, harvest	6 fl. oz.	90	20.0
Lots-A-Noodles, garden	7 fl. oz.	130	23.0
(Manischewitz)	6 fl. oz.	50	9.0
(Southland) frozen	⅓ of 16-oz. pkg.	60	12.0
*Mix, dietetic:			
Beef (Lipton) *Cup-A-Soup*, trim	6 fl. oz.	10	1.0
Beef noodle (Estee)	6 fl. oz.	20	3.0
Beefy tomato (Lipton) *Cup-A-Soup*, trim	6 fl. oz.	10	2.0

Food and Description	Measure or Quantity	Calories	Carbo-hydrates (grams)
Chicken (Lipton) *Cup-A-Soup*, trim	6 fl. oz.	10	1.0
Chicken noodle (Estee)	6 fl. oz.	25	4.0
Herb vegetable (Lipton) *Cup-A-Soup*, trim	6 fl. oz.	10	1.0
Mushroom, cream of (Estee)	6 fl. oz.	40	3.0
Onion (Estee)	6 fl. oz.	25	4.0
Tomato (Estee)	6 fl. oz.	40	5.0
SOUP GREENS (Durkee)	2½-oz. jar	216	43.0
SOUR CREAM (See CREAM, Sour)			
SOURSOP, raw (USDA):			
Whole	1 lb. (weighed with skin & seeds)	200	50.3
Flesh only	4 oz.	74	18.5
SOUSE (USDA)	1 oz.	51	.3
SOUTHERN COMFORT:			
80 proof	1 fl. oz.	79	3.4
100 proof	1 fl. oz.	95	3.5
SOYBEAN:			
(USDA):			
Young seeds:			
Raw	1 lb. (weighed in pod)	322	31.7
Boiled, drained	4 oz.	134	11.5
Canned:			
Solids & liq.	4 oz.	85	7.1
Drained solids	4 oz.	117	8.4
Mature seeds:			
Raw	1 lb.	1828	152.0
Raw	1 cup (7.4 oz.)	846	70.4
Cooked	4 oz.	147	12.2

(USDA): United States Department of Agriculture
(HEW/FAO): Health, Education and Welfare/Food and Agriculture Organization
* Prepared as Package Directs

Food and Description	Measure or Quantity	Calories	Carbo-hydrates (grams)
Oil roasted:			
(Soy Ahoy) regular, or garlic	1 oz.	152	4.8
(Soytown)	1 oz.	152	4.8
SOYBEAN CURD OR TOFU (USDA):			
Regular	4 oz.	82	2.7
Cake	4.2-oz. cake	86	2.9
SOYBEAN FLOUR (See **FLOUR**)			
SOYBEAN GRITS, high fat (USDA)	1 cup (4.9 oz.)	524	46.0
SOYBEAN MILK (USDA):			
Fluid	4 oz.	37	1.5
Powder	1 oz.	122	7.9
SOYBEAN PROTEIN (USDA)	1 oz.	91	4.3
SOYBEAN PROTEINATE (USDA)	1 oz.	88	2.2
SOYBEAN SPROUT (See **BEAN SPROUT**)			
SOY SAUCE (See **SAUCE**, Soy)			
SPAGHETTI (see also **NOODLE**). Plain spaghetti products are essentially the same in calorie value and carbohydrate content on the same weight basis. The longer the cooking, the more water is absorbed and this affects the nutritive and caloric value:			
Dry (Pritikin) whole wheat	1 oz.	110	18.0
Cooked (USDA):			
8–10 minutes, "Al Dente"	1 cup (5.1 oz.)	216	43.9
14–20 minutes, tender	1 cup (4.9 oz.)	155	32.2

Food and Description	Measure or Quantity	Calories	Carbo-hydrates (grams)
Canned, regular pack:			
(Franco-American):			
With meatballs in tomato sauce, *SpaghettiOs*	7⅜-oz. can	210	25.0
With meatballs, in tomato sauce	7⅜-oz. can	220	22.0
In meat sauce	7½-oz. can	210	26.0
With sliced franks in tomato sauce, *SpaghettiOs*	7⅜-oz. can	210	28.0
In tomato & cheese sauce, *SpaghettiOs*	7⅜-oz. can	170	34.0
In tomato sauce with cheese	7⅜-oz. can	190	36.0
(Hormel) *Short Orders:*			
& beef	7½-oz. can	260	25.0
& meatballs	7½-oz. can	210	26.0
(Libby's) & meatballs in tomato sauce	7½-oz. serving	189	27.5
Canned, dietetic:			
(Estee) & meatballs	7½-oz. serving	240	19.0
(Featherweight) & meatballs	7½-oz. serving	200	28.0
Frozen:			
(Banquet):			
Casserole, with meat sauce	8-oz. meal	270	35.0
Dinner, Family Favorites, & meatballs	9½-oz. meal	418	57.0
(Blue Star) *Dining Lite,* with beef & mushrooms	11-oz. meal	286	35.2
(Conagra) *Light & Elegant,* & meat sauce	10¼-oz. entree	290	40.0
(Green Giant) & meatballs, twin pouch	10-oz. entree	396	53.9
(Morton) & meatballs	10-oz. dinner	198	39.0
(Stouffer's):			
Regular:			
With meatballs	12⅝-oz. meal	380	42.0
With meat sauce	12⅞-oz. meal	370	49.0
Lean Cuisine, with beef & mushroom sauce	11½-oz. meal	280	38.0

(USDA): United States Department of Agriculture
(HEW/FAO): Health, Education and Welfare/Food and Agriculture
Organization
* Prepared as Package Directs

Food and Description	Measure or Quantity	Calories	Carbo-hydrates (grams)
(Swanson):			
Dinner	12½-oz. dinner	360	44.0
Entree, in tomato sauce			
with breaded veal	8¼-oz. meal	280	29.0
(Weight Watchers) with			
meat sauce	10½-oz. meal	280	36.0
SPAGHETTI SAUCE,			
canned:			
Regular pack:			
Beef (Prego Plus) ground			
sirloin, with onion	4-oz. serving	160	20.0
Garden Style (Ragú) chunky:			
Extra tomato, garlic &			
onion, green pepper &			
mushroom or mushroom			
& onion	¼ of 15½-oz. jar	80	14.0
Italian garden combination			
or sweet green & red			
bell pepper	¼ of 15½-oz. jar	80	12.0
Home style (Ragú):			
Plain or mushroom	4-oz. serving	70	12.0
Meat flavored	4-oz. serving	80	12.0
Marinara:			
(Prince)	4-oz. serving	80	12.4
(Ragú)	4-oz. serving	120	12.0
Meat or meat flavored:			
(Hunt's)	4-oz. serving	70	12.0
(Prego)	4-oz. serving	150	21.0
(Prince)	½ cup (4.9 oz.)	101	11.0
(Ragú):			
Regular	4-oz. serving	80	11.0
Extra Thick & Zesty	4-oz. serving	100	14.0
Meatless or plain:			
(Hain) Italian style	4-oz. serving	72	14.2
(Prego)	4-oz. serving	140	20.0
(Prince)	½ cup (4.6 oz.)	90	11.4
(Ragú):			
Regular	4-oz. serving	80	11.0
Extra Thick & Zesty	4-oz. serving	100	15.0
Mushroom:			
(Hain)	4-oz. serving	80	14.3
(Hunt's)	4-oz. serving	70	12.0
(Prego):			
Regular	4-oz. serving	140	21.0

Food and Description	Measure or Quantity	Calories	Carbo-hydrates (grams)
Prego Plus	4-oz. serving	130	18.0
(Prince)	4-oz. serving	77	11.3
(Ragú):			
Regular	4-oz. serving	90	9.0
Extra Thick & Zesty	4-oz. serving	110	13.0
Sausage & green pepper			
(Prego Plus)	4-oz. serving	170	19.0
Veal (Prego Plus) with sliced			
mushrooms	4-oz. serving	150	20.0
Dietetic pack:			
(Estee)	4-oz. serving	60	13.0
(Furman's) low sodium	½ cup	83	12.7
(Prego) plain, no salt added	4 oz.	100	10.0
(Pritikin) plain or mushroom	4-oz. serving	60	12.0
SPAGHETTI SAUCE MIX:			
*(Durkee):			
Regular	½ cup	45	10.4
With mushrooms	1⅓ cups	104	24.0
*(French's):			
Italian style	⅝ cup	100	15.0
With mushrooms	⅝ cup	100	13.0
Thick, homemade style	⅞ cup	170	24.0
(Lawry's):			
With imported mushrooms	1½-oz. pkg.	143	26.0
Rich & thick	1½-oz. pkg.	147	28.1
(McCormick)	1½-oz. pkg.	128	25.1
*(Spatini)	½ cup	84	8.4
SPAM, luncheon meat (Hormel):			
Regular, smoke flavored or			
with cheese chunks	1-oz. serving	85	0.
Deviled	1 T.	35	0.
SPANISH MACKEREL, raw			
(USDA):			
Whole	1 lb. (weighed whole)	490	0.
Meat only	4 oz.	201	0.

(USDA): United States Department of Agriculture
(HEW/FAO):   Health, Education and Welfare/Food and Agriculture
              Organization
* Prepared as Package Directs

Food and Description	Measure or Quantity	Calories	Carbo-hydrates (grams)
SPARKLING COOLER, CITRUS,			
La Croix, 3½% alcohol	12 fl. oz.	215	30.0
SPECIAL K, cereal (Kellogg's)	1 cup (1 oz.)	110	20.0
SPICES (See individual spice names)			
SPINACH:			
Raw (USDA):			
Untrimmed	1 lb. (weighed with large stems & roots)	85	14.0
Trimmed or packaged	1 lb.	118	19.5
Trimmed, whole leaves	1 cup (1.2 oz.)	9	1.4
Trimmed, chopped	1 cup (1.8 oz.)	14	2.2
Boiled (USDA) whole leaves, drained	1 cup (5.5 oz.)	36	5.6
Canned, regular pack:			
(USDA):			
Solids & liq.	½ cup (4.1 oz.)	21	3.5
Drained solids	½ cup	27	4.0
(Allen's) chopped, solids & liq.	½ cup	25	4.0
(Del Monte) solids & liq.	½ cup (4.1 oz.)	27	3.3
(Larsen) *Freshlike*, cut	½ cup (4.3 oz.)	25	4.0
(Libby's) solids & liq.	½ cup (4.2 oz.)	27	3.6
(Sunshine) whole leaf, solids & liq.	½ cup (4.1 oz.)	24	2.9
Canned, dietetic or low calorie:			
(USDA) low sodium:			
Solids & liq.	4 oz.	24	3.9
Drained solids	4 oz.	29	4.5
(Allen's) low sodium, solids & liq.	½ cup	25	4.0
(Blue Boy) solids & liq.	4-oz. serving	22	2.4
(Del Monte) No Salt Added, solids & liq.	½ cup	25	4.0
(Featherweight) low sodium	½ cup	35	4.0
(Larsen) *Fresh Lite,* cut, no salt added	½ cup (4.3 oz.)	20	4.0
Frozen:			
(Birds Eye):			
Chopped or leaf	⅓ of pkg. (3.3 oz.)	28	3.4

Food and Description	Measure or Quantity	Calories	Carbo-hydrates (grams)
Creamed	⅓ of pkg. (3 oz.)	60	4.9
& water chestnuts with selected seasonings (Green Giant):	⅓ of 10-oz. pkg.	32	5.0
Creamed	½ cup	70	8.0
Cut or leaf, in butter sauce	½ cup	50	6.0
Harvest Fresh	½ cup	30	4.0
(McKenzie) chopped or cut	⅓ of pkg.	25	3.0
(Stouffer's) creamed	½ of 9-oz. pkg.	170	7.0
SPINACH, NEW ZEALAND (USDA):			
Raw	1 lb.	86	14.1
Boiled, drained	4 oz.	15	2.4
SPINACH PUREE, canned (Larsen) no salt added	½ cup (4.3 oz.)	22	3.5
SPLEEN, raw (USDA):			
Beef & calf	4 oz.	118	0.
Hog	4 oz.	121	0.
Lamb	4 oz.	130	0.
SPLIT PEA (See **PEA, MATURE SEED**)			
SQUAB, pigeon, raw (USDA):			
Dressed	1 lb. (weighed with feet, inedible viscera & bones)	569	0.
Meat & skin	4 oz.	333	0.
Meat only	4 oz.	161	0.
Light meat only, without skin	4 oz.	142	0.
Giblets	1 oz.	44	.3
SQUASH PUREE, canned (Larsen) no salt added	½ cup (4.5 oz.)	35	7.5

(USDA): United States Department of Agriculture
(HEW/FAO):   Health, Education and Welfare/Food and Agriculture
              Organization
* Prepared as Package Directs

Food and Description	Measure or Quantity	Calories	Carbo-hydrates (grams)
SQUASH SEEDS, dry (USDA):			
In hull	4 oz.	464	12.6
Hulled	1 oz.	157	4.3
SQUASH, SUMMER:			
Fresh (USDA):			
Crookneck & straightneck, yellow:			
Whole	1 lb. (weighed untrimmed)	89	19.1
Boiled, drained:			
Diced	½ cup (3.6 oz.)	15	3.2
Slices	½ cup (3.1 oz.)	13	2.7
Scallop, white & pale green:			
Whole	1 lb. (weighed untrimmed)	93	22.7
Boiled, drained, mashed	½ cup (4.2 oz.)	19	4.5
Zucchini & cocazelle, green:			
Whole	1 lb. (weighed untrimmed)	73	15.5
Boiled, drained slices	½ cup (2.7 oz.)	9	1.9
Canned (Del Monte) zucchini, in tomato sauce	½ cup (4 oz.)	30	8.0
Frozen:			
(Birds Eye):			
Regular	⅓ of 10-oz. pkg.	22	3.9
Zucchini	⅓ of 10-oz. pkg.	19	3.3
(Larsen):			
Yellow crookneck	3.3-oz.	18	4.0
Zucchini	3.3-oz.	16	3.0
(McKenzie):			
Crookneck	⅓ of pkg. (3.3 oz.)	20	4.0
Zucchini	3.3 oz.	18	3.0
(Mrs. Paul's) sticks, batter dipped, french fried	⅓ of 9-oz. pkg.	180	23.1
(Southland):			
Crookneck	⅕ of 16-oz. pkg.	15	4.0
Zucchini	⅕ of 16-oz. pkg.	15	3.0
SQUASH, WINTER:			
Fresh (USDA):			
Acorn:			

Food and Description	Measure or Quantity	Calories	Carbo-hydrates (grams)
Whole	1 lb. (weighed with skin & seeds)	152	38.6
Baked, flesh only, mashed	½ cup (3.6 oz.)	56	14.3
Boiled, mashed	½ cup (4.1 oz.)	39	9.7
Butternut:			
Whole	1 lb. (weighed with skin & seeds)	171	44.4
Baked, flesh only	4 oz.	77	19.8
Boiled, flesh only	4 oz.	46	11.8
Hubbard:			
Whole	1 lb. (weighed with skin & seeds)	117	28.1
Baked, flesh only	4 oz.	57	13.3
Boiled, flesh only, diced	½ cup (4.2 oz.)	35	8.1
Boiled, flesh only, mashed	½ cup (4.3 oz.)	37	8.4
Frozen:			
(USDA) heated	½ cup (4.2 oz.)	46	11.0
(Birds Eye)	⅓ of pkg. (3.3 oz.)	43	9.2
(Southland) butternut	⅕ of 20-oz. pkg.	45	11.0
SQUID, raw (USDA) meat only	4 oz.	95	1.7
STARCH (See CORNSTARCH)			
START, instant breakfast drink	½ cup	51	12.7
STEAK & GREEN PEPPERS, frozen:			
(Green Giant) twin pouch, with rice & vegetables	9-oz. entree	250	32.0
(Swanson) in oriental style sauce	8½-oz. entree	200	11.0
STEAK UMM	2-oz. serving	180	0.

(USDA): United States Department of Agriculture
(HEW/FAO):   Health, Education and Welfare/Food and Agriculture
                        Organization
* Prepared as Package Directs

Food and Description	Measure or Quantity	Calories	Carbo-hydrates (grams)
STEW (See individual listings such as beef stew)			
STOCK BASE (French's):			
Beef	1 tsp. (4 grams)	8	2.0
Chicken	1 tsp. (3 grams)	8	3.0
STOMACH, PORK, scalded (USDA)	4 oz.	172	0.
STRAINED FOOD (See **BABY FOOD**)			
STRAWBERRY:			
Fresh (USDA):			
Whole	1 lb. (weighed with caps & stems)	161	36.6
Whole, capped	1 cup (5.1 oz.)	53	2.1
Canned (USDA) unsweetened or low calorie, water pack, solids & liq.	4 oz.	25	6.4
Frozen (Birds Eye):			
Halves:			
Regular	⅓ of 16-oz. pkg.	164	34.9
Quick thaw in lite syrup	½ of 10-oz. pkg.	68	15.8
Whole:			
Regular	¼ of 16-oz. pkg.	89	21.4
In lite syrup	¼ of 16-oz. pkg.	61	14.4
Quick thaw	1.2 of 10-oz. pkg.	125	30.1
STRAWBERRY DRINK (Hi-C):			
Canned	6 fl. oz.	89	22.0
*Mix	6 fl. oz.	68	17.0
STRAWBERRY FRUIT JUICE canned (Smucker's)	8 fl. oz.	120	30.0
STRAWBERRY JELLY:			
Sweetened (Smucker's)	1 T. (.7 oz.)	53	13.5
Dietetic:			
(Diet Delight)	1 T. (.6 oz.)	12	3.0
(Estee)	1 T.	18	4.8
(Featherweight)	1 T.	16	4.0

Food and Description	Measure or Quantity	Calories	Carbo-hydrates (grams)
STRAWBERRY KRISPIES, cereal (Kellogg's)	¾ cup (1 oz.)	110	25.0
STRAWBERRY NECTAR, canned (Libby's)	6 fl. oz.	60	14.0
STRAWBERRY PRESERVE OR JAM:			
Sweetened:			
(Smucker's)	1 T. (.7 oz.)	53	13.5
(Welch's)	1 T.	52	13.5
Dietetic or low calorie:			
(Estee)	1 T. (.6 oz.)	6	0.
(Featherweight): calorie reduced	1 T.	16	4.0
(Louis Sherry) wild	1 T. (.6 oz.)	6	0.
(S & W) *Nutradiet*, red label	1 T.	12	3.0
STRAWBERRY SHORTCAKE, cereal (General Mills)	1 cup (1 oz.)	110	25.0
STUFFING MIX:			
*Beef, *Stove Top*	½ cup	181	21.5
*Chicken:			
(Bell's)	½ cup	224	25.0
(Betty Crocker)	⅕ of pkg.	180	21.0
Stove Top	½ cup	178	20.2
Cornbread:			
*(Betty Crocker)	⅙ of pkg.	180	23.0
(Pepperidge Farm)	1 oz.	110	22.0
Stove Top	½ cup	174	21.6
Cube (Pepperidge Farm)	1 oz.	110	22.0
*Herb (Betty Crocker) seasoned	⅙ of pkg.	190	22.0
*New England Style, *Stove Top*	½ cup	180	20.8
*Pork, *Stove Top*	½ cup	176	20.3
*Premium Blend (Bell's)	½ cup	180	24.0
*Ready Mix (Bell's)	½ cup	224	25.0

(USDA): United States Department of Agriculture
(HEW/FAO):   Health, Education and Welfare/Food and Agriculture
                    Organization
* Prepared as Package Directs

Food and Description	Measure or Quantity	Calories	Carbohydrates (grams)
*San Francisco Style, *Stove Top*	½ cup	175	19.9
&Turkey, *Stove Top*	½ cup	177	20.7
White bread (Mrs. Cubbison's)	1 oz.	101	20.5
*With rice, *Stove Top*	½ cup	183	23.2
STURGEON (USDA)			
Raw:			
Section	1 lb. (weighed with skin & bones)	362	0.
Meat only	4 oz.	107	0.
Smoked	4 oz.	169	0.
Steamed	4 oz.	181	0.
SUCCOTASH:			
Canned, solids & liq.:			
(Comstock):			
Cream style	½ cup (4.4 oz.)	110	20.0
Whole kernel	½ cup (4.4 oz.)	80	15.0
(Larsen) *Freshlike*	½ cup (4.5 oz.)	80	18.0
(Libby's):			
Cream style	½ cup (4.6 oz.)	111	22.8
Whole kernel	¼ of 16-oz. can	82	16.0
(Stokely-Van Camp)	½ cup (4.5 oz.)	85	17.5
Frozen (Birds Eye)	⅓ of 10-oz. pkg.	104	20.7
SUCKER, CARP (USDA) raw:			
Whole	1 lb. (weighed whole)	196	0.
Meat only	4 oz.	126	0.
SUCKER, including **WHITE MULLET** (USDA) raw:			
Whole	1 lb. (weighed whole)	203	0.
Meat only	4 oz.	118	0.
SUET, raw (USDA)	1 oz.	242	0.
SUGAR, beet or cane (there are no differences in calories and carbohydrates among brands) (USDA): Brown:			

Food and Description	Measure or Quantity	Calories	Carbo-hydrates (grams)
Regular	1 lb.	1692	437.3
Brownulated	1 cup (5.4 oz.)	567	146.5
Firm-packed	1 cup (7.5 oz.)	791	204.4
Firm-packed	1 T. (.5 oz.)	48	12.5
Confectioner's:			
Unsifted	1 cup (4.3 oz.)	474	122.4
Unsifted	1 T. (8 grams)	30	7.7
Sifted	1 cup (3.4 oz.)	366	94.5
Sifted	1 T. (6 grams)	23	5.9
Stirred	1 cup (4.2 oz.)	462	119.4
Stirred	1 T. (8 grams)	29	7.5
Granulated	1 lb.	1746	451.3
Granulated	1 cup (6.9 oz.)	751	194.0
Granulated	1 T. (.4 oz.)	46	11.9
Granulated	1 lump (1⅛" × ¾" × ⅜", 6 grams)	23	6.0
Maple	1 lb.	1579	408.0
Maple	1¾" × 1¼" × ½" piece (1.2 oz.)	104	27.0
SUGAR APPLE, raw (USDA):			
Whole	1 lb. (weighed with skin & seeds)	192	48.4
Flesh only	4 oz.	107	26.9
SUGAR CORN POPS, cereal (Kellogg's)	1 cup (1 oz.)	110	26.0
SUGAR CRISP, cereal (Post)	⅞ cup (1 oz.)	112	25.6
SUGAR PUFFS, cereal (Malt-O-Meal)	⅞ cup (1 oz.)	110	26.0
SUGAR SMACKS cereal (Kellogg's)	¾ cup (1 oz.)	110	25.0
SUGAR SUBSTITUTE:			
(Estee) fructose	1 tsp.	12	3.0
Spoon for Spoon	1 tsp.	2	1.0

(USDA): United States Department of Agriculture
(HEW/FAO):   Health, Education and Welfare/Food and Agriculture Organization
* Prepared as Package Directs

Food and Description	Measure or Quantity	Calories	Carbo-hydrates (grams)
Sprinkle Sweet (Pillsbury)	1 tsp.	2	.5
Sweet 'N Low:			
Brown	1 tsp.	20	10.0
Granulated	1-gram packet	14	.9
Liquid	1 drop	0	0.
Sweet'n It (Estee) liquid	6 drops	0	0.
Sweet *10 (Pillsbury)	⅛ tsp.	0	0.
*SUKIYAKI DINNER, canned:			
(Chun King) stir fry	6-oz. serving	257	9.6
(La Choy)	¾ cup	210	9.0
SUNFLOWER SEED:			
(USDA):			
In hulls	4 oz. (weighed in hull)	343	12.2
Hulled	1 oz.	159	5.6
(Fisher):			
In hull, roasted, salted	1 oz.	86	3.0
Hulled, roasted:			
Dry, salted	1 oz.	164	5.6
Oil, salted	1 oz.	167	5.6
(Flavor House) dry roasted	1 oz.	179	4.0
(Frito-Lay's)	1 oz.	181	4.7
(Planter's):			
Dry roasted	1 oz.	160	5.0
Unsalted	1 oz.	170	5.0
SUNFLOWER SEED FLOUR, (See **FLOUR**)			
SUNSHINE PUNCH DRINK, canned (Johanna Farms) *Ssips*	8.45-fl.-oz. container	130	32.0
SURIMI (SEE CRAB, IMITATION)			
SUZY Q (Hostess):			
Banana	2¼-oz. piece	242	38.4
Chocolate	2¼-oz. piece	237	36.4

Food and Description	Measure or Quantity	Calories	Carbo-hydrates (grams)
SWAMP CABBAGE (USDA):			
Raw, whole	1 lb. (weighed untrimmed)	107	19.8
Boiled, trimmed, drained	4 oz.	24	4.4
SWEETBREADS (USDA):			
Beef:			
Raw	1 lb.	939	0.
Braised	4 oz.	363	0.
Calf:			
Raw	1 lb.	426	0.
Braised	4 oz.	363	0.
Hog (See **PANCREAS**)			
Lamb:			
Raw	1 lb.	426	0.
Braised	4 oz.	198	0.
SWEET POTATO:			
Baked (USDA) peeled after baking	5″ × 2″ potato (3.9 oz.)	155	35.8
Candied, home recipe (USDA)	3½″ × 2¼″ piece (6.2 oz.)	294	59.8
Canned:			
(USDA):			
In syrup	4-oz. serving	129	31.2
Vacuum or solid pack	½ cup (3.8 oz.)	118	27.1
(Trappey's) *Sugary Sam:*			
Cut, in light syrup	½ cup (4.3 oz.)	110	25.0
Mashed	½ cup (4.3 oz.)	100	25.0
Whole, in heavy syrup	½ cup (4.3 oz.)	130	30.0
Frozen:			
(Mrs. Paul's) candied:			
Regular	4-oz. serving	180	44.0
N' apples	4-oz. serving	150	36.0
(Stouffer's) & apples	5-oz. serving	160	31.0
SWEET POTATO PIE (USDA)			
home recipe	⅙ of 9″ pie (5.4 oz.)	324	36.0

(USDA): United States Department of Agriculture
(HEW/FAO):   Health, Education and Welfare/Food and Agriculture
                        Organization
* Prepared as Package Directs

Food and Description	Measure or Quantity	Calories	Carbo-hydrates (grams)
SWEET & SOUR PORK, frozen:			
(Chun King)	13-oz. entree	394	78.0
(La Choy)	12-oz. entree	360	64.0
(Van de Kamp's) & rice	11-oz. serving	460	61.0
SWISS STEAK, frozen:			
(Green Giant)	1 meal	350	37.0
(Swanson) 4-compartment dinner	10-oz. dinner	350	33.0
SWORDFISH (USDA):			
Raw, meat only	1 lb.	535	0.
Broiled, with butter or margarine	3″ × 3″ × ½″ steak (4.4 oz.)	218	0.
Canned, solids & liq.	4 oz.	116	0.
SYRUP (See also **TOPPING**):			
Regular:			
Apricot (Smucker's)	1 T. (.6 oz.)	50	13.0
Blackberry (Smucker's)	1 T. (.6 oz.)	50	13.0
Chocolate or chocolate-flavored:			
Bosco	1 T. (.7 oz.)	55	13.3
(Hershey's)	1 T. (.7 oz.)	40	9.0
(Nestlé) *Quik*	1 oz.	80	18.0
Cane (USDA)	1 T. (.7 oz.)	55	14.0
Corn, *Karo*, dark or light	1 T. (.7 oz.)	58	14.5
Maple:			
(USDA)	1 T. (.7 oz.)	50	13.0
Karo, imitation	1 T.	57	14.2
Pancake or waffle:			
(Aunt Jemima)	1 T. (.7 oz.)	53	13.1
Golden Griddle	1 T. (.7 oz.)	55	14.2
Karo	1 T. (.7 oz.)	60	14.9
Log Cabin	1 T. (.7 oz.)	56	14.0
Mrs. Butterworth's	1 T. (.7 oz.)	55	13.3
Strawberry (Smucker's)	1 T.	50	13.0
Dietetic or low calorie:			
Blueberry:			
(Estee)	1 T. (.5 oz.)	4	1.0
(Featherweight)	1 T.	14	3.0
Chocolate or chocolate-flavored:			

Food and Description	Measure or Quantity	Calories	Carbo-hydrates (grams)
(Estee) *Choco-Syp*	1 T.	6	1.0
(Diet Delight)	1 T. (.6 oz.)	8	2.0
(No-Cal)	1 T.	6	0.
Coffee (No-Cal)	1 T.	6	1.2
Cola (No-Cal)	1 T.	0	Tr.
Maple:			
(Cary's)	1 T.	6	2.0
(S&W) *Nutradiet*, imitation	1 T.	12	3.0
Pancake or waffle:			
(Aunt Jemima)	1 T. (.6 oz.)	29	7.3
(Diet Delight)	1 T. (.6 oz.)	6	4.0
(Estee)	1 T.	4	1.0

Food and Description	Measure or Quantity	Calories	Carbo-hydrates (grams)

T

TACO:
*(Ortega)	1 oz.	54	.9
*Mix:			
*(Durkee)	½ cup	321	3.7
(French's)	1¼-oz. pkg.	120	24.0
(McCormick)	1¼-oz. pkg.	123	23.7
(Old El Paso)	1 pkg.	100	20.7
Shell:			
(Gebhardt)	1 shell (.4 oz.)	30	4.0
(Lawry's)	1 shell	50	8.0
(Old El Paso)	1 shell (.4 oz.)	59	7.0
(Rosarita)	1 shell (.4 oz.)	45	6.0

TACO BELL RESTAURANTS:
Burrito:			
Bean:			
Green sauce	6¾-oz. serving	351	52.9
Red sauce	6¾-oz. serving	357	54.5
Beef:			
Green sauce	6¾-oz serving	398	37.7
Red sauce	6¾-oz. serving	403	39.1
Supreme:			
Regular:			
Green sauce	8½-oz. serving	407	45.2
Red sauce	8½-oz. serving	413	46.6
Double beef:			
Green sauce	9-oz. serving	451	40.3
Red sauce	9-oz. serving	456	41.7
Cinnamon crispas	1.7-oz. serving	259	27.5
Enchirito:			
Green sauce	7½-oz. serving	371	28.0
Red sauce	7½-oz. serving	382	30.9
Fajita:			
Chicken	4¾-oz. serving	225	19.8
Steak	4¾-oz. serving	234	19.5
Guacamole	¾-oz. serving	34	2.9

Food and Description	Measure or Quantity	Calories	Carbo-hydrates (grams)
Meximelt	3¾-oz. serving	266	18.7
Nachos:			
Regular	3 ¾-oz. serving	345	37.5
Bellgrande	10.1-oz. serving	648	60.6
Pepper, jalapeno	3½-oz. serving	20	4.0
Pico De Gallo	1-oz. serving	8	1.1
Pintos & cheese:			
Green sauce	4½-oz. serving	184	17.5
Red sauce	4½-oz. serving	190	18.9
Pizza, Mexican	7.9-oz. serving	575	39.7
Ranch dressing	2.6-oz. serving	235	1.5
Salsa	.3-oz. serving	18	3.6
Sour Cream	¾-oz. serving	46	.9
Taco:			
Regular	2¾-oz. serving	183	10.6
Bellgrande	5¾-oz. serving	355	17.6
Light	6-oz. serving	410	18.1
Soft:			
Regular	3¼-oz. serving	338	17.9
Supreme	4.4-oz. serving	275	19.1
Super combo	5-oz. serving	286	20.9
Taco salad:			
With shell	18.7-oz. serving	502	26.3
With salsa:			
Regular	21-oz. serving	941	63.1
Without shell	18.7-oz. serving	520	30.0
Taco sauce:			
Regular	.4-oz. packet	2	.4
Hot	.4-oz. packet	2	.3
Tostada:			
Green sauce	5½-oz. serving	237	25.1
Red sauce	5½-oz. serving	243	26.6
TACO JOHN'S:			
Burrito:			
Bean	5-oz. serving	197	37.0
Beef	5-oz. serving	303	25.0
Chicken:			
Regular	5-oz. serving	227	19.0

(USDA): United States Department of Agriculture
(HEW/FAO):   Health, Education and Welfare/Food and Agriculture
                Organization
* Prepared as Package Directs

Food and Description	Measure or Quantity	Calories	Carbo-hydrates (grams)
With green chili	12 ¼-oz. serving	344	29.0
Combo	5-oz. serving	250	31.0
Smothered:			
With green chili	12 ¼-oz. serving	367	40.0
With Texas chili	12 ¼-oz. serving	455	47.0
Super:			
Regular	8 ¼-oz. serving	389	51.0
With chicken	8 ¼-oz. serving	366	40.0
Chimichanga:			
Regular	12-oz. serving	464	67.0
With chicken	12-oz. serving	441	55.0
Mexican rice	8-oz. serving	340	59.0
Nachos:			
Regular	5-oz. serving	468	45.0
Super	11 ¼-oz. serving	669	60.0
Potato Ole, large	6-oz. serving	414	96.0
Taco:			
Regular	4 ¼-oz. serving	178	15.0
With chicken	4 ¼-oz. serving	140	12.0
Softshell:			
Regular	5-oz. serving	224	23.0
With chicken	5-oz. serving	180	20.0
Taco Bravo:			
Regular	6 ¾-oz. serving	319	42.0
Super	8-oz. serving	361	43.0
Taco burger	6-oz. serving	281	31.0
Taco salad:			
Regular:			
Without dressing	6-oz. serving	229	30.0
With dressing	8-oz. serving	359	35.0
Chicken:			
Without dressing	12 ¼-oz. serving	377	56.0
With dressing	14 ¼-oz. serving	507	61.0
Super:			
Without dressing	12 ¼-oz. serving	428	59.0
With dressing	14 ¼-oz. serving	558	65.0
TAMALE:			
Canned:			
(Hormel) beef:			
Regular	1 tamale	70	4.0
Hot & Spicy	1 tamale	70	4.5
Short Orders	7½-oz. can	270	17.0
Old El Paso, with chili gravy	1 tamale	96	8.2
Frozen (Hormel) beef	1 tamale (3.1 oz.)	130	13.0

Food and Description	Measure or Quantity	Calories	Carbo-hydrates (grams)
TAMARIND, fresh (USDA):			
Whole	1 lb. (weighed with peel, membrane & seeds) ½ cup (4.4 oz.)	104	24.6
Juice	½ cup (4.4 oz.)	51	12.0
TANG:			
Grape, regular	6 fl. oz.	93	23.2
Orange:			
Regular	6 fl. oz.	87	21.8
Dietetic	6 fl. oz.	2	.5
TANGELO, fresh (USDA):			
Whole	1 lb. (weighed with peel, membrane & seeds)	104	24.6
Juice	½ cup (4.4 oz.)	51	12.0
TANGERINE OR MANDARIN ORANGE:			
Fresh (USDA):			
Whole	1 lb. (weighed with peel, membrane & seeds)	154	38.9
Whole	4.1-oz. tangerine (2⅜″ dia.)	39	10.0
Sections (without membranes)	1 cup (6.8 oz.)	89	22.4
Canned, regular pack (Del Monte) solids & liq.	¼ of 22-oz. can	100	25.0
Canned, dietetic or low calorie, solids & liq.:			
(Diet Delight) juice pack	½ cup (4.3 oz.)	50	13.0
(Featherweight) water pack	½ cup	35	8.0
(S&W) *Nutradiet*	½ cup	28	7.0

(USDA): United States Department of Agriculture
(HEW/FAO):   Health, Education and Welfare/Food and Agriculture
Organization
* Prepared as Package Directs

Food and Description	Measure or Quantity	Calories	Carbo-hydrates (grams)
TANGERINE DRINK, canned (Hi-C)	6 fl. oz.	90	23.0
*TANGERINE JUICE, frozen (Minute Maid)	6 fl. oz.	85	20.8
TAPIOCA, dry, *Minute*, quick cooking	1 T. (.3 oz.)	32	7.9
TAQUITO, frozen shredded (Van de Kamp's) beef	8-oz. serving	490	45.0
TARO, raw (USDA):			
Tubers, whole	1 lb. (weighed with skin)	373	90.3
Tubers, skin removed	4 oz.	111	26.9
Leaves & stems	1 lb.	181	33.6
TARRAGON (French's)	1 tsp. (1.4 grams)	5	.7
TASTEEOS cereal (Ralston Purina)	1¼ cups (1 oz.)	110	22.0
TAUTUG or BLACKFISH, raw (USDA):			
Whole	1 lb. (weighed whole)	149	0.
Meat only	4 oz.	101	0.
*TEA:			
Bag:			
(Celestial Seasonings):			
After dinner:			
Amaretto Nights or *Cinnamon Vienna*	1 cup	<3	.3
Bavarian Chocolate Orange	1 cup	7	1.6
Caffeine free	1 cup	4	.8
Fruit & tea	1 cup	<3	1.0
Herb:			
Almond Sunset, Cinnamon Rose or *Cranberry Cove*	1 cup	3	<2.0

Food and Description	Measure or Quantity	Calories	Carbo-hydrates (grams)
Emperor's Choice, Lemon Zinger or *Raspberry Patch*	1 cup	4	<2.0
Mandarin Orange Spice or *Orange Zinger*	1 cup	5	<2.0
Roastaroma	1 cup	11	2.0
Premium black tea	1 cup	3	.4
(Lipton):			
Plain or flavored	1 cup	2	Tr.
Herbal:			
Almond pleasure, dessert mint, gentle orange or cinnamon apple	1 cup	2	0.
Quietly chamomile or toasty spice	1 cup	4	Tr.
(Sahadi):			
Herbal	6 fl. oz.	2	0.
Spearmint	6 fl. oz.	4	Tr.
Instant (Lipton) 100% tea or lemon flavored	8 fl. oz.	2	0.
TEA, ICED:			
Canned:			
Regular:			
(Johanna Farms) *Ssips* container	8.45 fl. oz.	100	26.0
(Lipton) lemon & sugar flavored	6 fl. oz.	70	18.0
(Shasta)	6 fl. oz.	61	16.5
Dietetic (Lipton) lemon flavored	6 fl. oz.	2	0.
*Mix:			
Regular:			
Country Time, sugar & lemon flavored	8 fl. oz.	121	30.2
(Lipton)	8 fl. oz.	60	16.0
(Nestea) lemon & sugar flavored	6 fl. oz.	70	9.0
Dietetic:			

(USDA): United States Department of Agriculture
(HEW/FAO):   Health, Education and Welfare/Food and Agriculture
                        Organization
* Prepared as Package Directs

Food and Description	Measure or Quantity	Calories	Carbo- hydrates (grams)
Crystal Light	8 fl. oz.	2	.2
(Lipton) lemon flavored	8 fl. oz.	2	0.
(Nestea) light	6 fl. oz.	4	1.0
TEAM, cereal (Nabisco)	1 cup (1 oz.)	110	24.0
TEQUILA SUNRISE COCKTAIL (Mr. Boston) 12% alcohol	3 fl. oz.	120	14.4
TERIYAKI, frozen:			
(Chun King) beef	13-oz. entree	379	68.0
(Conagra) *Light & Elegant*, beef	8-oz. entree	240	37.0
(La Choy) Fresh & Light, with rice & vegetables	10-oz. meal	240	39.9
(Stouffer's) beef, with rice & vegetables	9¾-oz. meal	290	33.0
TERIYAKI BASTE & GLAZE (Kikkoman)	1 T. (.8 oz.)	28	6.0
TERIYAKI MARINADE & SAUCE	1 oz.	30	5.0
***TEXTURED VEGETABLE PROTEIN**, *Morningstar Farms:*			
Breakfast link	1 link	73	1.3
Breakfast patties	1 patty (1.3 oz.)	100	3.5
Breakfast strips	1 strip (.3 oz.)	37	.6
Grillers	1 patty (2.3 oz.)	190	6.0
THURINGER:			
(Eckrich):			
Sliced	1-oz. slice	90	1.0
Smoky Tangy	1-oz. serving	80	1.0
(Hormel):			
Packaged, sliced	1 slice	80	0.
Whole:			
Regular or tangy, chub	1-oz.	90	0.
Beefy	1-oz. serving	100	0.
Old Smokehouse	1-oz. serving	90	1.0
(Louis Rich) turkey	1-oz. slice	50	Tr.
(Ohse):			
Regular	1 oz.	75	2.0
Beef	1 oz.	80	1.0

Food and Description	Measure or Quantity	Calories	Carbo-hydrates (grams)
(Oscar Mayer):			
Regular	.8-oz. slice	73	.2
Beef	.8-oz. slice	73	.5
THYME (French's)	1 tsp.	5	1.0
TIGER TAILS (Hostess)	2¼-oz. piece	227	38.9
TOASTED WHEAT AND RAISINS, cereal (Nabisco)	1 oz.	100	23.0
TOASTER CAKE OR PASTRY:			
Pop-Tarts (Kellogg's):			
Regular:			
Blueberry or cherry	1.8-oz. pastry	210	36.0
Brown sugar cinnamon	1¾-oz. pastry	210	33.0
Strawberry	1.8-oz. pastry	200	37.0
Frosted:			
Blueberry or strawberry	1 pastry	200	38.0
Brown sugar cinnamon	1 pastry	210	34.0
Cherry chocolate fudge	1 pastry	200	36.0
Chocolate-vanilla creme	1 pastry	210	37.0
Concord grape, dutch apple or raspberry	1 pastry	210	36.0
Toastees (Howard Johnson):			
Blueberry	1 piece	121	48.0
Corn	1 piece	112	51.3
Oatmeal	1 piece	95	53.2
Orange	1 piece	127	54.8
Raisin bran	1 piece	104	55.4
Toaster Strudel (Pillsbury):			
Blueberry	1 piece	190	28.0
Cinnamon	1 piece	190	26.0
Raspberry or strawberry	1 piece	190	27.0
Toastettes (Nabisco):			
Regular, any flavor	1 pastry	200	36.0
Frosted:			
Brown sugar cinnamon or strawberry	1 pastry	200	36.0
Fudge	1 pastry	200	35.0

Food and Description	Measure or Quantity	Calories	Carbohydrates (grams)
Toast-R-Cake (Thomas'):			
Blueberry	1 piece	108	18.0
Bran	1 piece	103	17.6
Corn	1 piece	120	19.2
TOASTIES, cereal (Post)	1¼ cups (1 oz.)	107	24.4
TOASTY O's, cereal (Malt-O-Meal)	1¼ cups (1 oz.)	110	20.0
TOFU (See SOYBEAN CURD)			
TOFUTTI:			
Frozen:			
Regular:			
Chocolate supreme	4 fl. oz.	210	20.0
Maple walnut	4 fl. oz.	230	20.0
Vanilla	4 fl. oz.	200	21.0
Vanilla almond bark	4 fl. oz.	230	23.0
Wildberry supreme	4 fl. oz.	210	22.0
Cuties:			
Chocolate	1 piece	140	21.0
Vanilla	1 piece	130	21.0
Lite Lite, chocolate-vanilla	4 fl. oz.	90	20.0
Love Drops	4 fl. oz.	230	26.0
Soft serve:			
Regular	4 fl. oz.	158	20.0
Hi-Lite:			
Chocolate	4 fl. oz.	100	18.0
Vanilla	4 fl. oz.	90	18.0
TOMATO:			
Fresh (USDA):			
Green:			
Whole, untrimmed	1 lb. (weighed with core & stem end)	99	21.1
Trimmed, unpeeled	4 oz.	27	5.8
Ripe:			
Whole:			
Eaten with skin	1 lb.	100	21.3
Peeled	1 lb. (weighed with skin, stem ends & hard core)	88	18.8

Food and Description	Measure or Quantity	Calories	Carbo-hydrates (grams)
Peeled	1 med. (2″ × 2½″, 5.3 oz.)	33	7.0
Peeled	1 small (1¾″ × 2½″, 3.9 oz.)	24	5.2
Sliced, peeled	½ cup (3.2 oz.)	20	4.2
Boiled (USDA)	½ cup (4.3 oz.)	31	6.7
Canned, regular pack, solids & liq.:			
(Contadina):			
Sliced, baby	½ cup (4.2 oz.)	50	10.0
Pear shape	½ cup (4.2 oz.)	25	6.0
Stewed	½ cup (4.3 oz.)	35	9.0
Whole, peeled	½ cup (4.2 oz.)	25	5.0
(Del Monte):			
Stewed	4 oz.	35	8.0
Wedges	½ cup (4 oz.)	30	8.0
Whole, peeled	½ cup (4 oz.)	25	5.0
(Hunt's):			
Crushed	½ cup	25	5.2
Stewed	4-oz. serving	35	8.0
Whole	4-oz. serving	20	5.0
(La Victoria) green, whole	1 T.	4	1.0
(Stokely-Van Camp) stewed	½ cup (4.2 oz.)	35	7.5
Canned, dietetic pack, solids & liq.:			
(Del Monte) No Salt Added	½ cup (4 oz.)	35	8.0
(Diet Delight) whole, peeled	½ cup (4.3 oz.)	25	5.0
(Furman's) crushed	½ cup	72	13.1
(Hunt's) no added salt:			
Stewed	4-oz. serving	35	8.0
Whole	4-oz. serving	20	5.0
(S&W) *Nutradiet*, green label:			
Stewed	½ cup	30	8.0
Whole	½ cup	25	5.0
TOMATO JUICE, CANNED:			
Regular pack:			
(Ardmore Farms)	6 fl. oz.	36	7.8
(Campbell)	6 fl. oz.	35	8.0
(Hunt's)	6 fl. oz.	30	7.0

(USDA): United States Department of Agriculture
(HEW/FAO):   Health, Education and Welfare/Food and Agriculture Organization
* Prepared as Package Directs

Food and Description	Measure or Quantity	Calories	Carbo-hydrates (grams)
(Ocean Spray)	6 fl. oz.	35	7.0
(Welch's)	6 fl. oz.	35	7.0
Dietetic pack:			
(Diet Delight)	6 fl. oz.	35	7.0
(Hunt's) no added salt	6 fl. oz.	30	7.0
(S&W) *Nutradiet*, green label	6 fl. oz.	35	8.0
TOMATO JUICE COCKTAIL,			
canned:			
(Ocean Spray) *Firehouse Jubilee*	6 fl. oz.	44	9.1
Snap-E-Tom	6 fl. oz. (6.5 oz.)	40	7.0
TOMATO PASTE, canned:			
Regular pack:			
(Contadina):			
Regular	6 oz.	150	35.0
Italian:			
Plain	6 oz.	210	36.0
With mushroom	6 oz.	180	36.0
(Del Monte)	6-oz. can	150	35.0
(Hunt's):			
Regular	2 oz.	45	11.0
Italian style	2 oz.	50	11.0
Dietetic (Hunt's) low			
sodium	2 oz.	45	11.0
TOMATO & PEPPER, HOT CHILI:			
(Old El Paso), Jalapeno	¼ cup	13	2.5
(Ortega) Jalapeno	1 oz.	10	2.6
TOMATO, PICKLED			
(Claussen) green	1 piece (1 oz.)	6	1.1
TOMATO PUREE, canned:			
Regular (Contadina)	½ cup (4.2 oz.)	50	11.0
Dietetic (Featherweight) low			
sodium	1 cup	90	20.0
TOMATO SAUCE, canned:			
(Contadina):			
Regular	½ cup (4.4 oz.)	45	9.0
Italian style	½ cup (4.4 oz.)	40	8.0
(Del Monte):			
Regular or No Salt Added	½ cup (4 oz.)	35	4.0
With onions	½ cup (4 oz.)	50	11.5

Food and Description	Measure or Quantity	Calories	Carbo-hydrates (grams)
(Furman's)	½ cup	58	9.8
(Hunt's):			
Regular or with bits	4 oz.	30	7.0
With cheese	4 oz.	45	8.0
Herb	4 oz.	80	11.0
Italian	4 oz.	60	11.0
With mushrooms	4 oz.	25	6.0
With onions	4 oz.	40	9.0
Special	4 oz.	35	8.0
TOMCOD, ATLANTIC, raw (USDA):			
Whole	1 lb. (weighed whole)	136	0.
Meat only	4 oz.	87	0.
TOM COLLINS (Mr. Boston)			
12½% alcohol	3 fl. oz.	111	10.8
***TOM COLLINS MIX**			
(Bar-Tender's)	6 fl. oz.	177	18.0
TONGUE (USDA):			
Beef, medium fat:			
Raw, untrimmed	1 lb.	714	1.4
Braised	4 oz.	277	.5
Calf:			
Raw, untrimmed	1 lb.	454	3.1
Braised	4 oz.	181	1.1
Hog:			
Raw, untrimmed	1 lb.	741	1.7
Braised	4 oz.	287	.6
Lamb:			
Raw, untrimmed	1 lb.	659	1.7
Braised	4 oz.	288	.6

(USDA): United States Department of Agriculture
(HEW/FAO): Health, Education and Welfare/Food and Agriculture Organization
* Prepared as Package Directs

Food and Description	Measure or Quantity	Calories	Carbo-hydrates (grams)
Sheep:			
Raw, untrimmed	1 lb.	877	7.9
Braised	4 oz.	366	2.7
TONGUE, CANNED:			
(USDA):			
Pickled	1 oz.	76	Tr.
Potted or deviled	1 oz.	82	.2
(Hormel) cured	1 oz.	63	0.
TONIC WATER (See SOFT DRINK, quinine or tonic water)			
TOPPING:			
Regular:			
Butterscotch (Smucker's)	1 T. (.7 oz.)	70	16.5
Caramel (Smucker's) hot	1 T.	75	14.0
Chocolate:			
(Hershey's) fudge	1 T.	50	9.0
(Smucker's):			
Regular	1 T.	65	13.5
Fudge:			
Regular	1 T.	65	15.5
Hot	1 T.	55	9.0
Milk	1 T.	70	15.5
Nut (Planters)	½ oz.	90	4.5
Peanut butter caramel (Smucker's)	1 T.	75	14.5
Pecans in syrup (Smucker's)	1 T.	65	14.0
Pineapple (Smucker's)	1 T. (.7 oz.)	65	16.0
Strawberry (Smucker's)	1 T.	60	15.0
Walnuts in syrup (Smucker's)	1 T.	65	13.5
Dietetic, chocolate (Diet Delight)	1 T. (.6 oz.)	16	3.6
TOPPING, WHIPPED:			
Regular:			
Cool Whip (Birds Eye):			
Dairy	1 T.	16	1.2
Non-dairy	1 T.	13	1.0
Dover Farms, dairy	1 T. (.2 oz.)	17	1.2
(Johanna) aerosol	1 T. (3 grams)	8	<1.0

Food and Description	Measure or Quantity	Calories	Carbo-hydrates (grams)
Lucky Whip, aerosol	1 T.	12	.5
Dietetic (Featherweight)	1 T.	3	.5
*Mix:			
Regular, *Dream Whip*	1 T. (.2 oz.)	9	.9
Dietetic (Estee)	1 T.	4	Tr.
TOP RAMEN, beef (Nissin Foods)	3-oz. serving	390	50.5
TORTELLINI, frozen:			
(Armour) *Classics Lite,* with meat	10-oz. dinner	250	8.0
(Buitoni):			
Cheese filled:			
Regular	2.6-oz. serving	222	29.8
Tricolor	2.6-oz. serving	221	29.7
Verdi	2.6-oz. serving	220	29.8
Meat filled:			
Plain	2.4-oz. serving	212	21.9
Entree	2.5-oz. serving	223	32.4
(Stouffer's):			
Cheese:			
Alfredo sauce	7⅞-oz. meal	600	32.0
Tomato sauce	9⅝-oz. meal	360	37.0
Vinaigrette	6⅞-oz. meal	400	24.0
Veal, in Alfredo sauce	8⅝-oz. meal	500	32.0
TORTILLA:			
(Amigos)	6″ × ⅛″ tortilla	111	19.7
Old El Paso, corn	1 oz.	76	15.3
TOSTADA, frozen (Van de Kamp's)	8½-oz. serving	530	37.0
TOSTADA SHELL:			
Old El Paso	1 shell (.4 oz.)	57	6.8
(Ortega)	1 shell (.4 oz.)	50	6.0

(USDA): United States Department of Agriculture
(HEW/FAO): Health, Education and Welfare/Food and Agriculture
               Organization
* Prepared as Package Directs

Food and Description	Measure or Quantity	Calories	Carbo-hydrates (grams)
TOTAL, cereal (General Mills):			
Regular	1 cup (1 oz.)	110	23.0
Corn	1 cup (1 oz.)	110	24.0
TOWEL GOURD, raw (USDA):			
Unpared	1 lb. (weighed with skin)	69	15.8
Pared	4 oz.	20	4.6
TRIPE:			
Beef (USDA):			
Commercial	4 oz.	113	0.
Pickled	4 oz.	70	0.
Canned (Libby's)	¼ of 24-oz. can	290	1.1
TRIPLE SEC LIQUEUR (Mr. Boston)	1 fl. oz.	79	8.5
TRIX, cereal (General Mills)	1 cup (1 oz.)	110	25.0
TROUT (USDA):			
Brook, fresh:			
Whole	1 lb. (weighed whole)	224	0.
Meat only	4 oz.	115	0.
Lake (See **LAKE TROUT**)			
Rainbow:			
Fresh, meat with skin	4 oz.	221	0.
Canned	4 oz.	237	0.
TUNA:			
Raw (USDA) meat only:			
Bluefin	4 oz.	164	0.
Yellowfin	4 oz.	151	0.
Canned in oil:			
(Bumble Bee):			
Chunk, light, solids & liq.	½ of 6½-oz. can	265	0.
Solid, white, solids & liq.	½ cup (3.5 oz.)	285	0.
(Carnation) solids & liq.	6½-oz. can	427	0.
(Star Kist) solid, white, solids & liq.	7-oz. serving	503	0.
Canned in water:			
(Breast O'Chicken)	6½-oz. can	211	0.

Food and Description	Measure or Quantity	Calories	Carbo-hydrates (grams)
(Bumble Bee):			
Chunk, light, solids & liq.	½ cup	117	0.
Solid, white, solids & liq.	½ cup	126	0.
(Featherweight) light, chunk	6½-oz. can	210	0.
(Star Kist) light	7-oz. can	220	0.
*TUNA HELPER			
(General Mills):			
Au gratin	⅕ of pkg.	300	21.0
Cheesy noodles 'n tuna	⅕ of pkg.	250	30.0
Cold salad	⅕ of pkg.	440	29.0
Creamy mushroom	⅕ of pkg.	250	28.0
Creamy noodles 'n tuna	⅕ of pkg.	270	32.0
Potpie	⅙ of pkg.	430	33.0
Tetrazzini	⅕ of pkg.	270	26.0
TUNA NOODLES CASSEROLE, frozen			
(Stouffer's)	10-oz. meal	310	31.0
TUNA PIE, frozen:			
(Banquet)	8-oz. pie	395	43.0
(Morton)	8-oz. pie	370	36.0
TUNA SALAD:			
Home recipe, (USDA) made with tuna, celery, mayonnaise, pickle, onion and egg	4-oz. serving	193	4.0
Canned (Carnation)	¼ of 7½-oz. can	100	3.3
TURBOT, GREENLAND			
(USDA) raw:			
Whole	1 lb. (weighed whole)	344	0.
Meat only	4 oz.	166	0.
TURKEY:			
Raw (USDA):			
Ready-to-cook	1 lb. (weighed with bones)	722	0.
Dark meat	4 oz.	145	0.

(USDA): United States Department of Agriculture
(HEW/FAO):   Health, Education and Welfare/Food and Agriculture
                        Organization
* Prepared as Package Directs

Food and Description	Measure or Quantity	Calories	Carbohydrates (grams)
Light meat	4 oz.	132	0.
Skin only	4 oz.	459	0.
Barbecued (Louis Rich) breast, half	1 oz.	40	0.
Roasted (USDA):			
Flesh, skin & giblets	From 13½-lb. raw, ready-to-cook turkey	9678	0.
Flesh & skin	From 13½-lb. raw, ready-to cook turkey	7872	0.
Flesh & skin	4 oz.	253	0.
Meat only:			
Chopped	1 cup (5 oz.)	268	0.
Diced	4 oz.	200	0.
Light	1 slice (4″ × 2″ × ¼″, 3 oz.)	75	0.
Dark	1 slice (2½″ × 1⅝″ × ¼″, .7 oz.)	43	0.
Skin only	1 oz.	128	0.
Giblets, simmered (USDA)	2 oz.	132	.9
Gizzard (USDA):			
Raw	4 oz.	178	1.2
Simmered	4 oz.	222	12.
Canned (Swanson) chunk	2½-oz. serving	120	0.
Packaged:			
(Carl Buddig) smoked:			
Regular	1 oz.	50	Tr.
Ham or salami	1 oz.	40	Tr.
Hebrew National, breast	1 oz.	37	<1.0
(Hormel) breast			
Regular	1 slice	30	0.
Smoked	1 slice	25	0.
(Louis Rich):			
Turkey bologna	1-oz. slice	60	1.0
Turkey breast:			
Oven roasted	1-oz. slice	30	0.
Smoked	.7-oz. slice	25	0.
Turkey cotto salami	1-oz. slice	50	Tr.
Turkey ham:			
Chopped	1-oz. slice	45	Tr.
Cured	1-oz. slice	35	Tr.
Turkey pastrami	1-oz. slice	35	Tr.

Food and Description	Measure or Quantity	Calories	Carbo-hydrates (grams)
(Ohse):			
Oven cooked or smoked breast	1 oz.	30	1.0
Turkey bologna	1 oz.	70	2.0
Turkey salami	1 oz.	50	1.0
(Oscar Mayer) breast, smoked	¾-oz. slice	19	.2
Smoked (Louis Rich):			
Breast	1 oz.	35	0.
Drumsticks	1 oz. (without bone)	40	Tr.
Wing drumettes	1 oz. (without bone)	45	Tr.
TURKEY DINNER OR ENTREE, FROZEN:			
(Armour) *Dinner Classics,* & dressing	11¼-oz. dinner	330	32.0
(Banquet):			
American Favorites	11-oz. dinner	320	41.0
Extra Helping	9-oz. dinner	723	98.0
(Conagra) *Light & Elegant,* sliced	8-oz. entree	230	25.0
(Green Giant) twin pouch with white & wild rice stuffing	9-oz. entree	460	34.0
(Le Menu) sliced breast, with mushrooms	11¼-oz. meal	460	34.0
(Morton)	10-oz. meal	226	28.0
(Stouffer's):			
Regular:			
Casserole with gravy & dressing	9¾-oz. meal	360	29.0
Tetrazzini	10-oz. meal	380	28.0
Lean Cuisine:			
Breast, sliced, in mushroom sauce	8-oz. meal	240	20.0
Dijon	9½-oz. meal	270	22.0
Right Course, sliced, in mild curry sauce with rice pilaf	8¾-oz. meal	320	40.0

(USDA): United States Department of Agriculture
(HEW/FAO):   Health, Education and Welfare/Food and Agriculture
                       Organization
* Prepared as Package Directs

Food and Description	Measure or Quantity	Calories	Carbohydrates (grams)
(Swanson):			
Regular:			
Dinner, 4-compartment	11½-oz. dinner	330	39.0
Entree	8¾-oz. entree	250	24.0
Hungry Man:			
Dinner	18½-oz. dinner	590	66.0
Entree	13¼-oz. entree	390	36.0
(Weight Watchers) stuffed breast	8½-oz. meal	260	21.0
TURKEY NUGGET, frozen (Empire Kosher)	¼ of 12-oz. pkg.	255	14.0
TURKEY PATTY, frozen (Empire Kosher)	¼ of 12-oz. pkg.	188	12.0
TURKEY PIE, frozen:			
(Banquet):			
Regular	8-oz. pie	526	32.0
Supreme	8-oz. pie	430	41.0
(Empire Kosher)	8-oz. pie	491	50.0
(Morton)	7-oz. pie	420	27.0
(Stouffer's)	10-oz. pie	540	35.0
(Swanson):			
Regular	8-oz. pie	430	41.0
Chunky	10-oz. pie	530	45.0
Hungry Man	16-oz. pie	740	66.0
TURKEY, POTTED (USDA)	1 oz.	70	0.
TURKEY SALAD, canned (Carnation)	¼ of 7½-oz. can	110	31.1
TURKEY TETRAZZINI, frozen (Stouffer's)	6-oz. serving	240	17.0
TURNIP (USDA):			
Fresh:			
Without tops	1 lb. (weighed with skins)	117	25.7
Pared, diced	½ cup (2.4 oz.)	20	4.4
Pared, slices	½ cup (2.3 oz.)	19	4.2
Boiled, drained:			
Diced	½ cup (2.8 oz.)	18	3.8
Mashed	½ cup (4 oz.)	26	5.6

Food and Description	Measure or Quantity	Calories	Carbo-hydrates (grams)
TURNIP GREENS, leaves & stems:			
Fresh (USDA):	1 lb. (weighed untrimmed)	107	19.0
Boiled (USDA):			
In small amount water, short time, drained	½ cup (2.5 oz.)	14	2.6
In large amount water, long time, drained	½ cup (2.5 oz.)	14	2.4
Canned:			
(USDA) solids & liq.	½ cup (4.1 oz.)	21	3.7
(Allen's) chopped, with diced turnips	½ cup	20	1.0
(Stokely-Van Camp) chopped	½ cup (4.1 oz.)	23	3.5
(Sunshine) solids & liq.:			
Chopped	½ cup (4.1 oz.)	19	2.5
& diced turnips	½ cup (4.1 oz.)	21	3.2
Frozen:			
(Birds Eye):			
Chopped	⅓ of 10-oz. pkg.	20	3.0
Chopped, with sliced turnips	⅓ of 10-oz. pkg.	20	3.0
(Frosty Acres)	3.3-oz. serving	20	4.0
(McKenzie or Seabrook Farms):			
Chopped	⅓ of 10-oz. pkg.	25	3.4
Diced	1-oz. serving	4	.8
(Southland):			
Chopped	⅕ of 16-oz. pkg.	20	4.0
With diced turnips	⅕ of 16-oz. pkg.	20	5.0
Mashed	⅓ of 11-oz. pkg.	30	9.0
TURNIP ROOT, frozen (McKenzie) diced	1 oz.	4	1.0
TURNOVER:			
Frozen (Pepperidge Farm):			
Apple	1 turnover	310	35.0
Blueberry	1 turnover	320	32.0
Cherry	1 turnover	310	32.0

(USDA): United States Department of Agriculture
(HEW/FAO): Health, Education and Welfare/Food and Agriculture
Organization
* Prepared as Package Directs

Food and Description	Measure or Quantity	Calories	Carbo-hydrates (grams)
Peach	1 turnover	320	34.0
Raspberry	1 turnover	320	37.0
Refrigerated (Pillsbury)	1 turnover	170	23.0
TURTLE, GREEN (USDA):			
Raw:			
In shell	1 lb. (weighed in shell)	97	0.
Meat only	4 oz.	101	0.
Canned	4 oz.	120	0.
TWINKIE (Hostess):			
Regular	1½-oz. piece	155	26.0
Devil's food	1½-oz. piece	150	24.7

Food and Description	Measure or Quantity	Calories	Carbo-hydrates (grams)

U

UFO'S, canned
  (Franco-American):

Regular	7½-oz. can	180	35.0
With meteors (meatballs)	7½-oz. can	240	30.0

(USDA): United States Department of Agriculture
(HEW/FAO): Health, Education and Welfare/Food and Agriculture
          Organization
* Prepared as Package Directs

Food and Description	Measure or Quantity	Calories	Carbo-hydrates (grams)

V

V-8 JUICE (See **VEGETABLE JUICE COCKTAIL**)

Food and Description	Measure or Quantity	Calories	Carbo-hydrates (grams)
VALPOLICELLA WINE (Antinori) red	3 fl. oz.	84	6.3
VANDERMINT, liqueur	1 fl. oz.	90	10.2
VANILLA EXTRACT (Virginia Dare) pure, 35% alcohol	1 tsp.	10	DNA
VEAL, medium fat (USDA):			
Chuck:			
Raw	1 lb. (weighed with bone)	628	0.
Braised, lean & fat	4 oz.	266	0.
Flank:			
Raw	1 lb. (weighed with bone)	1410	0.
Stewed, lean & fat	4 oz.	442	0.
Foreshank:			
Raw	1 lb. (weighed with bone)	368	0.
Stewed, lean & fat	4 oz.	245	0.
Loin:			
Raw	1 lb. (weighed with bone)	681	0.
Broiled, medium done, chop, lean & fat	4 oz.	265	0.
Plate:			
Raw	1 lb. (weighed with bone)	828	0.
Stewed, lean & fat	4 oz.	344	0.
Rib:			
Raw, lean & fat	1 lb. (weighed with bone)	723	0.

Food and Description	Measure or Quantity	Calories	Carbo-hydrates (grams)
Roasted, medium done, lean & fat	4 oz.	305	0.
Round & rump:			
Raw	1 lb. (weighed with bone)	573	0.
Broiled, steak or cutlet, lean & fat	4 oz. (weighed with bone)	245	0.
VEAL DINNER, frozen:			
(Armour) *Dinner Classics,* parmigiana	10¾-oz. meal	400	34.0
(Banquet) parmigiana:			
Dinner:			
Extra Helping	20-oz. dinner	1092	116.0
International Favorites	11-oz. dinner	413	43.0
Entree:			
Family Entrees	2-lb. pkg.	1410	105,0
Entrees For One	5-oz. pkg.	230	20.0
(Morton) parmegiana	10-oz. dinner	252	35.0
(Swanson) parmigiana:			
Regular, 4-compartment	12¾-oz. dinner	470	49.0
Hungry Man	20-oz. dinner	640	62.0
(Weight Watchers) patty, parmigiana	8¹⁄₁₆ meal	230	9.0
VEAL STEAK, frozen (Hormel):			
Regular	4-oz. serving	130	2.0
Breaded	4-oz. serving	240	13.0
VEGETABLE BOUILLON:			
(Herb-Ox):			
Cube	1 cube	6	.6
Packet	1 packet	12	2.2
(Wyler's) instant	1 tsp.	6	1.0

VEGETABLE FAT (See **FAT**)

(USDA): United States Department of Agriculture
(HEW/FAO):   Health, Education and Welfare/Food and Agriculture
                        Organization
* Prepared as Package Directs

Food and Description	Measure or Quantity	Calories	Carbo-hydrates (grams)
VEGETABLE FLAKES			
(French's)	1 T.	12	3.0
VEGETABLE JUICE COCKTAIL:			
Regular, *V-8*, regular or spicy hot	6 fl. oz.	35	8.0
Dietetic:			
(Featherweight) low sodium	6 fl. oz.	35	8.0
(S&W) *Nutradiet*, low sodium, green label	6 fl. oz.	35	8.0
V-8, low sodium	6 fl. oz.	40	9.0
VEGETABLE, MIXED:			
Canned, regular pack:			
(Del Monte) solids & liq.	½ cup (4 oz.)	40	7.0
(Chun King) chow mein, drained	½ of 8-oz. can	32	6.3
(La Choy) drained:			
Chinese	⅓ of 14-oz. can	12	2.0
Chop Suey	½ cup (4.7 oz.)	9	2.0
(Libby's) solids & liq.	½ cup (4.2 oz.)	40	9.8
(Veg-all) solids & liq.	½ cup	35	8.0
Canned, dietetic pack:			
(Featherweight) low sodium	½ cup (4 oz.)	40	8.0
(Larsen) *Fresh Lite*, no added salt	½ cup	35	8.0
Frozen:			
(Birds Eye):			
Regular:			
Broccoli, cauliflower & carrot in butter sauce	⅓ of 10-oz. pkg.	51	5.7
Broccoli, cauliflower & carrot in cheese sauce	⅓ of 10-oz. pkg.	72	7.9
Broccoli, cauliflower & red pepper	⅓ of 10-oz. pkg.	31	4.7
Carrot, pea & onion, deluxe	⅓ of 10-oz. pkg.	52	10.0
Medley, in butter sauce	⅓ of 10-oz. pkg.	62	9.7
Mixed	⅓ of 10-oz. pkg.	68	13.3
Mixed, with onion sauce	⅓ of 8-oz. pkg.	103	11.7
Pea & potato in cream sauce	⅓ of 8-oz. pkg.	164	15.6

Food and Description	Measure or Quantity	Calories	Carbo- hydrates (grams)
Farm Fresh:			
Broccoli, carrot & water chestnut	⅕ of 16-oz. pkg.	36	6.5
Broccoli, cauliflower & carrot strips	⅕ of 16-oz. pkg.	30	5.3
Broccoli, corn & red pepper	⅕ of 16-oz. pkg.	58	10.9
Broccoli, green bean, onion & red pepper	⅕ of 16-oz. pkg.	31	5.4
Brussels sprout, cauliflower & carrot	⅕ of 16-oz. pkg.	38	6.5
Cauliflower, green bean & carrot	⅕ of 16-oz. pkg.	42	8.1
Green bean, corn, carrot & pearl onion	⅕ of 16-oz. pkg.	49	10.1
Green bean, cauliflower & carrot	⅕ of 16-oz. pkg.	32	6.1
Pea, carrot & pearl onion	⅕ of 16-oz. pkg.	59	10.7
International:			
Bavarian style beans & spaetzle	⅓ of 10-oz. pkg.	112	11.5
Chinese style	⅓ of 10-oz. pkg.	85	8.4
Far Eastern style	⅓ of 10-oz. pkg.	84	8.4
Italian style	⅓ of 10-oz. pkg.	114	11.4
Japanese style	⅓ of 10-oz. pkg.	102	10.4
Mexican style	⅓ of 10-oz. pkg.	133	16.1
New England style	⅓ of 10-oz. pkg.	129	14.2
San Francisco style	⅓ of 10-oz. pkg.	99	10.9
Stir Fry:			
Chinese style	⅓ of 10-oz. pkg.	36	6.9
Japanese style	⅓ of 10-oz. pkg.	32	5.9
(Green Giant):			
Regular:			
Broccoli, carrot fanfare	½ cup	25	5.0
Broccoli, cauliflower & carrot in cheese sauce	½ cup	60	8.0
Broccoli, cauliflower supreme	½ cup	20	4.0

(USDA): United States Department of Agriculture
(HEW/FAO): Health, Education and Welfare/Food and Agriculture Organization
* Prepared as Package Directs

Food and Description	Measure or Quantity	Calories	Carbohydrates (grams)
Cauliflower, green bean festival	½ cup	16	3.0
Corn, broccoli bounty	½ cup	60	11.0
Mixed, butter sauce	½ cup	80	12.0
Mixed, polybag	½ cup	50	10.0
Pea, pea pod & water chestnut in butter sauce	½ cup	80	10.0
Pea & cauliflower medley	½ cup	40	7.0
Harvest Fresh	½ cup	60	13.0
Harvest Get Togethers:			
Broccoli-cauliflower medley	½ cup	60	10.0
Broccoli fanfare	½ cup	80	14.2
Cauliflower-carrot bonanza	½ cup	60	7.0
Chinese style	½ cup	60	7.0
Japanese style	½ cup	45	8.0
(Frosty Acres):			
Regular	3.3-oz. serving	65	13.0
Dutch style	3.2-oz. serving	30	5.0
Italian	3.2-oz. serving	40	8.0
Oriental	3.2-oz. serving	25	5.0
Rancho Fiesta	3.2-oz. serving	60	13.0
Soup mix	3-oz. serving	45	11.0
Stew	3-oz. serving	42	10.0
Swiss mix	3-oz. serving	25	5.0
(La Choy) stir fry	4-oz. serving	40	7.9
(Larsen):			
Regular	3.3-oz. serving	70	13.0
California or Italian blend	3.3-oz. serving	30	6.0
Chuckwagon blend	3.3-oz. serving	70	16.0
Midwestern blend	3.3-oz. serving	40	8.0
Oriental or winter blend	3.3-oz. serving	25	5.0
Scandinavian blend	3.3-oz. serving	45	9.0
For soup or stew	3.3-oz. serving	50	11.0
Wisconsin blend	3.3-oz. serving	50	12.0
(Southland):			
Gumbo	⅕ of 16-oz. pkg.	40	9.0
Soup	⅕ of 16-oz. pkg.	50	11.0
Stew	4 oz.	60	13.0

VEGETABLE IN PASTRY,
frozen (Pepperidge Farm):
Asparagus with mornay

Food and Description	Measure or Quantity	Calories	Carbo-hydrates (grams)
sauce or broccoli with cheese	½ of 7½-oz. pkg.	250	18.0
Broccoli with cheese	½ of 7½-oz. pkg.	250	19.0
Cauliflower & cheese sauce	½ of 7½-oz. pkg.	220	20.0
Mushroom dijon	½ of 7½-oz. pkg.	230	19.0
Spinach almondine	½ of 7½-oz. pkg.	260	19.0
Zucchini provencal	½ of 7½-oz. pkg.	210	21.0
VEGETABLE STEW, canned			
Dinty Moore (Hormel)	⅓ of 24-oz. can	170	20.0
"VEGETARIAN FOODS":			
Canned or dry:			
Chicken, fried (Loma Linda) with gravy	1½-oz. piece	70	2.0
*Chicken, supreme (Loma Linda)	¼ cup	50	4.0
Chili (Worthington)	½ cup (4.9 oz.)	177	13.2
Choplet (Worthington)	1 choplet (1.6 oz.)	50	1.7
Dinner cuts (Loma Linda) drained:			
Regular	1 piece (1.8 oz.)	55	2.0
No Salt Added	1 piece (1.8 oz.)	55	2.0
Dinner loaf (Loma Linda)	¼ cup (.6 oz.)	50	4.0
Franks, big (Loma Linda)	1.8-oz. frank	100	4.0
Franks, sizzle (Loma Linda)	1.2-oz. frank	85	1.5
FriChik (Worthington)	1 piece (1.6 oz.)	75	2.5
Granburger (Worthington)	1 oz.	96	5.8
Linkettes (Loma Linda)	1.3-oz. link	75	2.5
Little links (Loma Linda) drained	.8-oz. link	40	1.0
Non-Meatballs (Worthington)	1 meatball (.6 oz.)	32	1.9

(USDA): United States Department of Agriculture
(HEW/FAO):   Health, Education and Welfare/Food and Agriculture Organization
* Prepared as Package Directs

Food and Description	Measure or Quantity	Calories	Carbo- hydrates (grams)
Numete (Worthington)	½" slice (2.4 oz.)	145	7.1
Nuteena (Loma Linda)	½" slice (2.4 oz.)	160	5.0
*Ocean platter (Loma Linda)	¼ cup	50	5.0
*Patty mix (Loma Linda)	¼ cup	50	4.0
Peanuts & soya (USDA)	4 oz.	269	15.2
Prime Stakes	1 slice	171	7.8
Proteena (Loma Linda)	½" slice	144	6.5
Protose (Worthington)	½" slice	140	5.0
Redi-burger (Loma Linda)	½" slice (2.4 oz.)	130	5.0
Sandwich spread (Loma Linda)	1 T. (.5 oz.)	23	1.3
Savorex (Loma Linda)	1 tsp.	16	1.0
*Savory dinner loaf (Loma Linda)	1 slice (¼ cup dry)	110	4.0
Skallops (Worthington) drained	½ cup (3 oz.)	89	3.0
Soyagen (Loma Linda):			
All purpose or no sucrose	½ cup	65	7.0
Carob	½ cup	70	8.0
Soyameat (Worthington):			
Beef, sliced	1 slice (1 oz.)	44	2.6
Chicken, diced	1 oz.	40	1.4
Soyamel, any kind (Worthington)	1 oz.	120	12.2
Stew pack (Loma Linda) drained	2 oz.	70	4.0
Super Links (Worthington)	1 link (1.9 oz.)	110	3.7
Swiss steak with gravy (Loma Linda)	1 steak (2¾ oz.)	140	8.0
Taystee cuts (Loma Linda)	1 cut (1.3 oz.)	35	1.0
Tender bits (Loma Linda) drained	1 piece	20	1.0
Tender rounds (Loma Linda)	1-oz. piece	20	1.2
Vege-burger (Loma Linda):			
Regular	½ cup	110	4.0
No Salt Added	½ cup	140	4.0
Vegelona (Loma Linda)	½" slice (2.4 oz.)	100	6.0
Vega-links (Worthington)	1 link (1.1 oz.)	55	2.8
Veg-scallops (Loma Linda)	1 piece (.5 oz.)	12	.3
Vita-Burger (Loma Linda)	1 T. (¼ oz.)	23	2.3
Wheat protein (USDA)	4 oz.	170	10.8
Worthington 209	1 slice (1.1 oz.)	58	2.2
Frozen:			
Beef pie (Worthington)	8-oz. pie	278	41.8

Food and Description	Measure or Quantity	Calories	Carbo-hydrates (grams)
Bologna (Loma Linda)	1 oz.	75	2.5
Bolono (Worthington)	¾-oz. slice	23	1.0
Chicken (Loma Linda)	1-oz. slice	46	2.1
Chicken, fried (Loma Linda)	2-oz. serving	180	2.0
Chicken pie (Worthington)	8-oz. pie	346	37.5
Chic-Ketts (Worthington)	1 oz.	53	2.2
Chik-Nuggets (Loma Linda)	1 piece (.6 oz.)	45	3.4
Chik-Patties (Loma Linda)	1 patty (3 oz.)	226	15.0
Corn dogs (Loma Linda)	1 piece (2.6 oz.)	250	7.0
Corned beef, sliced (Worthington)	1 slice (.5 oz.)	32	1.9
Fillets (Worthington)	1½-oz. piece	90	4.6
FriPats (Worthington)	1 patty	204	5.2
Griddle Steak (Loma Linda)	1 piece (2 oz.)	190	5.0
Meatballs (Loma Linda)	1 meatball (.3 oz.)	63	.8
Meatless salami (Worthington)	¾-oz. slice	44	1.2
Ocean fillet (Loma Linda)	1 piece (2 oz.)	160	5.0
Olive loaf (Loma Linda)	1 slice (1 oz.)	59	2.7
Prosage (Worthington):			
Links	1 link	60	1.5
Patty	1.3-oz. piece	96	2.8
Roll	⅜" slice (1.2 oz.)	86	2.0
Roast beef (Loma Linda)	1 oz.	53	2.6
Salami (Loma Linda)	1 slice (1 oz.)	49	2.8
Sizzle burger (Loma Linda)	1 burger (2.5 oz.)	210	13.0
Smoked beef, slices (Worthington)	1 slice	14	1.1
Stakelets (Worthington)	3-oz. piece	164	9.4
Tuno (Worthington)	2-oz. serving	81	3.4
Turkey (Loma Linda)	1 slice (1 oz.)	47	2.3
Wahm roll (Worthington)	1 slice (.8 oz.)	36	1.9
VENISON (USDA) raw, lean, meat only	4 oz.	143	0.
VERMOUTH:			
Dry & extra dry (Lejon; Noilly Pratt)	1 fl. oz.	33	1.0

(USDA): United States Department of Agriculture
(HEW/FAO): Health, Education and Welfare/Food and Agriculture
Organization
* Prepared as Package Directs

Food and Description	Measure or Quantity	Calories	Carbo-hydrates (grams)
Sweet (Lejon; Taylor)	1 fl. oz.	45	3.8
VICHY WATER (Schweppes)	Any quantity	0	0.
VINEGAR:			
Cider:			
(USDA)	1 T. (.5 oz.)	2	.9
(USDA)	½ cup (4.2 oz.)	17	7.1
Distilled:			
(USDA)	1 T. (.5 oz.)	2	.8
(USDA)	½ cup (4.2 oz.)	14	6.0
Red, red with garlic or white wine (Regina)	1 T. (.5 oz.)	Tr.	Tr.
VINESPINACH or BASELLA			
(USDA) raw	4 oz.	22	3.9
VODKA, unflavored (See **DISTILLED LIQUOR**)			

Food and Description	Measure or Quantity	Calories	Carbo-hydrates (grams)

W

WAFFELOS, cereal
  (Ralston Purina) — 1 cup (1 oz.) — 110 — 25.0

WAFFLE:
  Home recipe (USDA) — 7" waffle (2.6 oz.) — 209 — 28.1
  Frozen:
    (Aunt Jemima) jumbo — 1 waffle — 86 — 14.5
    (Eggo):
      Regular — 1 waffle — 120 — 16.0
      Apple cinnamon — 1 waffle — 150 — 20.0
      Blueberry — 1 waffle — 130 — 16.0
      Buttermilk — 1 waffle — 110 — 15.0
      Home style — 1 waffle — 120 — 18.0
    Roman Meal:
      Regular — 1 waffle — 140 — 16.5
      Golden Delight — 1 waffle — 131 — 15.1

WAFFLE MIX (See also
  **PANCAKE & WAFFLE
  MIX**) (USDA):
  Complete mix:
    Dry — 1 oz. — 130 — 18.5
    *Prepared with water — 2.6-oz. waffle — 229 — 30.2
  Incomplete mix:
    Dry — 1 oz. — 101 — 21.5
    *Prepared with egg & milk — 2.6-oz. waffle — 206 — 27.2
    *Prepared with egg & milk — 7.1-oz. waffle (9" × 9" × ⅝", 1⅛ cups) — 550 — 72.4

Food and Description	Measure or Quantity	Calories	Carbohydrates (grams)
WAFFELOS, cereal (Ralston Purina)	1 cup (1 oz.)	110	25.0
WAFFLE:			
Home recipe (USDA)	7" waffle (2.6 oz.)	209	28.1
Frozen:			
(Aunt Jemima) jumbo	1 waffle	86	14.5
(Eggo):			
Regular	1 waffle	120	16.0
Apple cinnamon	1 waffle	150	20.0
Blueberry	1 waffle	130	16.0
Buttermilk	1 waffle	110	15.0
Home style	1 waffle	120	18.0
Roman Meal:			
Regular	1 waffle	140	16.5
Golden Delight	1 waffle	131	15.1
WAFFLE MIX (See also **PANCAKE & WAFFLE MIX**) (USDA):			
Complete mix:			
Dry	1 oz.	130	18.5
*Prepared with water	2.6-oz. waffle	229	30.2
Incomplete mix:			
Dry	1 oz.	101	21.5
*Prepared with egg & milk	2.6-oz. waffle	206	27.2
*Prepared with egg & milk	7.1-oz. waffle (9" × 9" × ⅝", 1⅛ cups)	550	72.4

(USDA): United States Department of Agriculture
(HEW/FAO):   Health, Education and Welfare/Food and Agriculture
                    Organization
* Prepared as Package Directs

Food and Description	Measure or Quantity	Calories	Carbo-hydrates (grams)
WAFFLE SYRUP (See **SYRUP**)			
WALNUT:			
(USDA):			
Black, in shell, whole	1 lb. (weighed in shell)	627	14.8
Black, shelled, whole	4 oz. (weighed whole)	712	16.8
Black, chopped	½ cup (2.1 oz.)	377	8.9
English or Persian, shelled, whole	1 lb. (weighed in shell)	1327	32.2
English or Persian, shelled, whole	4 oz.	738	17.9
English or Persian, halves	½ cup (1.8 oz.)	356	6.5
(California) halves & pieces	½ cup (1.8 oz.)	356	6.5
(Fisher):			
Black	½ cup (2.1 oz.)	374	8.8
English	½ cup (2.1 oz.)	389	9.5
WATER CHESTNUT, CHINESE:			
Raw (USDA):			
Whole	1 lb. (weighed unpeeled)	272	66.5
Peeled	4 oz.	90	21.5
Canned:			
(Chun King) drained:			
Sliced	½ of 8-oz. can	89	21.5
Whole	½ of 8-oz. can	85	22.9
(La Choy) drained, sliced	½ of 8-oz. can	32	7.8
WATERCRESS, raw (USDA):			
Untrimmed	½ lb. (weighed untrimmed)	40	6.2
Trimmed	½ cup (.6 oz.)	3	.5
WATERMELON, fresh (USDA):			
Whole	1 lb. (weighed with rind)	54	13.4
Wedge	4″ × 8″ wedge (2 lb. measured with rind)	111	27.3
Diced	½ cup	21	5.1

Food and Description	Measure or Quantity	Calories	Carbo-hydrates (grams)
WAX GOURD, raw (USDA):			
Whole	1 lb. (weighed with skin & cavity contents)	41	9.4
Flesh only	4 oz.	15	3.4
WEAKFISH (USDA):			
Raw, whole	1 lb. (weighed whole)	263	0.
Broiled, meat only	4 oz.	236	0.
WELSH RAREBIT:			
Home recipe	1 cup (8.2 oz.)	415	14.6
Frozen (Stouffer's)	5-oz. serving	350	8.0
WENDY'S:			
Bacon, breakfast	1 strip	55	Tr.
Bacon cheeseburger on white bun	1 burger	460	23.0
Breakfast sandwich	1 sandwich	370	33.0
Buns:			
Wheat, multi-grain	1 bun	135	23.0
White	1 bun	160	28.0
Chicken sandwich on multi-grain bun	1 sandwich	320	31.0
Chili:			
Regular	8 oz.	260	26.0
Large	12 oz.	390	39.0
Condiments:			
Bacon	½ strip	30	Tr.
Cheese, American	1 slice	70	Tr.
Ketchup	1 tsp.	6	1.0
Mayonnaise	1 T.	100	Tr.
Mustard	1 tsp.	4	Tr.
Onion rings	.3-oz. piece	4	Tr.
Pickle, dill	4 slices	1	Tr.
Relish	.3-oz. serving	14	3.0
Tomato	1 slice	2	Tr.
Danish	1 piece	360	44.0

(USDA): United States Department of Agriculture
(HEW/FAO): Health, Education and Welfare/Food and Agriculture Organization
* Prepared as Package Directs

Food and Description	Measure or Quantity	Calories	Carbo-hydrates (grams)
Drinks:			
Coffee	6 fl. oz.	2	Tr.
Cola:			
Regular	12 fl. oz.	110	29.0
Dietetic	12 fl. oz.	Tr.	Tr.
Fruit flavored drink	12 fl. oz.	110	28.0
Hot chocolate	6 fl. oz.	100	17.0
Milk:			
Regular	8 fl. oz.	150	11.0
Chocolate	8 fl. oz.	210	26.0
Non-cola	12 fl. oz.	100	26.0
Orange juice	6 fl. oz.	80	17.0
Egg, scrambled	1 order	190	7.0
Frosty dairy dessert:			
Small	12 fl. oz.	400	59.0
Medium	16 fl. oz.	533	78.7
Large	20 fl. oz.	667	98.3
Hamburger:			
Double, on white bun	1 burger	560	24.0
Kids Meal	1 burger	220	11.0
Single:			
On wheat bun	1 burger	340	20.0
On white bun	1 burger	350	27.0
Omelet:			
Ham & cheese	1 omelet	250	6.0
Ham, cheese & mushroom	1 omelet	290	7.0
Ham, cheese, onion & green pepper	1 omelet	280	7.0
Mushroom, onion & green pepper	1 omelet	210	7.0
Potato:			
Baked, hot stuffed:			
Plain	1 potato	250	53.0
Bacon & cheese	1 potato	570	57.0
Broccoli & cheese	1 potato	500	54.0
Cheese	1 potato	590	55.0
Chicken à la King	1 potato	350	59.0
Chili & cheese	1 potato	510	63.0
Sour cream & chives	1 potato	460	53.0
Stroganoff & sour cream	1 potato	490	60.0
French fries	regular order	280	35.0
Home fries	1 order	360	37.0
Salad Bar, *Garden Spot:*			
Alfalfa sprouts	2 oz.	20	2.0

Food and Description	Measure or Quantity	Calories	Carbohydrates (grams)
Bacon bits	⅛ oz.	10	Tr.
Blueberries, fresh	1 T.	8	2.0
Breadstick	1 piece	20	2.0
Broccoli	½ cup	14	2.0
Cantaloupe	1 piece (2 oz.)	4	1.0
Carrot	¼ cup	12	3.0
Cauliflower	½ cup	14	3.0
Cheese:			
American, imitation	1 oz.	70	1.0
Cheddar, imitation	1 oz.	90	1.0
Cottage	½ cup	110	3.0
Mozzarella, imitation	1 oz.	90	Tr.
Swiss, imitation	1 oz.	80	Tr.
Chow mein noodles	¼ cup	60	6.0
Cole slaw	½ cup	90	3.0
Cracker, saltine	1 piece	11	2.0
Crouton	1 piece	2	.2
Cucumber	¼ cup	4	1.0
Eggs	1 T.	14	Tr.
Mushroom	¼ cup	6	Tr.
Onions, red	1 T.	4	Tr.
Orange, fresh	1 piece	5	1.4
Pasta salad	½ cup	134	17.0
Peas, green	½ cup	60	9.0
Peaches, in syrup	1 piece	8	2.0
Peppers:			
Banana or mild			
pepperoncini	1 T.	18	4.0
Bell	¼ cup	4	1.0
Jalapeño	1 T.	9	2.0
Pineapple chunks in juice	½ cup	80	20.0
Sunflower seeds & raisins	¼ cup	180	12.0
Tomato	1 oz.	6	1.0
Turkey ham	¼ cup	46	1.0
Watermelon, fresh	1 piece (1 oz.)	1	Tr.
Salad dressing:			
Regular:			
Blue cheese	1 T.	60	Tr.
Celery seed	1 T.	70	3.0
French, red	1 T.	70	5.0

(USDA): United States Department of Agriculture
(HEW/FAO):   Health, Education and Welfare/Food and Agriculture
              Organization
* Prepared as Package Directs

Food and Description	Measure or Quantity	Calories	Carbo-hydrates (grams)
Italian, golden	1 T.	45	3.0
Oil	1 T.	130	Tr.
Ranch	1 T.	80	Tr.
Thousand Island	1 T.	70	2.0
Dietetic:			
Bacon & tomato	1 T.	45	2.0
Cucumber, creamy	1 T.	50	2.0
Italian	1 T.	25	2.0
Thousand Island	1 T.	45	2.0
Wine vinegar	1 T.	2	Tr.
Salad, Side, pick-up window	1 salad	110	5.0
Salad, taco	1 salad	390	36.0
Sausage	1 patty	200	Tr.
Toast:			
Regular, with margarine	1 slice	125	17.5
French	1 slice	200	22.5
WESTERN DINNER, frozen:			
(Banquet) American Favorites	11-oz. dinner	513	43.0
(Morton)	10-oz. dinner	289	29.0
(Swanson):			
Regular, 4-compartment dinner	12¼-oz. dinner	440	45.0
Hungry Man	17½-oz. dinner	750	71.0
WHEATENA, cereal	¼ cup	112	22.5
WHEAT FLAKES CEREAL			
(Featherweight) low sodium	1¼ cups (1 oz.)	100	23.0
WHEAT GERM:			
(USDA)	1 oz.	103	13.2
(Elam's) raw	1 T. (.3 oz.)	28	3.2
(Kretschmer)	1 oz.	110	13.0
WHEAT GERM CEREAL			
(Kretschmer):			
Regular	¼ cup (1 oz.)	110	13.0
Brown sugar & honey	¼ cup (1 oz.)	110	17.0
WHEAT HEARTS, cereal			
(General Mills)	1 oz. dry	110	21.0
WHEATIES, cereal			
(General Mills)	1 cup (1 oz.)	110	23.0

Food and Description	Measure or Quantity	Calories	Carbo-hydrates (grams)
WHEAT & OATMEAL CEREAL, hot (Elam's)	1 oz.	105	18.8
WHEAT, ROLLED (USDA):			
Uncooked	1 cup (3.1 oz.)	296	66.3
Cooked	1 cup (7.7 oz.)	163	36.7
WHEAT, SHREDDED, cereal (See **SHREDDED WHEAT**)			
WHEAT, WHOLE GRAIN (USDA) hard red spring	1 oz.	94	19.6
WHEAT, WHOLE-MEAL, cereal (USDA):			
Dry	1 oz.	96	20.5
Cooked	4 oz.	51	10.7
WHEY (USDA):			
Dry	1 oz.	99	20.8
Fluid	1 cup (8.6 oz.)	63	12.4
WHIPPED TOPPING (See **TOPPING, WHIPPED**)			
WHISKEY (See **DISTILLED LIQUOR**)			
WHISKEY SOUR COCKTAIL:			
(Mr. Boston) 12½% alcohol	3 fl. oz.	120	14.4
*Mix (Bar-Tender's)	3½ fl. oz.	177	18.0
WHITE CASTLE:			
Bun	.8-oz. bun	74	13.9
Cheeseburger	1 serving	200	15.5
Chicken sandwich	2¼-oz. sandwich	186	20.5
Fish sandwich without tartar sauce	2.1-oz. serving	155	20.9

(USDA): United States Department of Agriculture
(HEW/FAO): Health, Education and Welfare/Food and Agriculture Organization
* Prepared as Package Directs

Food and Description	Measure or Quantity	Calories	Carbo- hydrates (grams)
French fries	3.4-oz. serving	301	37.7
Hamburger	1 burger	161	15.4
Onion chips	1 serving	329	38.8
Onion rings	1 serving	245	26.6
Sausage & egg sandwich	1 sandwich	322	16.0
Sausage sandwich	1 sandwich	196	13.3
WHITEFISH, LAKE (USDA):			
Raw, meat only	4 oz.	176	0.
Baked, stuffed, home recipe, with bacon, butter, onion, celery & breadcrumbs	4 oz.	244	6.6
Smoked	4 oz.	176	0.
WHOPPER (See **BURGER KING**)			
WIENER (See **FRANKFURTER**)			
WIENER WRAP (Pillsbury)	1 piece	60	10.0
WILD BERRY DRINK, canned (Hi-C)	6 fl. oz.	92	22.5
WINCHELL'S DONUT HOUSE:			
Buttermilk:			
Bar	2.1-oz. piece	243	54.4
Old fashioned	2-oz. piece	249	56.0
Cake, devil's food, iced	2-oz. piece	241	54.0
Cinnamon crumb	2-oz. piece	240	60.1
Iced, chocolate	2-oz. piece	227	55.0
Raised, glaze	1¾-oz. piece	212	48.5
WINE (See individual listings)			
WINE, COOKING (Regina):			
Burgundy or sauterne	¼ cup	2	Tr.
Sherry	¼ cup	20	5.0
WINE COOLER (Bartles & Jaymes):			
White	6 fl. oz.	92	12.4

Food and Description	Measure or Quantity	Calories	Carbo-hydrates (grams)
Premium berry	6 fl. oz.	92	14.1
Premium peach	6 fl. oz.	92	13.8
Premium red	6 fl. oz.	97	13.0
Premium tropical	6 fl. oz.	111	18.6

(USDA): United States Department of Agriculture
(HEW/FAO):   Health, Education and Welfare/Food and Agriculture
                    Organization
* Prepared as Package Directs

Food and Description	Measure or Quantity	Calories	Carbo-hydrates (grams)

Y

YAM (USDA):
  Raw:

Whole	1 lb. (weighed with skin)	394	90.5
Flesh only	4 oz.	115	26.3

  Canned & frozen (See
   SWEET POTATO)

YAM BEAN, raw (USDA):

Unpared tuber	1 lb. (weighed unpared)	225	52.2
Pared tuber	4 oz.	62	14.5

YEAST:
  Baker's:
   Compressed:

(USDA)	1 oz.	24	3.1
(Fleischmann's)	1 cube	15	2.0

   Dry:

(USDA)	1 oz.	80	11.0
(USDA)	7-gram pkg.	20	2.7
(Fleischmann's)	1 packet	20	3.0

YOGURT:
  Regular:
   Plain:

(Bison)	8-oz. container	160	16.8
(Colombo):			
Regular	8-oz. container	150	13.0
Natural Lite	8-oz. container	110	17.0
(Dannon):			
Low fat	8-oz. container	140	16.0
Non-fat	8-oz. container	110	16.0
(Friendship)	8-oz. container	170	15.0
(Johanna) sundae style	8-oz. container	150	17.0

Food and Description	Measure or Quantity	Calories	Carbo-hydrates (grams)
(La Yogurt)	6-oz. container	140	12.0
Lite-Line (Borden)	8-oz. container	140	18.0
(Meadow Gold)	8-oz. container	160	16.0
(Mountain High)	8-oz. container	200	16.0
(Whitney's)	6-oz. container	150	13.0
Yoplait	6-oz. container	130	13.0
Apple:			
(Colombo) spiced	8-oz. container	240	39.0
(Dannon) dutch, Fruit-on-the-Bottom	8-oz. container	240	43.0
(New Country) crisp	8-oz. container	210	40.0
(Sweet'n Low) dutch	8-oz. container	150	33.0
Yoplait, Custard Style	6-oz. container	190	32.0
Apple-cinnamon, *Yoplait, Breakfast Yogurt*	6-oz. container	220	38.0
Banana (Dannon) Fruit-on-the-Bottom	8-oz. container	240	43.0
Berry:			
(Whitney's) wild	6-oz. container	200	33.0
Yoplait:			
Breakfast Yogurt	6-oz. container	230	40.0
Custard Style	6-oz. container	190	32.0
Blueberry:			
(Breyer's)	8-oz. container	260	44.0
(Dannon):			
Fresh Flavors	8-oz. container	200	34.0
Fruit-on-the-Bottom	4.4-oz. container	130	23.0
Fruit-on-the-Bottom	8-oz. container	240	43.0
(Friendship)	8-oz. container	230	44.0
(Mountain High)	8-oz. container	220	31.0
(Whitney's)	6-oz. container	200	33.0
Yoplait:			
Regular	6-oz. container	190	32.0
Custard Style	6-oz. container	190	30.0
Boysenberry:			
(Dannon) Fruit-on-the-Bottom	8-oz. container	240	43.0
(Whitney's)	6-oz. container	200	33.0
Yoplait, Custard Style	6-oz. container	190	32.0

(USDA): United States Department of Agriculture
(HEW/FAO): Health, Education and Welfare/Food and Agriculture
Organization
* Prepared as Package Directs

Food and Description	Measure or Quantity	Calories	Carbo-hydrates (grams)
Cherry:			
(Breyer's) black	8-oz. container	270	47.0
(Colombo) black	8-oz. container	230	34.0
(Dannon) Fruit-on-the-Bottom	8-oz. container	240	43.0
(Friendship)	8-oz. container	230	44.0
(Sweet'n Low)	8-oz. container	150	33.0
(Whitney's)	6-oz. container	200	33.0
Yoplait:			
Breakfast Yogurt, with almonds	6-oz. container	210	37.0
Custard Style	6-oz. container	190	32.0
Cherry-vanilla, *Lite-Line* (Borden)	8-oz. container	240	45.0
Citrus, *Yoplait, Breakfast Yogurt*	6-oz. container	250	43.0
Coffee:			
(Dannon) Fresh Flavors	8-oz. container	200	34.0
(Friendship)	8-oz. container	210	35.0
(Johanna) sundae style	8-oz. container	220	17.0
(Whitney's)	6-oz. container	200	28.0
Yoplait, Custard Style	6-oz. container	180	30.0
Exotic fruit (Dannon) Fruit-on-the-Bottom	8-oz. container	240	43.0
Lemon:			
(Dannon) Fresh Flavors	8-oz. container	200	34.0
(Johanna) sundae style	8-oz. container	220	17.0
(Whitney's)	6-oz container	200	28.0
Yoplait:			
Regular	6-oz. container	190	32.0
Custard Style	6-oz. container	190	30.0
Mixed Berries (Dannon):			
Extra Smooth	4.4-oz. container	130	24.0
Fruit-on-the-Bottom	4.4-oz. container	130	23.0
Fruit-on-the-Bottom	8-oz. container	240	43.0
Orange, *Yoplait Custard Style*	6-oz. container	190	32.0
Orchard, *Yoplait, Breakfast Yogurt*	6-oz. container	240	40.0
Peach:			
(Breyer's)	8-oz. container	270	46.0
(Dannon) Fruit-on-the-Bottom	8-oz. container	240	43.0
(Friendship)	8-oz. container	230	44.0
Lite-Line (Borden)	8-oz. container	230	42.0
(Whitney's)	6-oz. container	200	33.0

Food and Description	Measure or Quantity	Calories	Carbo- hydrates (grams)
Yoplait, Custard Style	6-oz. container	190	32.0
Pina colada:			
(Dannon) Fruit-on-the- Bottom	8-oz. container	240	43.0
(Friendship)	8-oz. container	230	44.0
Yoplait, Custard Style	6-oz. container	190	32.0
Pineapple:			
(Breyer's)	8-oz. container	270	45.0
(Light N' Lively)	8-oz. container	240	48.0
Yoplait, Custard Style	6-oz. container	190	32.0
Raspberry:			
(Breyer's) red	8-oz. container	260	44.0
(Colombo)	8-oz. container	250	39.0
(Dannon):			
Extra Smooth	4.4-oz. container	130	24.0
Fresh Flavors	8-oz. container	200	34.0
Fruit-on-the-Bottom	4.4-oz. container	130	23.0
Fruit-on-the-Bottom	8-oz. container	240	43.0
(Friendship)	8-oz. container	230	44.0
(Light N' Lively) red	8-oz. container	230	43.0
(Meadow-Gold) sundae style	8-oz. container	250	42.0
(Whitney's)	6-oz. container	200	33.0
Yoplait:			
Regular	6-oz. container	190	32.0
Custard Style	6-oz. container	180	32.0
Strawberry:			
(Breyer's)	8-oz. container	270	46.0
(Dannon):			
Extra Smooth	4.4-oz. container	130	24.0
Fresh Flavors	8-oz. container	200	34.0
Fruit-on-the-Bottom	4.4-oz. container	130	23.0
Fruit-on-the-Bottom	8-oz. container	240	43.0
(Friendship)	8-oz. container	230	44.0
Lite-Line (Borden)	8-oz. container	240	46.0
(Whitney's)	6-oz. container	200	33.0
Yoplait:			
Regular	6-oz. container	190	32.0
Breakfast Yogurt, with almonds	6-oz. container	210	38.0

(USDA): United States Department of Agriculture
(HEW/FAO): Health, Education and Welfare/Food and Agriculture Organization
* Prepared as Package Directs

Food and Description	Measure or Quantity	Calories	Carbo-hydrates (grams)
Custard Style	6-oz. container	190	30.0
Strawberry-banana:			
(Dannon):			
Fresh Flavors	8-oz. container	200	34.0
Fruit-on-the-Bottom	4.4-oz. container	130	23.0
Fruit-on-the-Bottom	8-oz. container	240	43.0
(Light N' Lively)	8-oz. container	260	52.0
(Sweet'n Low)	8-oz. container	190	33.0
(Whitney's)	6-oz. container	200	33.0
Yoplait:			
Breakfast Yogurt	6-oz. container	240	43.0
Custard Style	6-oz. container	190	32.0
Strawberry colada (Colombo)	8-oz. container	230	36.0
Tropical, *Yoplait, Breakfast Yogurt*	6-oz. container	230	41.0
Tropical fruit (Sweet'N Low)	8-oz. container	150	33.0
Vanilla:			
(Breyer's)	8-oz. container	230	31.0
(Dannon):			
Fresh Flavors	4.4-oz. container	110	20.0
Fresh Flavors	8-oz. container	220	34.0
(Friendship)	8-oz. container	210	35.0
(La Yogurt)	6-oz. container	160	26.0
(Whitney's)	6-oz. container	200	28.0
Yoplait, Custard Style	6-oz. container	180	30.0
Wild berries (Whitney's)	6-oz. container	200	33.0
Frozen, hard:			
Banana (Dannon)			
Danny-in-a-Cup	8-oz. cup	210	42.0
Boysenberry (Dannon)			
Danny-On-A-Stick, carob coated	2½-fl.-oz. bar	140	15.0
Boysenberry swirl (Bison)	¼ of 16-oz. container	116	24.0
Chocolate:			
(Bison)	¼ of 16-oz. container	116	24.0
(Colombo) bar, chocolate coated	1 bar	145	17.0
(Dannon):			
Danny-in-a-Cup	8-fl.-oz. cup	190	32.0
Danny-On-A-Stick:			
Uncoated	2½-fl.-oz. bar	60	10.0
Chocolate coated	2½-fl.-oz. bar	130	12.0
Mocha (Colombo) bar	1 bar	80	14.0

Food and Description	Measure or Quantity	Calories	Carbo-hydrates (grams)
Pina colada:			
(Colombo)	4-oz. serving	110	20.0
(Dannon):			
Danny-in-a-Cup	8-oz. cup	230	44.0
Danny-On-A-Stick, uncoated	2½-fl.-oz. bar	65	14.0
Raspberry, red (Dannon):			
Danny-in-a-cup	8-oz. container	210	42.0
Danny-On-A-Stick, chocolate coated	2½-fl.-oz. bar	130	15.0
Raspberry swirl (Bison)	¼ of 16-oz. container	116	24.0
Strawberry:			
(Bison)	¼ of 16-oz. container	116	24.0
(Colombo):			
Regular	4-oz. serving	110	20.0
Bar	1 bar	80	14.0
(Dannon):			
Danny-in-a-Cup	8-fl.-oz. container	210	42.0
Danny-On-A-Stick, chocolate coated	2½-fl.-oz. bar	130	15.0
Vanilla:			
(Bison)	¼ of 16-oz. container	116	24.0
(Colombo):			
Regular	4-oz. serving	110	20.0
Bar, chocolate coated	1 bar	145	17.0
(Dannon):			
Danny-in-a-Cup	8 fl. oz.	180	33.0
Danny-On-A-Stick	2½-fl.-oz. bar	60	11.0
Frozen, soft-serve (Baskin-Robbins): Banana, cheesecake, Jamocha, orange, peach, pineapple, raspberry, strawberry			

(USDA): United States Department of Agriculture
(HEW/FAO):   Health, Education and Welfare/Food and Agriculture
                    Organization
* Prepared as Package Directs

Food and Description	Measure or Quantity	Calories	Carbo-hydrates (grams)
or vanilla	1 fl. oz.	31	6.0
Chocolate	1 fl. oz.	35	6.1
Coconut	1 fl. oz.	36	5.5
Peanut butter	1 fl. oz.	37	5.8

Food and Description	Measure or Quantity	Calories	Carbo-hydrates (grams)

Z

ZINFANDEL WINE (Louis M. Martini):
Red, 12½% alcohol	3 fl. oz.	67	Tr.
White, 11% alcohol	3 fl. oz.	58	1.5

ZINGERS (Dolly Madison):
Devil's food or white	1¼-oz. piece	140	23.0
Raspberry	1¼-oz. piece	130	20.0

ZITI, FROZEN:
(Morton) Light	11-oz. dinner	280	43.0
(Weight Watchers)	11¼-oz. meal	290	32.0

ZWEIBACK:
(USDA)	1 oz.	120	21.1
(Gerber)	7-gram piece	30	5.1
(Nabisco)	1 piece	30	5.0

(USDA): United States Department of Agriculture
(HEW/FAO): Health, Education and Welfare/Food and Agriculture
Organization
* Prepared as Package Directs

CANADIAN SUPPLEMENT

Food and Description	Measure or Quantity	Calories	Carbo-hydrates (grams)

A

*AWAKE (General Foods)
  orange | 4 fl. oz. | 52 | 13.3 |

B

BACON BITS, *Bac-O-Bits* (General Mills)	1 oz.	119	8.0
BEAN, BAKED, canned (Campbell) in tomato sauce	8-oz. serving	251	44.0
BEAN, GREEN, frozen (McCain):			
French style	⅓ of 10-oz. pkg.	29	5.6
Whole	3.3-oz. serving	34	.6
BEAN, LIMA, frozen (McCain)	3.3-oz. serving	107	18.6
BEAN, YELLOW OR WAX, frozen (McCain)	⅓ of 10.6-oz. pkg.	34	6.8
BEEF DINNER OR ENTREE, frozen (Swanson):			
Regular, sliced	8½-oz. entree	248	16.4
Hungry Man, sliced	17-oz. dinner (482 gms.)	631	67.5

Food and Description	Measure or Quantity	Calories	Carbo-hydrates (grams)
TV Brand:			
Chopped sirloin	10-oz. dinner (283 gms.)	445	39.9
Sliced	11½-oz. dinner	433	34.0
BEEF PIE, frozen (Swanson):			
Regular	8-oz. pie (227 grams)	443	37.0
Hungry Man	16-oz. pie (454 grams)	631	51.3
BEEF STEW:			
Canned, regular pack (Bounty)	8-oz. serving	180	15.9
Frozen (EfficienC)	8-oz. entree (227 grams)	202	15.8
BROCCOLI, frozen (McCain):			
Chopped	⅓ of 10.6-oz. pkg.	36	5.2
Spears	⅓ of 10.6-oz. pkg.	40	5.7
BRUSSELS SPROUT, frozen (McCain)	⅓ of 10.6-oz. pkg.	68	11.2
BUTTER, dietetic, *Meadowlight*	1 T. (14 grams)	51	.2
BUTTERSCOTCH CHIPS (Baker's)	6.2-oz. pkg.	915	103.0

C

Food and Description	Measure or Quantity	Calories	Carbo-hydrates (grams)
CAKE, frozen:			
Banana (McCain)	⅛ of 19-oz. cake	218	35.5
Banana-nut loaf (Pepperidge Farm)	⅙ of 11½-oz. cake	199	28.3

(USDA): United States Department of Agriculture
(HEW/FAO): Health, Education and Welfare/Food and Agriculture Organization
* Prepared as Package Directs

Food and Description	Measure or Quantity	Calories	Carbo-hydrates (grams)
Carrot-nut loaf (Pepperidge Farm)	⅙ of 11½-oz. cake	227	24.4
Chocolate:			
(McCain):			
Regular	⅛ of 19-oz. cake	199	28.9
Fiesta	⅛ of 19-oz. cake	249	29.9
(Pepperidge Farm)	⅙ of 13-oz. cake	213	30.2
Coconut (Pepperidge Farm)	⅙ of 13-oz. cake	230	31.3
Devil's food (Pepperidge Farm)	⅙ of 13-oz. cake	223	32.0
Maple spice (Pepperidge Farm)	⅙ of 13-oz. cake	213	32.2
Marble (McCain)	⅛ of 19-oz. cake	219	34.2
Neapolitan Fiesta (McCain)	⅛ of 19-oz. cake	252	29.7
Pound (Pepperidge Farm)	⅙ of 10.4-oz. cake	198	24.0
Shortcake (McCain):			
Raspberry	⅛ of 25-oz. cake	269	44.4
Strawberry	⅛ of 25-oz. cake	207	37.6
Vanilla:			
(McCain)	⅛ of 18-oz. cake	211	31.7
(Pepperidge Farm) layer	⅙ of 13-oz. cake	222	32.0
CAKE ICING, regular (General Mills):			
Chocolate	¹⁄₁₂ of container	162	25.0
Vanilla	¹⁄₁₂ of container	166	28.0
*CAKE ICING MIX, regular (General Mills):			
Chocolate, fudge	¹⁄₁₂ of pkg.	134	28.6
White:			
Fluffy	¹⁄₁₂ of pkg.	58	14.9
Traditional	¹⁄₁₂ of pkg.	140	29.8
*CAKE MIX, regular (General Mills):			
Angel food:			
Regular	¹⁄₁₆ of cake	111	26.2
Confetti	¹⁄₁₆ of cake	114	26.8
Raspberry	¹⁄₁₆ of cake	115	27.0
Cherry chip, layer	¹⁄₁₂ of cake	198	37.6
Chocolate, layer:			
German	¹⁄₁₂ of cake	200	35.9
Milk	¹⁄₁₂ of cake	199	35.0

Food and Description	Measure or Quantity	Calories	Carbo-hydrates (grams)
Sour cream, fudge	¹⁄₁₂ of cake	195	35.4
Devil's food, layer	¹⁄₁₂ of cake	199	35.8
Lemon, layer	¹⁄₁₂ of cake	202	36.1
Orange, layer	¹⁄₁₂ of cake	201	36.8
Pound, golden	¹⁄₁₂ of cake	210	28.0
White, layer:			
Regular	¹⁄₁₂ of cake	190	34.5
Sour cream	¹⁄₁₂ of cake	191	34.1
CANDY, regular (Rowntree Mackintosh):			
Aero:			
Regular	1.4-oz. bar	206	23.5
Peppermint	1.1-oz. bar	168	18.1
Chocolate bar with whole almonds	1.1-oz. bar	171	16.2
Coffee Crisp	1.7-oz. bar	246	28.1
Crispettes, coffee or orange	15-gram piece	79	9.6
Kit Kat	1.5-oz. bar (42 grams)	222	26.6
Maple Buds	1.1-oz. bar (31 grams)	162	18.9
Mint, chocolate covered, *After Eight*	.3-oz. piece (8.4 grams)	37	6.2
Mirage	1.4-oz. bar (39 grams)	208	23.5
Smarties	1.5-oz. bar (44 grams)	207	32.1
Toffee	2-oz. serving	255	40.1
CARROT, frozen (McCain):			
Diced, sticks or whole	3½-oz. serving	34	7.1
Sliced	3½-oz. serving	48	9.6
CAULIFLOWER, frozen (McCain)	3½-oz. serving	77	13.2
CEREAL (General Mills):			
Boo*Berry	1 cup (1 oz.)	111	24.0

(USDA): United States Department of Agriculture
(HEW/FAO): Health, Education and Welfare/Food and Agriculture Organization
* Prepared as Package Directs

Food and Description	Measure or Quantity	Calories	Carbo-hydrates (grams)
Cherrios:			
Regular	1¼ cups (1 oz.)	109	20.2
Honey nut	¾ cup (1 oz.)	110	23.0
Cocoa Puffs	1 cup (1 oz.)	107	24.2
Corn flakes, *Country*	1¼ cups (1 oz.)	109	24.0
Count Chocula	1 cup (1 oz.)	105	24.1
Frankenberry	1 cup (1 oz.)	110	24.5
Golden Grahams	1 cup (1 oz.)	110	23.6
Lucky Charms	1 cup (1 oz.)	112	24.4
Total	1¼ cups (1 oz.)	100	23.0
Trix	1 cup (1 oz.)	107	24.4
Wheaties	1¼ cups (1 oz.)	100	23.0
CHICKEN A LA KING, frozen:			
(EfficienC)	7-oz. entree (198 grams)	257	9.3
(Swanson)	9¾-oz. entree	284	9.9
CHICKEN DINNER OR ENTREE, frozen (Swanson):			
Regular	7-oz. entree	410	27.0
Hungry Man:			
Boneless	19-oz. dinner	685	60.4
Fried	15-oz. dinner	1058	96.9
TV Brand	11½-oz. entree	575	44.7
CHICKEN PIE, frozen (Swanson):			
Regular	8-oz. pie (227 grams)	503	52.9
Hungry Man	16-oz. pie (454 grams)	731	57.7
CHICKEN STEW:			
Canned (Bounty)	8-oz. serving	186	15.5
Frozen (EfficienC)	8-oz. entree	238	12.9
CHILI OR CHILI CON CARNE, canned, with beans (Bounty)	8-oz. serving	270	21.8
CHOCOLATE, BAKING (Baker's):			
Unsweetened	1-oz. square	143	8.8

Food and Description	Measure or Quantity	Calories	Carbo-hydrates (grams)
Milk, chips	6.2-oz. pkg.	857	115.0
Semi-sweet:			
Regular	1-oz. square	136	16.8
Chips	6.2-oz. pkg.	798	120.0
Sweet	1-oz. square	138	18.8
CLAMATO JUICE DRINK,			
canned (Mott's)	6 fl. oz.	75	18.0
COCOA:			
Dry, unsweetened (Fry's)	1 T. (5 grams)	23	2.8
*Mix, regular (Cadbury's)			
instant	6 fl. oz.	116	23.0
COCONUT, packaged (Baker's):			
Angel Flake	½ of 7-oz. pkg.	438	44.4
Premium Shred	½ of 7-oz. pkg.	453	46.0
***COFFEE,** instant,			
General Foods International			
Coffee:			
Amaretto	6 fl. oz.	46	DNA
Irish Mocha Mint	6 fl. oz.	46	6.4
Orange Cappucino	6 fl. oz.	55	9.5
Suisse Mocha	6 fl. oz.	49	6.8
Vienna Royale	6 fl. oz.	57	10.0
COOKIE OR BISCUIT, regular:			
Animal (Christie's) *Barnum*	1 piece (2.7 grams)	13	2.1
Arrowroot (Christie's)	1 piece (6.6 grams)	29	5.3
Chew Chews (Christie's)	1 piece (.7 oz.)	93	15.7
Chocolate:			
(Cadbury's):			
Fingers	1 oz.	148	20.0
Wafer	1 oz.	162	18.2
(Christie's) wafer	1 piece (4.5 grams)	20	3.5

(USDA): United States Department of Agriculture
(HEW/FAO):   Health, Education and Welfare/Food and Agriculture
                Organization
* Prepared as Package Directs

Food and Description	Measure or Quantity	Calories	Carbo-hydrates (grams)
Chocolate chip (Christie's) *Chips Ahoy!*	1 piece (.5 oz.)	76	10.3
Coffee Break (Christie's)	1 piece (11.2 grams)	53	7.7
Date Lunch (Christie's)	1 piece (.6 oz.)	60	13.2
Fig Newtons (Christie's)	1 piece (.6 oz.)	60	13.4
Fudgee-O (Christie's)	1 piece (13 grams)	60	9.0
Hey-Days (Christie's)	1 piece (.7 oz.)	81	10.8
Hoo-Rays (Christie's)	1 piece (.6 oz.)	78	11.3
Jelly shortcake (Christie's)	1 piece (.4 oz.)	44	6.7
Lemon puff (Christie's)	1 piece (6.5 grams)	35	4.0
Maple leaf creams (Christie's)	1 piece (.4 oz.)	53	7.3
Midget snaps (Christie's)	1 piece (5.3 grams)	21	4.5
Miniatures (Christie's)	1 piece (.3 oz)	40	6.4
Mint (Christie's):			
Cream	1 piece (.4 oz.)	58	7.6
Sandwich	1 piece (.6 oz.)	92	12.4
Neapolitan wafer (Christie's)	1 piece (4 grams)	21	2.8
Oatmeal (Christie's)	1 piece (.4 oz.)	53	8.0
Oreo (Christie's)	1 piece (.4 oz.)	57	8.3
Pantry (Christie's)	1 piece	55	9.9
Pirate (Christie's)	1 piece (10.6 grams)	53	7.2
Sandwich (Cadbury's):			
Chocolate	1 oz.	153	18.5
Coffee	1 oz.	155	18.9
Orange	1 oz.	154	19.4
Social Tea (Christie's)	1 piece (4.5 grams)	20	3.6
Soft (Christie's):			
Apple or raspberry	1 piece (.7 oz.)	89	13.8
Date	1 piece (.7 oz.)	89	14.2
Granola	1 piece (.7 oz.)	86	13.4
Sugar (Christie's) raisin	1 piece (.5 oz.)	65	9.3
Sultana (Christie's)	1 piece (.4 oz.)	43	9.7
Tea Treats (Christie's)	1 piece (.2 oz.)	25	3.8
Vanilla Wafer (Christie's)	1 piece (3.7 grams)	17	2.6
CORN, frozen (McCain) whole kernel	¼ of 12.4-oz. pkg.	74	14.7

Food and Description	Measure or Quantity	Calories	Carbo-hydrates (grams)
CRACKERS, PUFFS & CHIPS:			
Bacon Dipper (Christie's)	1 piece (2.1 grams)	10	1.3
Bits & Bites (Christie's):			
Regular	1 piece (.4 grams)	2	.3
Cheese flavor	1 piece (.3 grams)	1	.2
Bugles (General Mills)	1 piece (.9 grams)	5	.5
Canadian Harvest (Christie's)	1 piece (.1 oz.)	14	1.8
Cheese or cheese flavored:			
Cheddees (Christie's)	1 piece (.5 grams)	3	.2
Cheese Bits (Christie's)	1 piece (.8 grams)	3.6	.5
Cheese Willikers (General Mills)	1 piece (1.1 grams)	6	.6
& green onion (Christie's)	1 piece (.1 oz.)	14	1.8
Nips (Christie's)	1 piece (1.1 grams)	5	.6
Premium Plus (Christie's)	1 piece (3.2 grams)	13	2.1
Swiss cheese (Christie's)	1 piece (2 grams)	10	1.2
Tid Bits (Christie's)	1 piece (.3 grams)	1	.2
Corn chip (Christie's)	1 piece (.9 grams)	6	.6
Crisp-I-Taters (General Mills)	1 piece (.6 grams)	3	.3
Escort (Christie's)	1 piece (4.4 grams)	23	2.6
Flings (Christie's)	1 piece (.8 grams)	5	.3
Graham (Christie's):			
Country Maid	1 piece (5.5 grams)	25	3.9
Honey Maid	1 piece	27	4.8

(USDA): United States Department of Agriculture
(HEW/FAO): Health, Education and Welfare/Food and Agriculture Organization
* Prepared as Package Directs

Food and Description	Measure or Quantity	Calories	Carbo-hydrates (grams)
Montclair	1 piece (.3 oz.)	39	6.8
Hovis Cracker (Christie's)	1 piece (5.7 grams)	28	3.4
Meal Mates (Christie's)	1 piece (5.3 grams)	23	3.7
Milk Lunch (Christie's)	1 piece (7.2 grams)	31	5.2
Mini chips (Christie's)	1 piece (.4 grams)	2	.3
Onion crisp (Christie's) with sesame	1 piece (3.8 grams)	17	2.5
Onion, french, thins (Christie's)	1 piece (2.1 grams)	10	1.4
Pizza Cracker (Christie's)	1 piece (.1 oz.)	7	1.1
Ritz (Christie's):			
Regular	1 piece (.1 oz.)	17	2.2
Cheese	1 piece (.1 oz.)	14	1.9
Rusk, Holland (Christie's)	1 piece (9.2 grams)	36	7.0
Rye, buffet (Christie's)	1 piece (3.4 grams)	16	2.4
Saltine, *Premium* (Christie's):			
Old fashioned	1 piece (6.6 grams)	30	4.4
Plus, with or without salt	1 piece (.1 oz.)	13	2.1
Sociables (Christie's)	1 piece (2.6 grams)	13	1.6
Sour cream & chive (Christie's)	1 piece	12	1.6
Tortilla chip (Christie's) nacho or taco flavor	1 piece (2.2 grams)	11	1.4
Triangle thins (Christie's)	1 piece (1.7 grams)	8	1.0
Triscuit Wafers (Christie's)	1 piece (4.7 grams)	21	3.3
Triticale Crackers (Christie's)	1 piece (.1 oz.)	15	1.8
Vegetable thins (Christie's)	1 piece (1.7 grams)	8	1.1
Wheat thins (Christies):			
Regular	1 piece (2.1 grams)	10	1.4

Food and Description	Measure or Quantity	Calories	Carbo-hydrates (grams)
Ground	1 piece (5.8 grams)	24	4.5
Wheatsworth (Christie's)	1 piece (3.4 grams)	16	2.0
Whistles (General Mills)	1 piece (.8 grams)	4	.7
CRANAPPLE JUICE DRINK (Ocean Spray)	8 fl. oz.	180	44.0
CRANBERRY JUICE COCKTAIL, canned (Ocean Spray)	8 fl. oz.	160	40.0
CRANBERRY SAUCE, canned (Ocean Spray) jellied or whole	2 fl. oz. serving	90	22.0

D

DOUGHNUT, frozen (McCain) chocolate iced	¼ of 9-oz. pkg.	266	24.1

F

FIDDLEHEAD GREENS, frozen (McCain)	⅓ of 10½-oz. pkg.	26	3.3
FLOUR:			
Bisquick (General Mills)	¼ cup	126	19.9
Five Roses:			
All-purpose or unbleached	¼ cup	104	21.0
Whole wheat	¼ cup	105	21.3
(Swansdown) cake	½ cup (2 oz.)	204	44.4

(USDA): United States Department of Agriculture
(HEW/FAO): Health, Education and Welfare/Food and Agriculture Organization
* Prepared as Package Directs

Food and Description	Measure or Quantity	Calories	Carbo-hydrates (grams)

G

*GELATIN DESSERT MIX:
Regular (Jell-O)	½ cup	81	19.4
Dietetic (D-Zerta):			
Lemon	½ cup	8	0.
Orange or strawberry	½ cup	9	.1
Raspberry	½ cup	9	0.
GRAPE DRINK, canned,			
Welch's	8 fl. oz. (8.4 oz.)	112	30.0
GRAPE JUICE, canned,			
Welch's, purple or white	8 fl. oz.	160	40.0
GRAPEFRUIT JUICE, canned (Ocean Spray)	8 fl. oz.	95	21.0
GRAVY, canned (Franco-American):			
Beef	2-oz. serving	44	3.6
Chicken	2-oz. serving	50	3.1
Mushroom	2-oz. serving	28	2.8
Onion	2-oz. serving	40	2.7

H

*HAMBURGER HELPER (General Mills):
Beef flavored dinner	1 cup	328	26.2
Cheeseburger	1 cup	334	35.2
Chili tomato dinner	1 cup	334	35.2
Hash	1 cup	300	26.8
Lasagna	1 cup	332	35.2
Noodle Romanoff	1 cup	241	26.4
Potato Stroganoff	1 cup	323	28.5
Short cut spaghetti	1 cup	330	24.7
Tomato Roma	1 cup	334	35.2

Food and Description	Measure or Quantity	Calories	Carbo-hydrates (grams)
HAM DINNER OR ENTREE, frozen (Swanson) *TV Brand*	10½-oz. dinner	365	42.0

I

ICE CREAM CONE (Christie's):			
Regular	1 piece (4.5 grams)	19	3.7
Sugar	1 piece (12.5 grams)	49	10.3
ICE CREAM CUP (Christie's)	1 cup (5.8 grams)	23	4.7
ICE MAGIC (General Foods) chocolate or chocolate mint	.6-oz. serving	111	6.0

J

JELL-O PUDDING POPS (General Foods):			
Chocolate	2.1-oz. pop	88	16.7
All other flavors	2.1-oz. pop	87	15.9

K

***KOOL-AID** (General Foods):			
Regular, sugar added after bought	8 fl. oz.	106	28.0
Pre-sweetened, with sugar:			
All except lemonade, orange and sunshine punch	8 fl. oz.	86	22.3

(USDA): United States Department of Agriculture
(HEW/FAO): Health, Education and Welfare/Food and Agriculture Organization
* Prepared as Package Directs

Food and Description	Measure or Quantity	Calories	Carbo-hydrates (grams)
Lemonade	8 fl. oz.	85	22.1
Orange	8 fl. oz.	85	22.2
Sunshine punch	8 fl. oz.	85	22.3
Dietetic, sugar free:			
Cherry, grape or strawberry	8 fl. oz.	2	.2
Orange	8 fl. oz.	3	.3
Tropical Punch	8 fl. oz.	2	.3

L

LASAGNA, frozen:			
(EfficienC)	9.2-oz. entree	325	30.5
(Swanson)	12-oz. entree	445	39.4
LEMONADE, canned, *Country Time*	10 fl. oz.	248	29.5

M

MACARONI:			
Dry (Catelli)	3 oz.	306	63.8
Canned (Franco-American) and beef	8-oz. serving	225	25.0
Frozen (Swanson) and beef	8-oz. casserole	211	24.4
MACARONI & CHEESE:			
Canned (Franco-American)	8 oz.	220	25.0
Frozen:			
(EfficienC)	8-oz. entree	308	64.5
(Swanson)	8-oz. casserole	328	29.2
Mix (Catelli)	3 oz.	425	77.4
MEATBALL, frozen (Swanson) and gravy	9-oz. entree	378	17.6
*MUFFIN MIX (General Mills):			
Apple cinnamon	1 muffin	159	26.4
Blueberry	1 muffin	118	19.3
Butter pecan	1 muffin	159	21.3

Food and Description	Measure or Quantity	Calories	Carbo-hydrates (grams)
Corn	1 muffin	156	24.8
Honey bran	1 muffin	154	26.2

N

NOODLE, dry (Catelli):			
Egg	3 oz.	316	61.3
Lasagna, spinach	3 oz.	304	63.2

O

ONION, frozen (McCain) rings, battered or breaded	3 oz.	167	24.1

P

PANCAKE, frozen (EfficienC)	1.7-oz. pancake	112	17.8
PATTY SHELL, frozen (Pepperidge Farm) regular	1.7-oz. shell (47.2 grams)	215	13.4
PEA, green, frozen (McCain)	¼ of 12.4-oz. pkg.	72	11.9
PEA & CARROT, frozen (McCain)	⅓ of 10½-oz. pkg.	65	11.6
PIE, frozen (McCain):			
Banana cream	⅙ of 14-oz. pie	149	20.3

(USDA): United States Department of Agriculture
(HEW/FAO):   Health, Education and Welfare/Food and Agriculture
                    Organization
* Prepared as Package Directs

Food and Description	Measure or Quantity	Calories	Carbo-hydrates (grams)
Chocolate cream	⅙ of 14-oz. pie	197	22.5
Coconut cream	⅙ of 14-oz. pie	201	19.9
Lemon cream	⅙ of 14-oz. pie	210	29.0
Mincemeat	⅛ of 24-oz. pie	237	35.0
Pecan	⅛ of 20-oz. pie	307	36.4
Pumpkin	⅛ of 22-oz. pie	168	19.1
Raisin	3½-oz. serving	277	42.7
*PIE CRUST MIX:			
(Christie's) graham	1 shell (14.1 oz.)	2097	243.2
(General Mills)	⅙ of double-crust shell	302	24.1
*PIE MIX (General Mills)			
Boston cream	⅛ of pie	265	47.9
PIZZA, frozen (McCain):			
Deluxe:			
Regular	5″ pie (15 oz.)	268	29.0
Tendercrisp	5″ pie (17 oz.)	269	29.0
Pepperoni, regular or tendercrisp	5″ pie	293	29.0
PORK DINNER OR ENTREE, frozen (Swanson) *TV Brand,* loin of	11-oz. dinner	505	44.5
POTATO, frozen (McCain):			
Country style	2-oz. serving	83	12.4
Diced, all-purpose	2-oz. serving	42	9.9
French fries	2-oz. serving	83	12.4
Hashbrowns, western style	2-oz. serving	129	16.5
Puffs	⅓ of 8.8-oz. pkg.	157	20.9
Superfries	2-oz. serving	41	11.8
PRETZELS (Christie's) *Mr. Salty:*			
Sticks	1 piece (3.9 grams)	15	3.1
Twists	1 piece (6.9 grams)	26	5.4
PRUNE NECTAR, canned, *Welch's*	8 fl. oz. (8.6 oz.)	200	45.0

Food and Description	Measure or Quantity	Calories	Carbo-hydrates (grams)
PUDDING OR PIE FILLING:			
Canned, regular pack (Laura Secord):			
Chocolate:			
Regular	5-oz. serving	199	32.4
Fudge	5-oz. serving	199	32.7
Vanilla	5-oz. serving	192	29.4
*Mix:			
Regular:			
Banana cream (Jell-O):			
Regular	½ cup	150	27.7
Instant	½ cup	163	30.9
Butter pecan (Jell-O):			
Regular	½ cup	147	27.2
Instant	½ cup	159	28.7
Butterscotch (Jello-O):			
Regular	½ cup	168	32.8
Instant	½ cup	169	32.8
Caramel (Jell-O):			
Regular	½ cup	168	32.8
Instant	½ cup	169	32.7
Chocolate (Jell-O):			
Plain:			
Regular	½ cup	163	31.0
Instant	½ cup	165	31.5
Cream, regular	½ cup	158	28.4
Fudge, instant	½ cup	162	30.6
Coconut cream (Jell-O) regular	½ cup	159	25.0
Custard (Bird's)	½ cup	98	17.0
Lemon (Jell-O) instant	½ cup	163	31.3
Pistachio (Jell-O) instant	½ cup	166	30.3
Tapioca:			
(Jell-O) instant	½ cup	149	27.7
Minit (General Foods)	½ cup	140	21.9
Vanilla (Jell-O):			
Regular	½ cup	150	27.7
Instant	½ cup	149	27.6
Dietetic (D-Zerta):			
Butterscotch	½ cup	68	11.8

(USDA): United States Department of Agriculture
(HEW/FAO):   Health, Education and Welfare/Food and Agriculture
                      Organization
* Prepared as Package Directs

Food and Description	Measure or Quantity	Calories	Carbo-hydrates (grams)
Chocolate	½ cup	77	13.3
Vanilla	½ cup	69	11.9

Q

QUENCH (General Foods):
  Canned
    Regular:

Fruit punch	9.5 fl. oz.	115	30.2
Grape	9.5 fl. oz.	139	37.0
Lemonade	9.5 fl. oz.	111	29.5
Orange	9.5 fl. oz.	121	33.0

  Dietetic:

Fruit punch or grape	8½ fl. oz.	5	.5
Lemonade	8½ fl. oz.	8	.9
Orange	8½ fl. oz.	7	.7

  *Mix, regular:

Fruit punch	8½ fl. oz.	116	30.4
Grape or lemonade	8½ fl. oz.	115	30.4
Lemon-lime	8½ fl. oz.	115	30.5
Orange	8½ fl. oz.	115	30.2

R

ROLL OR BUN, frozen
  (McCain):

Danish, iced	2-oz. serving	241	25.3
Honey	2-oz. serving	121	28.0

S

SALISBURY STEAK, frozen:
  (EfficienC)

	5¾-oz. entree	274	5.4

  (Swanson):

Regular	5½-oz. entree	330	26.6
Hungry Man	17-oz. dinner	805	65.1
TV Brand	11½-oz. dinner	427	37.8

Food and Description	Measure or Quantity	Calories	Carbo-hydrates (grams)
*SOUP, canned, regular pack:			
Asparagus (Campbell)			
condensed, cream of	7-oz. serving	71	9.3
Bean (Campbell) condensed,			
with bacon	7-oz. serving	133	17.0
Beef (Campbell) condensed:			
Broth	7-oz. serving	22	1.9
Mushroom	7-oz. serving	51	4.5
Noodle	7-oz. serving	58	7.2
With vegetables & barley	7-oz. serving	86	9.1
Celery (Campbell) condensed,			
cream of	7-oz. serving	66	6.4
Cheddar cheese (Campbell)			
condensed	7-oz. serving	124	8.4
Chicken (Campbell) condensed:			
Alphabet	7-oz. serving	64	8.1
Broth	7-oz. serving	27	.7
Cream of:			
Made with milk	7-oz. serving	144	11.1
Made with water	7-oz. serving	76	3.6
Creamy, & mushroom	7-oz. serving	77	7.3
Gumbo	7-oz. serving	48	7.3
Noodle	7-oz. serving	54	7.1
NoodleOs	7-oz. serving	59	7.8
With rice	7-oz. serving	42	4.9
& stars	7-oz. serving	49	6.1
Vegetable	7-oz. serving	60	7.6
Chowder, clam (Campbell)			
condensed:			
Manhattan style	7-oz. serving	64	9.1
New England style	7-oz. serving	71	9.4
Consomme (Campbell)			
condensed	7-oz. serving	29	2.3
Meatball alphabet (Campbell)			
condensed	7-oz. serving	53	8.8
Minestrone (Campbell)			
condensed	7-oz. serving	71	9.1
Mushroom (Campbell)			
condensed:			
Cream of	7-oz. serving	114	7.5

(USDA): United States Department of Agriculture
(HEW/FAO):   Health, Education and Welfare/Food and Agriculture
                        Organization
* Prepared as Package Directs

Food and Description	Measure or Quantity	Calories	Carbo-hydrates (grams)
Golden	7-oz. serving	70	6.8
Noodle (Campbell) condensed, & ground beef	7-oz. serving	80	8.1
Onion (Campbell) condensed:			
Regular	7-oz. serving	36	2.9
Cream of, made with water	7-oz. serving	74	8.6
Ox Tail (Campbell) condensed	7-oz. serving	83	8.7
Oyster stew (Campbell) condensed	7-oz. serving	31	2.7
Pea, French Canadian style (Campbell) condensed	7-oz. serving	139	20.1
Pea, green:			
(Campbell) condensed	7-oz. serving	115	18.4
(Habitant)	1 cup (259 grams)	176	24.2
Potato (Campbell) condensed, cream of, made with water	7-oz. serving	58	9.1
Scotch broth (Campbell) condensed	7-oz. serving	74	8.6
Shrimp (Campbell) condensed	7-oz. serving	74	6.2
Tomato (Campbell) condensed:			
Regular	7-oz. serving	69	12.2
Bisque of	7-oz. serving	101	18.3
& rice, old fashioned	7-oz. serving	87	14.6
Turkey (Campbell) condensed:			
Noodle	7-oz. serving	63	6.5
Vegetable	7-oz. serving	64	7.0
Vegetable:			
(Campbell) condensed:			
Regular	7-oz. serving	67	11.0
Beef	7-oz. serving	62	6.3
Country style	7-oz. serving	50	6.7
Cream of, made with water	7-oz. serving	91	8.4
Hearty	7-oz. serving	81	15.6
Old fashioned	7-oz. serving	61	7.8
Vegetarian	7-oz. serving	62	10.3
(Habitant)	1 cup (9 oz.)	74	13.2
SPINACH, frozen (McCain)	⅓ of 12-oz. pkg.	37	4.3
SPAGHETTI, canned (Franco-American):			
& ground beef	8-oz. serving	218	32.7
In tomato sauce	8-oz. serving	159	31.4

Food and Description	Measure or Quantity	Calories	Carbo-hydrates (grams)
SpaghettiOs	8-oz. serving	173	32.9
SQUASH, frozen (McCain)	¼ of 14-oz. pkg.	25	4.7
STRUDEL, frozen (Pepperidge Farm): Apple	⅙ of strudel (2.3 oz.)	78	10.0
Blueberry	⅙ of strudel (2.3 oz.)	93	11.0
SWISS STEAK DINNER OR ENTREE, frozen (Swanson) *TV Brand*	11¼-oz. dinner	374	38.2

T

Food and Description	Measure or Quantity	Calories	Carbo-hydrates (grams)
***TANG** (General Foods):* Apple	4.2 fl. oz.	69	18.2
Grapefruit	4.2 fl. oz.	52	14.6
Orange	4.2 fl. oz.	56	15.0
Orange & grapefruit	4.2 fl. oz.	55	14.6
Pineapple & grapefruit	4.2 fl. oz.	66	17.4
TOMATO SAUCE, canned, regular pack (Catelli): Plain	½ cup (80 grams)	44	5.9
With meat	½ cup (80.5 grams)	71	4.5
TOPPING, WHIPPED, frozen, *Cool Whip* (General Foods)	1 T. (.1 oz.)	13	1.0
TURKEY DINNER OR ENTREE, frozen: (EfficienC) sliced	5.2-oz. entree	157	4.4

(USDA): United States Department of Agriculture
(HEW/FAO):   Health, Education and Welfare/Food and Agriculture
                        Organization
* Prepared as Package Directs

Food and Description	Measure or Quantity	Calories	Carbo-hydrates (grams)
(Swanson):			
Regular	8¾-oz. entree	304	28.7
Regular, sliced	9¼-oz. entree	265	22.5
Hungry Man	19-oz. dinner	647	67.9
TV Brand	11½-oz. dinner	397	43.3
TURKEY PIE, frozen			
(Swanson):			
Regular	8-oz. pie	442	40.1
Hungry Man	16-oz. pie	608	53.1
TURNOVER, frozen:			
Apple:			
(McCain)	2-oz. serving	122	18.9
(Pepperidge Farm)	2.7-oz. piece	258	23.9
Blueberry (Pepperidge Farm)	2.7-oz. piece	263	26.0
Blueberry/raspberry (McCain)	2-oz. serving	123	19.4
Raspberry (Pepperidge Farm)	2.7-oz. piece	274	28.9
Strawberry (Pepperidge Farm)	2.7-oz. piece	267	27.2

V

Food and Description	Measure or Quantity	Calories	Carbo-hydrates (grams)
VEGETABLE, MIXED, frozen (McCain):			
Regular	⅓ of 10.6-oz. pkg.	67	12.6
Florentine style	⅕ of 17.6-oz. pkg.	41	7.2
Parisienne style	3-oz. serving	37	6.6
V-8 JUICE:			
Regular	6 fl. oz.	36	6.5
Spicy hot	6 fl. oz.	38	DNA

W

Food and Description	Measure or Quantity	Calories	Carbo-hydrates (grams)
WHIP'N CHILL (Jell-O):			
Chocolate	½ cup	131	18.6
Lemon	½ cup	129	18.1

Food and Description	Measure or Quantity	Calories	Carbo-hydrates (grams)
Strawberry	½ cup	129	17.7
Vanilla	½ cup	129	18.0

Y

YOGURT, regular
(Laura Secord):

Blueberry	4.5-oz. serving	120	19.5
Peach	4.5-oz. serving	119	19.1
Raspberry	4.5-oz. serving	120	19.4
Strawberry	4.5-oz. serving	122	18.3

(USDA): United States Department of Agriculture
(HEW/FAO):   Health, Education and Welfare/Food and Agriculture
             Organization
* Prepared as Package Directs